The Covid Survival Guide

What The Virus Is, How To Avoid It, How To Survive It

At Home ◆ At Work ◆ Traveling

The Covid Survival Guide by David M Rowell
© Copyright 2020 David M Rowell. All Rights Reserved
Contact : Book@TheCovidSurvivalGuide.com or B@Cov.cx

Book website : https://TheCovidSurvivalGuide.com or https://cov.cx/covid
Author website : https://DavidMRowell.com or https://cov.cx/dmr

Published by Aramoana Publishing, December 2020
17321 NE 31st Ct, Redmond WA 98052 USA
www.aramoana.pub or https://cov.cx/ara

ISBN 978-1-7362002-0-9 (eBook)
        978-1-7362002-1-6 (Trade Paperback – Printed in the USA)
Library of Congress Control Number: 2020924677

Edition 1 Update 0 Published 21 December 2020

Disclaimer
I am not a doctor. Nothing in this book is intended as medical advice. Every person's medical situation is different and medical issues and conditions can be complex. You should consult with your physician before adopting any of the medical issues discussed herein. Information on the Covid-19 virus is rapidly changing and you should always check for the most recent information. We neither endorse nor guarantee the content of external links.

Dedication

They say it takes a village to raise a child. It surely took a large community of supporters to create this book. Even those who disagreed with some of its content helped strengthen its presentation and the robustness of the material now offered and explained to you.

Everyone who has interacted with me during the development of this book deserves and is gladly given many thanks and much appreciation.

In a similar context, our ability to avoid infection – individually, as a nation, and globally, depends on us both individually and collectively. That too takes a village.

So, mixing an element of hope with an element of appreciation, thank **you***, too – yes, you, the reader – for choosing to become well-informed and hopefully for choosing to make responsible decisions about how to avoid and survive this pandemic.*

Table of Contents

How to Best Use This Book

Yes, I know. It is a bit sad when it is necessary to explain how to read a book, isn't it! Maybe I'm guilty of over-engineering things.

But there are several things I want to advise about.

- *Footnotes and Links*

As well as the main text, the book has 780 footnotes, and within those footnotes are over 620 links to websites.[1] This makes the book a "cross-over" between a traditional book (either in print or in eBook/Kindle format) and a webpage where you can click on links effortlessly.

Some of these footnotes are not just citing sources, but also provide helpful additional content, and by all means, visit some of the links to better understand and make your own decisions, especially about the more contentious issues to do with the virus.

I've made the footnotes appear on the page they relate to rather than at the very end of the book. This makes it easier for you to follow both the main text and immediately see the footnotes, rather than needing to be endlessly flipping backward and forwards.

---

[1] Here's the very first footnote. I try to provide sources and proof for everything I say and felt it easiest to put these in footnotes rather than to have the main narrative interrupted by such things.

If you have this book in print form, when you want to visit links, you'd normally have the challenge of having to type long strings of text into a computer, tablet, or phone. Yes, I know - that's a terrible hassle. If you have this as an eBook, you still might find it awkward to be swapping programs between a Kindle reader and a web browser, and there's the potential of losing your place as you jump backward and forwards.

For people reading the printed book, I've done two things for you. **Firstly**, I've created a link shortener and reduced all the links to short links. For example, instead of typing in a long website name, you can just type a short name that redirects to the actual website and page. Keep in mind, in most browsers, you don't even need to type the https:// part, just type cov.cx/abcd or whatever. That makes things very much easier, I hope. I show both the regular and the short links everywhere, so you know where the short links go.

Possibly even easier is if you go to the https://cov.cx website. On the home page is a simple form where you only need to type in the five or fewer character short link code, which will open up the linked page in a new tab. When you're done, close that new tab, and you're back at the cov.cx home page and able to type in a new code for the next link, and so on. I hope that makes it about as easy as possible!

Secondly, I've put a page of links up on the book's companion website[2] that has all the footnotes from this book, using the same footnote numbering as in the book. Whether you're reading a print edition, or have the eBook on one screen and the webpage links on another, you can easily go to the footnote you want, and click the link – no need to type anything at all.

I hope this helps and encourages you to dive "deeply" into the footnotes and links as well as to better enjoy the main material.

• *Abbreviations*

Most abbreviations are either explained in the text or are well-known and don't need explaining.

In addition, a complete list of abbreviations appears as one of the appendices at the end of the book.

• *Color*

It is a huge regret that the cost makes color printing prohibitive (the book would almost quadruple in cost!). Most of the charts, text headings and footnote

---

[2] See https://thecovidsurvivalguide.com/footnotes/ or https://cov.cx/fn

links, are better seen in color. This is possible in the Kindle eBook version when viewed on a color capable device like a tablet, phone, or computer.

Apologies for the slight loss of reader-friendliness in this print version.

- *Gender*

Rather than write "he or she" and all other variations of the third person pronouns every time, I'm using the masculine form throughout when talking about people in general, and, as they say in legal interpretation, "the masculine shall include the feminine". I guess these days it also needs to include, ahem, all the more modern genders, too!

Book Updates

The situation with the virus is changing every day. Some days see small changes, others see major discoveries. It has been very hard to publish this book – for month after month, every day I was about to publish, then something new and important came out, and so I'd update the book to reflect that, then the next day, another new thing would come out, and so on in a Sisyphean type never-ending process.

So now I'm publishing in as up-to-date a fashion as possible, and then I will do two things to help you keep up to date.

First, I publish (usually) twice-weekly updates on the book's website. You can choose to have those sent to you for free if you simply join the mailing list.[3]

Second, I will occasionally update the *eBook* for free. I believe I can create a "discount price:" for the eBook and print book combined – if I can, I will, to make it easier to have both and therefore, the best of both worlds.

If you have your Amazon update option set, you'll get updates automatically. If you have it set for manual updates, you'll see information about updates when you list your digital content on Amazon. I'll also show this on the book's website, and will mention it in the twice-weekly updates.

Amazon's policy on updates is that I can provide free updates until more than 10% of the book has changed, or if something fundamental/major changes. I expect you should be able to get several updates before that happens.

---

[3] See the form on the top right of the website home page, https://thecovidsurvivalguide.com/ or https://cov.cx/covid

Quick Start **Guide**

I f you're in a hurry and don't have the time to read the whole book while needing some urgent answers, here are some "frequently asked questions" to start with. Please keep in mind that these pages summarize what is covered in 100 times as many following pages. Many details will be skipped here but are available in the full coverage that follows.

- *What is Covid-19*

Covid-19 (often now referred to simply as Covid) is the name given to the respiratory illness caused by a coronavirus formally known as SARS-CoV-2. This virus is believed to have first appeared in China in late 2019 and spread to other countries in early 2020.

The actual origin of the virus is controversial, and of little relevance to how we respond to it now.

- *What are the Chances of Becoming Infected*

That's impossible to answer. It depends on what risks and precautions you take, and the period of time you're considering, as well as a certain element of random chance.

As of mid-December, just over 5.3% of the US population are known to have had a Covid infection. About an additional 0.06% of the population are getting infected each day.

In other words, if you are careful (and we tell you how, in great detail), your odds of avoiding it, at least for the next few months, seem good.

- ### *How Can I Avoid Becoming Infected*

The three most important things are to wear a mask, to keep away from other people, and to surround yourself with fresh air (outdoors) or a great filtered/fresh air system (indoors).

Many other strategies exist (eg handwashing) but these are the three most important.

- ### *How Do I Know if I am Infected*

Symptoms of an infection typically appear 4 – 6 days after you have been infected. There is no exact set of symptoms that everyone gets, but the two most common symptoms are a fever of over 100.4°F (38.0°C) (experienced in 88% of cases) and a dry cough (2/3 of infected people experience a dry cough). Fatigue, and congestion or a runny nose affect 1/3 of people.

Getting a formal test is a good idea. Keep in mind it usually takes 5 – 8 days from when you were infected until when a test will detect your infection.

- ### *What Should I Do if I Get Infected*

The official answer is nothing other than drink lots of fluids, take it easy and relax. If your symptoms worsen (mainly shortness of breath/difficulty breathing/lower blood oxygen level) you should go to a hospital, otherwise recuperate at home.

The unofficial answer is there are many promising and legal but not official treatments (at least, not in the US) and actions that some doctors are recommending and which some studies seem to validate. We discuss the most promising of these in chapters 14 and 15 in Part Four of the book.

- ### *How Long Is a Quarantine*

People are being told they should self-isolate as much as possible for 10 days after the date of possible infection.

If no symptoms are experienced after that time, you are probably okay, and neither have the virus yourself nor are infectious for others.

- ### *How Long Does it Take to Get Better*

If you have a fever, it typically lasts 8 – 11 days. In general, it is common for all symptoms to go away after two weeks.

But, as in all things to do with the virus, there is a huge range of experienced and outcomes. President Trump seemed to go from well to very sick to recovered, all in less than a week. Other people might take six weeks to recover, and some are still not recovered after three months.

- ## *Will I Die if I get the Virus*

That depends on your general state of health, your age (the older you are, the greater your risk), and various other "comorbidity" factors such as your weight, if you're diabetic, your gender (men die more than women), and assorted other things.

It also depends on the healthcare and treatment plan you receive. Some of the newer and some of the still-experimental treatments seem to make major improvements in survival rates. We discuss these later in the book.

Currently, fewer than 2% of all people who get the virus die. If you're under 40 and with no comorbidities, your chances of surviving are excellent. If you're over 80, and with comorbidities, your chances drop substantially.

- ## *Will I Get the Virus a Second Time*

Originally the hope was, like with many other viruses, after getting Covid once, you'd acquire immunity and not get it a second time.

Now it seems acquired immunity might be weak rather than strong and fade over time; indeed people who previously had the virus are now being advised to be vaccinated. For now, the hope is that most people will have effective immunity for at least three months, and perhaps as long as a year, but there's not yet any clear understanding of how long immunity might extend because it is still so new.

- ## *What are the Cures/Treatments/Vaccines for the Virus*

There is nothing yet in the category of "take one pill a day for a week and you'll be for sure recovered". There are a number of treatments that seem to make appreciable improvements to your survival chances and greatly reduce the possibility of needing to be hospitalized and potentially worse. Although in use in some countries, none of these are yet officially approved in the US.

There are also a number of treatments, some not yet officially approved, for people who do need to go to a hospital and get extra care and help.

We're hopeful survival rates will continue to improve. We write about the most promising of these treatments further on in the book.

As for a vaccine, the good news is over 100 vaccines are being developed all around the world, and about a dozen of those are already in "Phase Three Trials". If their Phase Three Trials are successful, the next step is then to request official

FDA approval. The Pfizer and Moderna vaccines have already applied for that, and Emergency Use Authorization for both might be granted in December 2020. Britain approved the Pfizer vaccine in early December and started vaccinating people on 8 December.

There are already approved (by their respective governments, but not yet by other major countries) Russian and Chinese vaccines too. There are some worries that these vaccines have been rushed through testing in less time than is normally required to credibly be certain of their safety and effectiveness, indeed the Russian vaccine was approved before it had even started its Phase Three trial.

There is no understanding of how long a vaccine will last before you'll need a booster shot. Maybe every year, maybe more (and also, of course, maybe less) often than that.

It is unlikely any of these vaccines will be readily available to most US residents until perhaps Spring of 2021.

• *When Will the Virus Go Away and Life Return to Normal*

Some optimists originally believed the virus might just disappear, all by itself. That now is clearly not going to be the case.

Other optimists believe herd immunity will eventually cause the virus to stop spreading. But herd immunity requires 60% or more of the population to have been infected, and in mid-December we were at about 5.3%. No-one wants to wait however many years for that to rise to over 60%. Plus there's a concern that herd immunity will wear off after some months, making it much less beneficial.

A vaccine will help greatly, of course. And while easy simple treatments won't get rid of the virus, they would make its presence less impactful and life-threatening.

How long for all this to happen? That's anyone's guess. Once a vaccine becomes reasonably available and the number of people vaccinated starts to become substantial, the harsh edge of concern will be removed for many of us.

We expect things will improve in the second or third quarter of 2021. Attitudes will probably shift to a more optimistic view of the future before then - once a vaccine has been identified, doses are starting to be distributed, and our case and death curves, rather than relentlessly rising, starts to steadily drop.

• *What Should I Buy Now for "Just in Case" Future Needs*

Obviously, plenty of toilet paper!

Beyond that, think about what might happen if you needed to quarantine and/or became bedridden for a couple of weeks with an actual case of the virus. Sure, home delivery services can get most things to you the same day you order them, or the next day if not. But if you're truly unwell, you might find it hard to concentrate and have the energy to work your way around websites and do the ordering.

Try and have enough basic essentials and easily prepared foods to see you through much or all of a two-week isolation period, so that is one less thing you'll need to worry about.

Also consider any medications or medical equipment you might need during that time. With occasional surges in buying, some of these items are not always in stock, and sometimes things are taking a week or longer to be delivered.

Buy the things you think you might want or need now. Don't wait until the last moment. Happily, most of the supplies you might choose to stock up on are inexpensive.

Introduction

When Covid-19 first started to become an issue – before it had even been given an official name – it was embarrassingly easy to accept two assumptions. Most of us did.

The first assumption – just like other recent respiratory virus threats (SARS, MERS, Swine 'flu, and so on) this too would be another flash-in-the-pan scare and not amount to anything serious.

The second assumption – of all the countries in the world, we in the US would most benefit from our highly sophisticated healthcare system and general infrastructure, and quickly minimize any potential impact and disruption, better than other countries.

When it became clearer the virus was indeed going to be a challenge, it still seemed the threat and problems posed would be something that could be addressed and quickly resolved by a unanimity of purpose and plan, guided by scientific methodology, analysis, and leadership and implemented by a populace eager to rid themselves of this viral scourge.

Hmmm....

Most people have been slow to gradually accept the steadily worsening reality. When, on 21 February, I canceled the international group tours I was planning to operate in May (France), June (Scotland), September (Kazakhstan), and December (European Christmas Markets) of 2020, disappointed potential tour members accused me of being overly pessimistic. Some said they'd go on their own, regardless.

Clearly, such attitudes have been shown to be tragically optimistic rather than pessimistic.   Never mind the political optimism, which is perhaps understandable.[4] Even intelligent, well-educated, and well-informed people were also distinctly optimistic to start with. For example, in early April, and after a steady barrage of anxious articles and information from me about the growing extent and implacable nature of the virus, a survey of my Travel Insider readers showed that on average, they expected life would be back to normal by August (ie within four months of the survey).

A repeat of the survey in early May showed a shift in expectations.   On average, readers then expected it would no longer be August, but February 2021 for things to get back to normal. When August came and the virus was infecting people at rates twice as high as in April and killing over a thousand people a day, a new survey of readers showed they are expecting a return to normalcy early in the second half of 2021 – a year or more after the survey date.

---

[4] Remember how there were hopes to "re-open" the country in time for Easter (12 April)? Then in time for May Day, Memorial Day (25 May), and 4 July? Alas, the virus is unpersuaded by three-day weekends.

Mere weeks before the election, President Trump was still maintaining there'd be a vaccine announced before the election. That never happened, but subsequently, it turned out that Trump may have finally been correct – Pfizer had very positive news about its vaccine candidate, which it chose to delay announcing until five days after the election. See https://blog.thetravelinsider.info/2020/11/why-did-pfizer-delay-their-vaccine-announcement-so-long.html or https://cov.cx/tia1 A week after Pfizer's announcement, Moderna made a similar announcement.

(Aug) We'll be back to normal by :

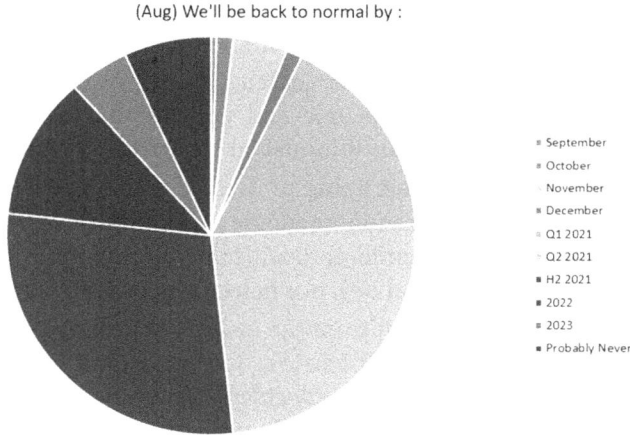

- September
- October
- November
- December
- Q1 2021
- Q2 2021
- H2 2021
- 2022
- 2023
- Probably Never

Figure 1 Changing expectations about the virus

That's an expectation that is withstanding the passing of time. A different survey in early December largely mirrored the results above with most readers expecting (hoping!) the third quarter of 2021 will be when it is safe to start traveling again.

Are people becoming more realistic, or is there still a stubborn unwillingness to accept the reality of the virus? Will the vaccines, now tantalizingly close to being approved, fulfill their promises of effectiveness? What happens if they don't?

Most of all, are we doing the right things now?

It is difficult for any of us, alone, to shape public policy about the virus, but I hope this book will help you – the person directly reading this now – understand and implement some of the critical issues you are personally facing, today, from the narrow perspective of what is most relevant and beneficial to you. What should you do to minimize your risk of personally getting infected by the virus? What would happen if you did get infected, and what should you do in such a case to ensure the easiest experience and most certain and full recovery?

These are questions that demand clear (and – please! – correct) answers. They are literally life and death questions. On 17 December, the US passed through 317,000 people "officially" dying of the virus, and possibly many more "unofficially",[5] and an unknown number of the other 17.5+ million people who

---

[5] We discuss the difficulties in counting deaths later on. Surprisingly, something as seemingly obvious as the number of deaths is vague and unclear, but there are reasons

(continued on next page)

have acquired the virus will either die prematurely or never fully recover, due to lasting damage to their heart, lungs, brain, and other organs.

It is not my intention to now search for and negatively shovel generous helpings of blame to all the people and policies that have utterly failed our country and aided rather than diminished the virus' spread and the problems arising from it.[6] I'm also not going to dwell either on issues about where the virus came from and if it was manmade or a naturally occurring virus. None of that resurrects the quarter-million dead (many of them unnecessary victims of bad public health policies to date), nor helps us plan for our future.

But, "those who don't learn from the lessons of history are doomed to repeat them" and it is interesting to at least try to understand how it is that so many seemingly clever experts can be so spectacularly wrong, and how public opinion has fractured into many different and conflicting viewpoints on matters that surely should seem simple and straightforward to answer with a clear unequivocal yes or no. To mask, or not to mask? Open schools or keep them closed? And so on.

So before directly answering these questions (but skip ahead if you wish), it is helpful to understand why these issues are open and controversial questions, rather than having universally understood and accepted answers. Isn't science supposed to be exact and objective, not vague and subjective?

In the possibly five minutes it has taken you to read to this point of the introduction, perhaps 750 – 900 more people have become infected by the Covid-19 virus, in the US alone. More grimly, maybe ten more people have died from it.[7] This is all very real, all very serious.

I'm not a doctor, and you're probably not one either. But I am certain both of us can gain a sufficient understanding of the underlying issues – some medical,

---

why this is so. This article is a helpful explainer and suggests that the true count, in early December, might be almost 400,000 – about a third more than the official count of 274,000. See https://www.mediaite.com/news/staggering-new-cdc-data-suggests-true-coronavirus-death-toll-is-now-near-400000/ or https://cov.cx/a1f59

[6] The problems, while definitely reflecting very poorly on the Trump Administration, date back to the previous Administration, and to several previous ones too. The problem further has to be shared between the Administration – wrong priorities – and the Congress – lack of budget funding. No-one, of any political persuasion, can feel proud of their record. And we, the voters, need to share in that complicity too.

[7] Assuming a rate of about 2500 deaths/day, as is the December seven-day average rate of US deaths – see https://www.msn.com/en-gb/news/us/1-american-is-dying-of-covid-19-every-30-seconds/ar-BB1bBckt or https://cov.cx/a1f60 and https://www.worldometers.info/coronavirus/country/us/ or https://cov.cx/a1a11 for whatever the rate is when you are reading this.

some social, some statistical. Sure, at the molecular and cellular level, viruses are complicated, but at the public policy level, their effects and our responses become less "medical" and more sociological/statistical/political/economic, rather than complex medical matters.[8]

With some understanding, we can all contribute to the public policy debate about how to respond as a society and nation, and make informed decisions about how we should respond, personally.

That is why I'm offering this to you now. I hope it proves helpful.

And please, let me know if there is more I can add to any part of what is already a very lengthy and detailed book.

Here's a hope and prayer for all of us and our safe survival through this scourge

David M Rowell.

David@TheCovidSurvivalGuide.com

---

[8] You don't need to understand how a car engine operates to drive a car well and we can all participate in public debates about what speed limits and other traffic rules should be. Similarly, you don't need to understand "virus spikes" and "receptor cells" to see the good sense in taking medications that help speed recovery, you don't need to understand the properties of aerosols to know that wearing a mask and keeping your distance is sensible, and so on.

PART ONE : Public Health and Policy

1. An Unfortunate and Unnecessary Controversy

T his part, and this chapter in particular, is essentially "a book within a book". But it is important and may give you new skills to understand and interpret not just issues to do with the coronavirus but many other things in life too. If you want to get straight to the "good stuff", then by all means skip on to the next chapter or even all the way to the second part.

If you're still here, let's start with a fundamental consideration. I am not a doctor. Some people have insisted that disqualifies me from any role in discussing Covid issues, and of course, they're saying that you too should not and can not contribute either. Obviously, I disagree.

I feel compelled to comment on this point, because if these critics are correct, this entire book is invalid, and by direct extension, you should have no ability to express your opinion either.[9]

If these people are correct, much of the world needs to be changed. Politicians could no longer pass laws on anything they didn't have advanced degrees in,

---

[9] In my case, even if I am not to be allowed to provide original findings, that shouldn't be a problem. Very little in this book is original "out of nowhere" material. Instead, I collate and present to you the best of the findings and expert opinions, and provide sources to substantiate every point I make. Critics should not "shoot the messenger". They shouldn't attack me for presenting such information – they should attack the underlying sources of anything they disagree with.

personal knowledge of, and hands-on experience of. Similarly, judges could no longer rule on any cases about which they didn't have in-depth qualifications to support their analysis. Travel agents could no longer recommend a vacation for you unless they had degrees in sociology, anthropology, history, and geography to best understand each destination, plus a degree in psychology and counseling to best understand exactly your stated and unstated needs, and had personally visited and experienced every offered product, and further experienced all competing products too.

Are there any topics, of any kind, that aren't based on special knowledge and complex data?

There are four different issues all being mixed together.

(a) Who Can Conduct Original Research?

None of the material I'm presenting to you is my own original research, so this is a question we can avoid.

But, in general terms, I'm okay with anyone conducting original research. As long as the methodology and results are clearly and correctly presented and reproducible (essential ingredients of the "scientific method"), people of all knowledge levels are then free to make their own evaluation of the research and form their own decisions based on the data presented to them.

This is vividly illustrated by a 14-year-old middle-school girl in Texas. In October 2020 she won a $25,000 award for a discovery that could lead to a Covid cure.[10]

Some of the most ignorant periods in history have been marked by restrictions on who is allowed to conduct scientific research, and on what topics. Some of the biggest scientific breakthroughs trespassed into what was, at the time, "forbidden knowledge" with the researchers having no official credentials and risking death by their studies and findings.

Science should be all about the data, not about who is presenting it. Let's not retreat back to the Dark Ages.

(b) Who Can Report Issues and Facts?

If only scientists are allowed to report their research and findings, we'd miss out on a lot of helpful information and public understanding.

---

[10] See https://www.cnn.com/2020/10/18/us/anika-chebrolu-covid-treatment-award-scn-trnd/index.html or https://cov.cx/a1a12

For example, consider this scientific paper and a "for the public" summary/restatement.

Here is the scientific paper :

https://www.frontiersin.org/articles/10.3389/fpubh.2020.00473/full or https://cov.cx/a1g12

It has the subject heading "Modeling the Onset of Symptoms of Covid-19". How many people do you think are likely to read through the 8,850 words and dense scientific shorthand that it comprises? And how many of those people are likely to accurately understand it?

Now compare that scientific paper with this article that writes up the paper for public consumption :

https://www.studyfinds.org/coronavirus-symptoms-order/   or https://cov.cx/aq1g13

The article's heading is "Coronavirus symptoms tend to begin in certain order: Fever first, then cough, muscle pain". That pretty much summarizes both its own 584 plain English words as well as the entirety of the original 8,850-word paper. This article fairly translates the scientific paper into everyday language and concepts that are easily understood by most people.

Is that harmful? Should it be forbidden? The article includes links to the original paper, so anyone who wishes to understand more or to check for the fairness and accuracy of the article can do so.

We feel this should be encouraged. A better-informed public can better understand and accept the policies being formulated and implemented.

This is much of what I am doing in the pages that follow. It is what most journalists do, most of the time. If you were to take out the "translations" of topics from the media, many publications would entirely disappear, leaving us only with "safe" articles about the Kardashians and their ilk.

Yes, there is the ever-present possibility that, accidentally or deliberately, a paraphrased simplification may be misleading or incomplete or incorrect or biased in its presentation. But is that possibility any greater than the possibility that if people had to read the original article, they'd either not do so at all, or they'd misunderstand what they were seeing?

In this case, guarding against the possibility of mistake is best solved not by seeking to forbid such popularizations, but by encouraging them so there is a fair and full range of interpretations presented. Truth is best exposed by shining multiple lights at an issue, not by restricting the perspective and evaluation to only officially approved people and viewpoints. Truth is best affirmed by challenging it, not by mandated acceptance.

One more point. Much important research only appears in subscription-only professional publications – and the cost of an annual subscription can cost many thousands of dollars.[11] Official research is often not open or accessible to us – like it or not, we must rely on popularizations.

(c) Who Can Criticize Scientific Research?

An analogy might be helpful here. Let's say Steven Spielberg directs a new movie starring Meryl Streep.

When it is released, film critics all start publishing their opinions. There are hundreds, even thousands, of such professional critics, and of course, millions of filmgoers, all of whom decide whether or not to attend the film, and afterward, if to recommend it on to their friends or not. We are all critics, to a greater or lesser degree.

No-one has ever said that only other directors who have also won four Oscars should be permitted to express opinions on Spielberg's latest movie. No-one has ever said that only other actresses with three Oscar awards can express opinions on Streep's performance in a movie.

You might say "Oh yes, but anyone can direct or act". That may or may not be true, but even if it is, how about, then, a composer of music? Or an author – can only other mega-best-selling middle-aged female authors in Scotland criticize a new work by J K Rowling? Can only other people who also lived in 16th century England express opinions on Shakespeare's work?

You might say "Well, these are subjective things which everyone can have an opinion on", and that is partially true, although much criticism is also technically based, and there are plenty of actors and directors who disagree with you when their work is challenged, whether on technical or artistic or "just because" grounds.

So what is scientific research and is it challengeable? Isn't scientific research supposed to be objective statements of data and theories/hypotheses that are derived and supported or contradicted by the data reported? While it might take special skills to develop the

---

[11] See https://pubs.acs.org/pb-assets/documents/infocentral/2018%20Institutional%20Print%20Subscription%20Rates.pdf or https://cov.cx/a1a13

theories/hypotheses (or medicines, etc) that are being tested, isn't the act of evaluating the results of tests *a totally different process*, requiring logical and statistical type skills, rather than requiring the specialist skills to develop the material, product, or process being tested?

Think of a trial of a new drug that is said to cure Covid-19. Sure, it takes special skills to develop the drug (skills that I don't have and never will develop), but what special skills are required to then evaluate the bottom-line finding "995 patients got better and 5 did not after taking this drug, while of patients not taking the drug, 300 got better and 700 did not"?[12]

The heart of the "scientific method" is creating robust findings that can be and are critically challenged and which can withstand such challenges.

Clearly, we think anyone should be allowed to share their analysis of such studies/trials, and you should be allowed to see the analysis and decide for yourself what is most persuasive.

Furthermore, there comes a point when we shift from the pure science of an issue to the broader social framework and values of what we are prepared to accept and the tradeoffs associated with outcomes. That's a point where we all have voices that count.

(d) The Issue is Mainly Public Policy, Not Medical Science

The last point is important, too. Most of the concepts in Part One of this book, and many in the other parts, are to do with public policy and notions of fairness and balance – who should suffer and make sacrifices, and who should be compensated and how much.

Those are matters more of public policy than of medical science, and surely in a democracy, we can all equally participate in that debate.

Maybe the preceding comments are sufficient to encourage you to keep reading. I hope so. But if you'd like a bit more explanation about the specifics of what I'm providing and why it is currently controversial, please continue through the rest of this section. I hope you'll find it interesting and helpful, not just in terms of how to evaluate this book, but how to evaluate scientific data and its analysis in general.

---

[12] This is of course an enormous simplification of how trial results are presented, but the ultimate point of any trial write-up should be one of three things –

(1) The trial persuasively shows a positive result
(2) The trial persuasively shows a negative result
(3) The trial is unpersuasive by itself and more research/trialing is required

Even though I'm no stranger to any of this, I should open what follows by telling you how astonished I have been, over the last eight months, to see just how subjective rather than objective, and sometimes downright error-prone, the science and its interpretation has been.[13] There are some reasons why this can sometimes happen, and traps that are easy both for original scientists and subsequent analysts to fall into.

Most of the information in the pages that follow is a collation of data from sources who usually are doctors or research scientists in the relevant fields. I've chosen the content that seems, to me, to be most valid and valuable, shaped by my own non-medical opinions, and based on the underlying research and data. If two scientists are allowed (by the shadowy forces who seek to censor and limit comment) to publish two different papers showing two different interpretations on an issue, surely other people must then be allowed to prefer one or the other of the two conflicting sets of findings and to explain their preferences or to view the differing interpretations as evidence that more research is required to more authoritatively resolve the matter one way or the other.

Other people may – and some indeed do – disagree with my conclusions and selected recommendations. That is to be expected and is why I provide links to the sources so you can form your own opinion, too. But these disagreements extend beyond what you and I might think and continues on to what the "experts" think, too. Surprisingly (perhaps) and dismayingly (definitely), not even all

---

[13] The most extreme example of extraordinarily wrong data has been just about every early projection about the extent of the spread of the disease and the number of people who would die.

Even more amusing are the studies that initially showed what seemed like enormously high numbers of infections and deaths that were then hastily changed by their authors (the highest-profile example being the Imperial College London projection in mid-March, projecting 2.2 million people would die in the US over the next few months – see https://www.theatlantic.com/health/archive/2020/03/how-many-americans-are-sick-lost-february/608521/ or https://cov.cx/a1a14), sometimes reducing by 20-fold their projections, with lots of excuse/explanation about how they were right to start with, but are now more right with their 20x lower numbers.

The tragically amusing part is that now we are getting closer to the original numbers which they rushed to disown, but in a very different scenario to the one that they earlier based their projections on.

It is true and fair to say that the early models and their projections were wrong due to a lack of hard data on which to base the models, but those weaknesses were only minimally featured in the model results and findings.

One last thing about models. There's a truism – "all models are wrong, but some are useful".

doctors agree on the best approach to combating the SARS-CoV-2 coronavirus and the Covid-19 illness it causes.[14]

Worse still, some people wonder if part of the current opinions and views have been shaped by the massive public relations and lobbying budgets of big pharma companies, and then further distorted when overlaid by political considerations (greatly magnified by the timing of the election recently held) and public health "we know best" attitudes.[15]

Sometimes a key question that needs to be asked when viewing any article and its findings/recommendations is "Who Benefits and How?". This is even recognized in formal scientific paper-writing protocols, where the authors of a study are required to disclose financial interests, funding, and conflicts.

For the record, I have no investments in any pharmaceutical or medical/health companies, and I'm receiving no money from anyone to write this book. My wish is that the answer to the question "Who benefits and how" as it applies to this book is "**You** will benefit from a better understanding and as a result will be able to better manage **your** lifestyle and approach to the Covid-19 virus".

It is no great surprise that our political leaders have not done a great job in leading the response to the Covid-19 crisis. We might variously disagree with what they should have done, but we can definitely agree that what has been done has been inadequate! The numbers speak for themselves.

Sadly, it isn't only our political leaders who are open to criticism. So too are the public health officials. For example, they outright lied to us originally, telling us there was no reason to wear masks. Public health authorities decided to

---

[14] This issue is one of the most important ones of all. The CDC says newly infected Covid-19 patients should do nothing except stay at home and hope for the best. Most doctors are adopting that advice without question. Only a minority are pointing out the ludicrous concept of doing nothing when it is easiest and least costly to defeat the virus, and waiting until an infection has become severe before responding. Imagine if the same approach was adopted for cancer treatments!

Here's a great article that supports early intervention and treatment, by a physician who is also the Executive Director of the Association of American Physicians and Surgeons. https://aapsonline.org/lessons-from-the-9-month-covid-emergency/ or https://cov.cx/a1f79

[15] For every opinion/theory that the Democrats are deliberately shaping the crisis to their advantage, there is a similar theory that the Republicans are doing the same for their advantage. I guess I'm either too naïve or too cynical and tend to ascribe the political mismanagement as much to incompetence as to venality, failings shared equally on each side.

discourage public mask-wearing, because there was a critical shortage of masks[16] and they wanted to hoard all the masks they could for healthcare workers. [17] But they didn't tell us that. Instead, they lied to us about masks not being necessary.[18] "Lie" is a strong word, but it seems appropriate, although if you'd prefer "gravely mistaken" that's fine, too. The proof this was a lie or at least gravely mistaken is seen in how there is now a near unanimity of public health voices all demanding we wear masks, and in many cases, state mandates making them compulsory.

_____

[16] Which in itself is an appalling situation that both public health officials and politicians should never have allowed to happen.

[17] At the risk of stating the obvious, it was always easy for adroit public health officials and government regulation to corner the market in officially approved highest quality "medical grade" N95 and similar masks. There was never a reason to lie to us.

Furthermore, the current encouragement for people to make their own masks of any style or shape/size, and from any material at all, could have been promulgated right from the start. A decision to lie to us back then has terribly diminished the trust and confidence we have now in what public health authorities are telling us.

[18] Even the venerated Dr Fauci tried to "square the circle" in the early days (March 8), when he said that mask-wearing was important for infected people, but not as a preventative measure for normal people. Here's a short video clip in which he waffles a bit but says "....in the United States people should not be walking around with masks". The interviewer asked him if he was sure about that, and Dr Fauci repeated the same statement. But later in the short clip, he then referred to other countries where up to 85% of the population are wearing masks and said, seemingly dismissively, "I'm not against it" and then revealed the big issue – "it could lead to a shortage of masks for the people who really need it". See https://www.youtube.com/watch?v=PRa6t_e7dgl or https://cov.cx/a1f87

Now flash forward to September, where the truth couldn't have changed more. The director of the CDC, Dr Robert Redfield, says in a Senate hearing "Facemasks are the most important powerful public health tool we have, and I will continue to appeal for all Americans to embrace these face coverings". He went on to say "we have clear scientific evidence they [disposable cheap face masks] work and they are our best defense". If that wasn't strong enough, he then said a face mask was better protection against the virus than a vaccine. Here's a short video clip : https://www.youtube.com/watch?v=NYRAZxcp_hU or https://cov.cx/a1f88

At the same time, public health authorities focused on the risk of being infected by touching an infected surface – a risk which has now been deemed to be the least significant risk and means of becoming infected.[19]

A more recent astonishing reversal in public policy is even harder to understand, explain, or justify than the other examples. On 25 August, the CDC changed its policy on who should be given Covid-19 tests. Famously, in the early stages of the outbreak, President Trump and other national health-care leaders promised us "If you want a test, you can get a test". That has sadly never been so (and even when tests are available, results have sometimes been so delayed as to be meaningless by the time they were finally received), but the promise has remained more or less intact, with apologies and excuses being offered up for the failure to honor it.

Another example is equally perplexing. After a major Mayo Clinic study and other lesser inputs, the FDA gave an Emergency Use Authorization for the use of convalescent plasma to treat severely suffering Covid patients.[20] But…. Two days later, the NIH issued a contradictory statement saying that convalescent plasma should *not* be used as a treatment.[21] Two branches of the US Government are now at war with each other, with contradictory statements. To the people who say "only doctors can discuss this matter", my question becomes – "when the doctors themselves disagree so fundamentally, how do we know which doctors to listen to?".

As you'll see further in this book, when we talk about testing, rapid testing of anyone who suspects they might have the virus is an essential part of controlling the spread of the virus, as is also preventative type testing of everyone else, too. It has been suggested that at least 40% of infected – and infectious – people have no symptoms but may still be infectious to others, and for people who do develop symptoms, they are infectious and a risk to other people before developing any

---

[19] The slowness to appreciate the risk presented by the aerosolized spread of virus particles is very puzzling. Was it related to the decision to downplay the value of masks, or was it a separate failing?

[20] See https://www.fda.gov/news-events/press-announcements/fda-issues-emergency-use-authorization-convalescent-plasma-potential-promising-covid-19-treatment or https://cov.cx/a1a15

[21] A relevant page on the NIH site now seems to have disappeared. Discussed from about the 18-minute point in this podcast : https://www.youtube.com/watch?v=fdbwTNNsF1E or https://cov.cx/a1a16 The NIH now seems more neutral about convalescent plasma use https://www.covid19treatmentguidelines.nih.gov/immune-based-therapy/blood-derived-products/convalescent-plasma/ or https://cov.cx/a1a17

symptoms. So testing asymptomatic people is as important as testing people with symptoms.

How can we now understand and reconcile the CDC's new statement that public testing might not be necessary? Barely a month ago, the CDC's director was stating "Anyone who thinks they may be infected -- independent of symptoms -- should get a test." Now the CDC is telling us "Don't bother, stay away".[22]

The strangest part of a very strange reversal of policy is that finally, now, we are starting to get fast and inexpensive tests that cost as little as $5 (retail), can be done at home, and give results in 15 minutes. Why were we urged to be tested if we thought we might be at risk when testing was unavailable, slow, and expensive; but now that testing is becoming more common, fast, and inexpensive, we're told not to bother?

So clearly, the experts and authorities are not infallible.[23] What are they lying to us about now, or if not lying again, simply wrong about?[24]

Maybe lying is too strong a word. Choose the word you prefer and the underlying reason for the incomplete and sometimes wrong advice, but we don't think there is any acceptable excuse for promulgating guidelines that place more people at gratuitous risk than would be the case if the guidelines were more

---

[22] See https://www.msn.com/en-us/news/politics/in-stunning-reversal-cdc-abruptly-changes-position-on-when-to-get-tested/ar-BB18oiTf or https://cov.cx/a1a18 and https://www.msn.com/en-us/news/us/trump-administration-defends-inexplicable-changes-to-coronavirus-testing-guidelines/ar-BB18p6yr or https://cov.cx/a1a19

[23] Here's an article headed "Health agencies' credibility at risk after week of blunders" – see : https://apnews.com/b9b6dc204d780fac7e6a79c1dbf21b8d or https://cov.cx/a1a20 . Maybe this is due to political meddling, but that is almost irrelevant. The point is that, for whatever reason, sometimes the public health leaders who we necessarily must place the highest degree of trust in are telling us things that don't survive scrutiny and which end up being reversed. We need to preserve and encourage such scrutiny, not seek to forbid it.

[24] Some apologists say that public health officials have been pressured into making incorrect policy statements by their political masters. That may or may not be true, but it is not an excuse. The excuse of "just following orders" didn't help many Germans at the Nuremberg trials after WW2, and is not allowed as a defense in our Armed Forces now. It shouldn't be a defense for public health officials either.

accurately stated. Here's an interesting and lengthy article about some of the CDC failings.[25]

Other leaders have done things that have killed hundreds or even thousands of Americans – for example, sending infected older people back to care homes, where they then proceeded to infect other aged residents,[26] causing the disease to spread around facilities that were never designed to offer isolation and containment of highly transmittable virus infections.[27]

Doctors themselves are far from infallible and are not always above reproach, either.[28]

And one final point. Just because we see a well-credentialed senior executive making a statement on a matter, it does not necessarily mean that he is sharing his personal research and analysis. Sure, he may have reviewed and even helped shape the material he is sharing, but then again, maybe he is blindly sharing

---

[25] See https://www.propublica.org/article/inside-the-fall-of-the-cdc or https://cov.cx/a1a21

[26] It is almost irrelevant whether this decision was made out of utter ignorance or because of trying to protect scarce hospital beds for people who were "more deserving" of treatment (ie would live longer). It was medically wrong and morally suspect and is another example where public policy is not necessarily reflective of the best practices, and another reason why we all deserve both to be given full information and to be allowed to participate in such policy discussion and formation.

[27] There's also a cogent case to be made that as a result of re-opening the country too early and being too permissive in terms of social distancing restrictions, tens of thousands of Americans have died who would not otherwise have been infected. The brutal reality is that the US is the third-worst country in the world (ignoring small countries) in terms of overall infection rate, and the 6th worst in terms of death rate. Canada to the north and Mexico to the south have had only one fifth and one quarter as many cases as us. Canada has one third the death rate, Mexico has slightly less than our death rate.
There are probably many factors giving rise to that, but our public health policies and virus response actions have to be considered a major influencer.

[28] For example, see https://www.npr.org/2020/10/01/914433778/web-of-wellness-doctors-promote-injections-of-unproven-coronavirus-treatment or https://cov.cx/a1a22 and https://www.nbcnews.com/news/us-news/oregon-doctor-s-license-revoked-over-refusal-wear-mask-during-n1250092 or https://cov.cx/a1f84

information from more junior members of his staff, blindly trusting it to be accurate and appropriate.[29]

Lessons from the Hydroxychloroquine Controversy

How can the value of medicines be so controversial? Like you, I'd hoped it might be a simple yes/no thing – does this drug work or not?

Of course, it has never been a simple yes/no issue. Determining the appropriateness of any drug has always been a more complicated evaluation of multiple issues such as "how well does this work, and for how many of the people does it work, and what are the related side-effects and downsides". Another consideration that we all prefer to overlook but which is a factor is "how much does the drug cost, and how much do the related support services add to that cost".

But, even with a more nuanced approach looking at all these factors, hydroxychloroquine seemed to have a lot in its favor. Astonishingly, the controversy that ensued about hydroxychloroquine seems to be driven by two issues that should be irrelevant – first being the recommendation by President Trump that people should look at the potential of this drug,[30] and secondly, because hydroxychloroquine ("HCQ") is a "public domain" drug, with expired patents, made at very low cost and even lower profit by many different drug

---

[29] I don't know if this lady – the Associate Chief Medical Officer of Health for Ontario, Canada, and her boss, the Chief Medical Officer, are joking or serious when, as you can see and hear in this video, she says "I don't know why I bring all these papers, I never look at them. I just say whatever they write down for me" and he appears to say, after some interaction, "Yeah, same". See https://twitter.com/OnCall4ON/status/1338933683592556544 or https://cov.cx/a1g11

[30] I've viewed the video of his conference where he first mentioned HCQ. He merely said that some people were reporting good results, that it seemed promising, and that it should be looked into. He never stated as a fact "HCQ is a for sure guaranteed way of curing Covid-19".

companies,[31] there is no orchestrated campaign of high-profile supporters and lobbyists to tell its story positively.[32]

To start with the negative, most "establishment" type organizations in the US have all recommended against using HCQ as a Covid treatment, including the FDA, CDC, and AMA. So why, in the face of such apparent agreement, does the debate about using HCQ continue?

Some of the research to "prove" that HCQ is useless or even harmful has been verging on dishonest and deceitful, so much so that it has been subsequently withdrawn by the refereed journals who had originally been too trusting and rushed to publish HCQ critiques for commercial rather than public health reasons.[33] And some of the organizations making these negative statements about HCQ seem – astonishingly – unable to explain why or to back up their

---

[31] More recently there has been a suggestion that President Trump only decided to promote HCQ because he has shares in a mutual fund that in turn has shares in a French company, Sanofi, that makes HCQ tablets, and so he decided to recommend it to make money for himself.

Ignoring the fact that any of us with mutual fund holdings probably indirectly have shares in half the companies listed on the stock market, there is very little likelihood that any company would get rich from making and selling HCQ, because it is made by so many different companies, already, all around the world, and at extremely low costs – I just checked and the Sanofi Plaquenil brand is selling at a price of 10c/tablet in US discount drugstores such as Kroger. If a drug is being sold, at retail, for 10c each, and you only need a dozen or so tablets for a course of treatment, how will anyone, anywhere, get ridiculously rich on that transaction?

[32] Is it a coincidence that the only "Emergency Use Authorization" treatments for Covid are very expensive drugs made by large pharmaceutical companies; while low-cost expired-patent medicines are now being used successfully in many other countries to treat their Covid sufferers but remain unacknowledged and unapproved in the US?

Rather than having deep-pocketed supporters and lobbyists pushing for HCQ use, it almost appears that the companies who do have the deep pockets and supporters may have been keen to argue against HCQ for fear that it would harm their efforts to promote their alternate and very much more expensive drugs.

[33] The highest-profile example is an article that was published to great acclaim by the once highly regarded British journal, The Lancet. Within a few days, the data used was exposed as being fraudulent. The Lancet has no explanation for how its peer-review process failed to notice the obvious data inconsistencies that even I saw, and has now retracted the article. https://www.thelancet.com/journals/lancet/article/PIIS0140-6736(20)31180-6/fulltext or https://cov.cx/a1a23 A similar reliance on unreliably sourced data caused the NEJM to somewhat ungraciously retract an article too – see https://www.sciencemag.org/news/2020/06/two-elite-medical-journals-retract-coronavirus-papers-over-data-integrity-questions or https://cov.cx/a1g09

negative evaluation with a comprehensive review of all the literature, including over 100 positive articles showing benefits from HCQ use, many in refereed journals.[34] Instead, they'll focus exclusively on one or two negative studies and ignore the 100+ positive studies.

The FDA, when called upon by Senators Johnson, Lee, and Cruz in August to provide evidence to prove their claim that HCQ use has no effect and may be harmful" was unable to do so (but didn't apologize or rescind their claim).[35]

It is also true that some of the material that supports the positive claims about HCQ and other low-cost drugs does not conform to the highest standards of double-blind fully-randomized trials. But many of the trials *do* conform to the highest standards and of the 205 studies known in mid-December, 139 have been peer-reviewed.   As such, the evidence in support of HCQ use appears overwhelming, and overwhelmingly positive. I don't believe there is any other drug that has been so exhaustively studied for Covid use as HCQ, and with such generally positive outcomes when used in the proper context (early treatment, not late treatment, and in conjunction with zinc being the key considerations).[36]

Even the less sophisticated studies have some value – the reality of the results should not be ignored. I find reports from small family medicine practices saying "we don't know what is causing this, but we've given 100 (or whatever other number) of Covid-infected patients (some drug combination) and none of them have needed to be admitted to hospital" to be credible and persuasive.[37]

There is no deceit, no sophistry, and no vested interest or ulterior motivation in such statements. Maybe there's not an abundance of statistical rigor, either, but whether the outcome is a placebo effect, the result of the drugs given, or purely random chance matters not to me. I know that if I get a Covid-19 infection, I want to similarly avoid going to a hospital, and if taking a safe but not yet

---

[34] See https://c19study.com/ or https://cov.cx/a1a24

[35] See this excellent testimony to a December Senate Committee
https://www.hsgac.senate.gov/imo/media/doc/Testimony-Orient-2020-12-08.pdf or
https://cov.cx/a1g06

[36] See https://c19study.com/ or https://cov.cx/a1a24

[37] While the "Who Benefits and How?" question/test shouldn't be the sole element of evaluating findings, we are touched by the obvious altruism and open honesty present in some of the quietly shared findings by individual doctors and their practices.

approved for Covid treatment drug may shift the odds in my favor, then I'm all for it. [38]

When you look at the arguments by people against HCQ use, you'll see they invariably cherry-pick one or two of the 205 studies (which can usually be critiqued for not studying HCQ use in the manner it is best suited for, and therefore, by design, predestined to show a negative but irrelevant outcome), and say "these studies clearly show HCQ is of no use", while ignoring both the limited nature of the studies they are citing and the many dozens of other studies that show HCQ to have major positive impacts on people in the early stages of a Covid infection.[39]

How to describe these people who ignore more than 100 positive studies, and focus only on one or two negative studies that don't even relate to the advocated use of HCQ? The words "honest" and "ethical" seem very inappropriate to such people and their opinions.

More than that, why are they so desperate to "prove" HCQ is no good?[40] If there is some valid doubt as to if it works or not, then as long as there is a chance

---

[38] This is often termed, sometimes derisively, as "Real World" results. A new act, passed in 2016, the "Cures" Act, encourages the FDA to give more credence to real world data, rather than only considering "gold standard" double-blind random clinical trials.

[39] We acknowledge that not all studies are equal, and trying to evaluate the evidence for/against HCQ (or anything else) based simply on counting the studies for and against is terribly over-simplistic and potentially misleading.

But when the imbalance between the "pro" and the "con" articles is so strongly in favor of the "pro" articles, it is perhaps an acceptable short-cut, prior to further examination of all articles, as a way of establishing there is probably something important and positive to be evaluated. This is especially true when so many of the "pro" articles are published in refereed journals and so can be considered, *prima facie*, as being of high quality and persuasive.

Limitations notwithstanding, we suggest a simple count is no worse and probably better than simply picking and choosing one or two articles to support the "con" view and not even looking at any of the many refereed articles that support the "pro" view.

[40] One of my pre-publication physician readers, who strongly disagrees with me about HCQ, challenged me that the better question is why I am so keen to prove that HCQ is good. I'm happy to answer that. I have no dog in this fight whatsoever and don't stand to profit. Amazingly, some physicians have even suggested that bad doctors are wanting to profit by promoting HCQ to their patients. That is impossible. Doctors don't sell medicines, pharmacies do, and the cost of HCQ is very low in any event.

(continued on next page)

that it might help, shouldn't we give it a chance to help us? They have an answer for that – "HCQ is too dangerous". That's the most specious of all statements. HCQ is being taken, every day in the US, by millions of people for lupus and rheumatoid arthritis. It is one of the most commonly prescribed drugs in the entire world, and has been for many decades. The very minor chance of heart irregularities is insignificant (although greater caution is required if used in conjunction with azithromycin), and can be tested for and evaluated before and during taking the HCQ.

Furthermore, a recent peer-reviewed published study showed no evidence of any harm experienced by patients taking HCQ for Covid-19, and indeed, rather than being a heart-risk, there was some suggestion that HCQ may have had some beneficial outcomes.[41]

We discuss hydroxychloroquine further in our chapter on 16. Medicines, Supplements, Vitamins, etc, starting on page 356. The specific section on HCQ starts on page 375.

What makes the way the establishment has reacted to the potential of HCQ all the more astonishing is the contrast in attitudes when it comes to another possible Covid treatment, remdesivir.

At the same time as heaping negativity on HCQ, an orchestrated campaign of support for remdesivir has been 180° opposite to how HCQ has been treated. Perhaps this is because remdesivir has big pharma (Gilead) pushing it with their lobbying and public relations teams, and promises huge profits (a drug that costs about $9 for a course of six doses is being sold for $3,120). We'd also point out that the US Government is believed to have fronted $70.5 million in R&D subsidies over five years to Gilead, helping them fund the development of

---

My only interest is in protecting myself and my loved ones. By helping you too, I'm in turn reducing the risk of you becoming infected, passing the infection on to someone else, who then passes it on to me or a member of my family. I see in HCQ a classic case of all upside, no downside. That is what I'm keen about – that we don't reject it "just because", but rather we give it a balanced and fair appraisal.

I'm writing this book to try and help us all, and in HCQ I see a drug that might help us. Many credible studies are suggesting it does help, and few studies to the contrary. I also note that everyone who says to me "HCQ is no good" – with a look of absolute certainty on their face – refuses to look at the huge number of positive studies. I don't know why, which brings me back to the "why are they so desperate to prove HCQ is bad" puzzle.

[41] See https://www.sciencedirect.com/science/article/pii/S2052297520300998 or https://cov.cx/a1d94

remdesivir.[42] Where now is the benefit and return to us, the taxpayers, for our investment in this drug? Why isn't Gilead selling the drug more cheaply to the US than to other countries – or, at the very least, at the same price? Instead, many other countries are being offered the drug at a lower price (although this pricing discrimination is far from unique to remdesivir), even though their governments didn't contribute anything to the drug's development.

Remdesivir may shorten the amount of time a person with a moderately severe Covid-19 case spends in hospital. It isn't claimed to save lives (although there have been hints and suggestions that it does), nor does it keep people out of hospital. At best, it just reduces the time a person who has needed to be admitted to a hospital will spend there. That's surely a welcome thing if it is you who gets to leave hospital some days sooner than otherwise, but compare that to HCQ which might keep people out of hospitals entirely, save their lives, and at the cost of a dollar or two of HCQ (plus all the savings of the many thousands of dollars a day of hospital stay).

Much has been made of the alleged (but shown not to exist in studies) danger of taking HCQ. But there is little discussion about the possible side-effects of taking remdesivir. As seen here,[43] remdesivir has a selection of severe side-effects.

After being initially approved under an "Emergency Use Authorization", remdesivir was given full approval on 28 October. This was a very strange decision because just a couple of weeks earlier, a large international study coordinated by WHO published its results showing that *remdesivir gave no benefit at all to the patients who were given it.*[44] Whereas HCQ has now had 205 different studies written up about its efficacy, remdesivir has had 12. According to this site[45], four have inconclusive results, six have positive results, and two have negative results.

---

[42] See https://www.citizen.org/news/the-public-already-has-paid-for-remdesivir/ or https://cov.cx/a1a25

[43] See https://www.webmd.com/drugs/2/drug-179015/remdesivir-intravenous/details/list-sideeffects or https://cov.cx/a1g10

[44] This article, and the linked article in Science Magazine, set out the puzzling nature of the remdesivir approval and would give most reasonable readers cause for concern. https://www.trialsitenews.com/remdesivirs-sordid-regulatory-history-calls-efficacy-into-question/ or https://cov.cx/a1a26 and https://www.sciencemag.org/news/2020/10/very-very-bad-look-remdesivir-first-fda-approved-covid-19-drug or https://cov.cx/a1a27

[45] See https://c19rmd.com/ or https://cov.cx/a1a28

So we have two controversial drugs. One – HCQ - costs pennies, has a long history of safe use, and has 205 different studies (as of mid-December, almost certainly more by the time you read this) showing generally positive results on its value for Covid-sufferers, but given the thumbs down by the authorities. The other, a new drug, remdesivir, has been thinly studied, with a major study showing a negative result, is very expensive, but has been approved. Does that make sense to you?

To be fair, while President Trump *might* be right about HCQ, he is definitely wrong about other elements of the Covid-19 pandemic, in particular, his repeated hopes that the virus will just disappear on its own. There was and still is no underlying reason to believe this at all, just wishful thinking.

Talking about wishful thinking, how about the statement by the head of the FDA, lauding the benefits of convalescent plasma, that was made on a Sunday and had to be walked back two days later as having been overstated? How do things like that ever happen?[46]

What follows is based on my view of the issues to do with the virus and the problems of becoming infected by it, as best I can determine from reading through some (but not all) studies. I try to explain my thinking so you can independently form your own conclusions.

I have no hidden agenda underlying my commentary. I am preparing this first for my own personal benefit, so I know what to do for myself and for the loved ones who rely on me.[47] Secondarily, your health impacts on my health. I want you to be healthy too, because if you are healthy, you won't infect your friend, who won't infect their friend, who then, somewhere down the "six degrees of separation" chain might end up infecting me.

If we are both healthy, our contributions to and participation in the national economy are less harmed. The healthcare system is less overloaded. We all benefit, we all win.

So, for the most sincere and selfish of reasons, I want to help you.

---

[46] See https://apnews.com/a7f0e8aac34a860ad502912564681b7c or https://cov.cx/a1a29 . Some of my pre-publication readers have suggested this is all political rather than medical. That may be true, but it is not a positive explanation. If we can't trust the FDA to tell us the medical truth rather than the political spin, and if this is an example of that, what shred of credibility do they have on any topic?

[47] Well, maybe I do have an agenda item. My travel business was zeroed out entirely by the virus. The sooner the world beats it, the sooner I can return to my "day job". So I've a vested interest in helping everyone beat the virus, allowing my own life to return to normal.

The Logical Fallacy of Restricting Discussion to Doctors

As I've already said, I am not a doctor. But you don't need to be a doctor to understand the methodology, the data and the statistics of what the virus is doing, and the methodology of the drug trials and tests being developed to hopefully combat the virus.

Indeed, I'll guess that few doctors have taken the requisite advanced courses in data analysis and statistics to allow them to sensibly understand, evaluate and interpret the results of some of the trials that claim variously to prove or disprove some of the treatments being considered.[48] It is also likely that few working doctors (other than those directly in the virology field) have the time to keep up with the barrage of often conflicting studies and reports being published every day at present.[49]

I'm not a doctor, but I do understand a bit about sampling, statistics, and data analysis. I've passed under-grad university subjects in (among other subjects) chemistry, physics, information systems, and applied maths, and post-graduate classes in data techniques and statistics (earning "A" grade passes at New Zealand's best business school). I've used these skills regularly in the decades subsequently.

I'm not boasting, and in any event I don't believe there is an automatic link between academic distinction (especially in my case, with my qualifications having been earned four decades ago[50]) and the ability to analyze data accurately and write up the results correctly.

---

[48] Actually, I'm not just guessing. Here's an interesting open letter from initially 37, now 42 American, British, and Brazilian professors, statisticians, mathematicians, and doctors pointing out basic errors in statistical analysis in some of the published studies about Covid-19 treatments. They refer also to similar errors being found present in 51% of all similar papers. See https://veja.abril.com.br/saude/especialistas-contestam-estudos-que-nao-viram-beneficios-na-cloroquina/amp/ or https://cov.cx/a1a30 and https://drive.google.com/file/d/1NZOJ57fM0RTaHD1t_9w2iua7lUJhOgWT/view or https://cov.cx/a1a31

[49] It can easily take an hour to fully read and analyze a single study and to understand how it was conducted and why, and then to consider its conclusions and seek to identify any unstated weaknesses or omissions.

We can't guess how many studies there are being published every week, but we'll guess more than 10, possibly even more than 100, some weeks.

[50] So if I were to go on and ridiculously say "I've forgotten more about statistics than you've ever learned" that would be a confession of my latter-day inadequacy rather than a boast!

There's something surprising when you see so many eminently respectable people, all viewed as experts in their fields, disagreeing so fundamentally on aspects of this virus and how we should be responding to it.

If degrees alone gave people insight, the more degreed people became, the more their thinking would converge into a unanimous single opinion. This is not the case. One should ponder why it isn't and what it implies.

Back to doctors and their expertise and ability to evaluate virus treatments and cures.

Sure, doctors know an enormous amount about medicine in general, and that's not surprising. They've studied for ten or more years before being able to practice, including serving an intensive "apprenticeship" in hospitals, matching the theory they've learned to the reality of actual illnesses and how they play out. They know all about the number of nerves in your body; they can name most of your bones, and they understand the logic of how to diagnose common illnesses and ailments and the generally recommended treatments for them.[51] They fully deserve our respect.

Beyond those general points, medical professionals quickly move to siloed areas of specialization,[52] with a general practitioner or family doctor's main skill shifting to knowing which specialists to then refer a patient to, and an ability to speak the general language of medicine with specialists and hopefully providing an oversight and coordination role, making sure the specialists in their silos are interacting appropriately.

Not all of this knowledge and experience is essential when it comes to evaluating new treatments for a new illness. New treatments are often evaluated by measures as simple as "did the patient live or die" or "how many days did they spend in a hospital before being discharged". You don't need to be a doctor to understand such outcomes, but you need statistical analytics to determine if there is a significant change in the number of patients who live or die, or whatever other criteria are used.

I am absolutely not saying that doctors do not have valuable opinions to offer to the discussion, but I am saying theirs should not be the only voices in that

---

[51] Yes, they know very many other things, too! This is not a complete list.

[52] It isn't just medicine in which the "funnel effect" occurs – specialists and experts become more and more knowledgeable, but about less and less, eventually ending up with people proudly knowing almost everything, but about almost nothing! A similar concept is "when the only tool you have is a hammer, every problem looks like a nail" – there is definitely validity in experts and their contributions, but they then need to be carefully interfaced into the general world in which they have to be applied. We need "Renaissance men" generalists as well as experts.

discussion, and the mere presence or absence of the letters "MD" after a person's name should not be given overriding importance when considering their commentary and opinions.[53]

This is doubly the case when it comes to public health policy issues, which are, at their core, *social issues not medical ones*. Public health policy strives to find a difficult balance between the cost and impact/disruption of healthcare policies, and the efficacy of the outcomes such policies create. In the ultimate, it boils down to awkward issues that some people prefer to pretend don't exist like "how much money should you spend to save a human life"? We all like to think that human life – and our own in particular – is priceless, but when formulating public policy, a very different view is taken.[54]

We understand and accept such differences of opinion; indeed, we welcome them. Open public discussion is the crucible in which effective public policy is formed. But we don't understand and greatly regret the disagreements over seemingly factual matters – does mask-wearing help reduce the spread of the virus? How many people are dying of the virus? And so on.

As you read through this, you should do two things. The **first** is balance my views and perspective, and those of the underlying sources I've relied upon, with those of other people and other sources. It is surprising there is such a diversity of opinions on what is appropriate and inappropriate in terms of responding to the threat of the Covid-19 virus. But diversity there is, and I am not pretending to be the person with the most correct view of all of these subjective issues. By all means, consider my preferred opinions and try to understand why I advocate

---

[53] In any event, just about every shade of opinion and approach to anything to do with Covid-19 is supported by some doctors and opposed by others. Should we put these issues to a vote? No, because science isn't a popularity contest, and most of science's currently accepted fundamental tenets were once unpopular and denigrated.

It is only by allowing and considering ideas that are first lambasted as being unpopular, unlikely, and unusual that ultimately sees science advancing.

[54] This concept is used as guidance by the government when deciding what new safety measures to mandate. Does the cost of the measure outweigh the benefit in terms of lives saved? Currently, it seems the value of a life is thought to be about $10 million. See https://www.npr.org/transcripts/835571843 or https://cov.cx/a1a32 and https://www.wired.com/story/how-much-is-human-life-worth-in-dollars/ or https://cov.cx/a1a33

them,[55] but at the end of the day, make your own decisions about yourself and your situation.

The **second** is, whether you agree or not, adapt my thoughts, other people's thoughts, and your own to your situation. Every person, their situation, and their values are different. Your personal risk tolerance may be higher or lower than mine. You might be in an elevated category of severe risk, or you might be young and robustly healthy. You might have readily available access to the highest quality unlimited healthcare and doctors who will patiently take as long as it takes to conversationally talk to you, discuss the issues and options, and involve you in the decision-making. Or you might not. And so on.

As regards the specific treatments being mentioned for your consideration, you should also modify them to reflect your particular medical situation. For example, as you age, things like immune system responses, kidney efficiency, and drug half-lives become more of an issue.

Plus there may be potential interactions with other drugs you are already taking. Maybe you're allergic to one of these things. And who only knows what else (answer – your doctor might know,[56] and if not, could find out[57]).

To restate. I am not recommending you should adopt anything I'm writing about. I'm merely offering up some thoughts for you to incorporate into your own evaluation and decisions about what is best for you.

If you need additional advice and guidance, please turn to your doctor. But insist he explains his reasoning to you – that's only fair.

---

[55] Generally, I try and support everything I say either with detailed reasoning or links to articles. But, even with this book now exceeding 400 pages, sometimes I edit out things that perhaps should be left in. So if there's something you don't understand and want to understand, please let me know. That will help me to know what is important and helpful to you, and I'll update the book to include additional explanation for the benefit of all readers.

[56] So too might your pharmacist.

[57] A sad emphasis needs to be placed on the "could". I know Covid-19 sufferers who were forced to "doctor-shop" in trying to find a doctor who would agree to at least have an open discussion with them about the pluses and minuses of HCQ and other drug use. Regrettably, most doctors recoiled in horror at the thought and refused to discuss the matter at all.

Why Are So Many Doctors So Risk-Averse?

A friend with two high-risk modifiers (he was elderly and overweight) came down with a Covid-19 infection. He was concerned about what might happen, with other family members relying on him for support, and of course, neither he nor they wished his experience to be any more than the mildest possible.

So he decided to try any and all possible cures that had been identified in the literature as maybe improving a person's chance of survival.

But he couldn't find a doctor, anywhere, to write him the prescriptions he needed for the medicines he wanted to take. Most doctors refused to even talk about the subject with him and treated him disdainfully as if he was a drug addict asking for a prescription for narcotics. Those who would at least interact had 100% closed minds and refused to enter into an engaged discussion of the studies and their findings, merely repeating mechanically either that the treatments he wanted would not work, or the possible strategies that showed promise were not officially approved and so would not be allowed.[58]

Many of us have a somewhat idealized notion of a doctor as being someone who will move heaven and earth and do everything possible to help a patient get cured of whatever afflicts them. But, in California, my friend's experience in July failed to find a single doctor who was willing to think independently or creatively, or even to read and evaluate trials that seemed to indicate possibly promising treatments. Most of all, they refused to prescribe drugs "off-label" that they lawfully could prescribe and which had no side-effects of concern, and which possibly might help reduce the severity of a Covid infection, and lied to him about why they wouldn't do so.

Why are doctors so risk-averse?

There are probably six reasons for this, and, to be fair, much/most of the time, their risk-aversion is the right thing.

The **obvious reason** is that in their experience in the past, they have seen too many not-yet-officially-approved treatments fail to live up to their initial promise. Think of all the "miracle" cancer cures that come and go, and the sometimes deliberate fake "quackery" medicine and snake oil treatments that are occasionally offered by fraudsters.

---

[58] The doctors were debatably wrong on the first point, and totally wrong on the second point. Yes, to be clear and blunt, I am saying the doctors lied directly to this person when they said they were not allowed to prescribe medicines for off-label use (discussed subsequently in this book). Doctors that lie to you? .....

The vastest part of non-mainstream medicine and the advice offered through such alternate channels is of very low value and accuracy.[59] So of course, they're going to be very cautious in all such cases.

When you've been repeatedly disappointed by past possible cures that have totally failed to live up to expectations, you become less open-minded when greeted with yet another treatment that promises much but has not yet gone through the rigorous testing and trials to meet full formal FDA and other approvals.

There are five other reasons doctors prefer to be "safe rather than sorry".

The **first** is doctors might be risking their professional accreditation and may have their license to practice revoked if they start egregiously prescribing medicines for purposes the medicines have not been officially certified as being appropriate for. Alternatively, they might be employed by a large institutionalized healthcare company, with rigorous rules and restrictions on how flexible and creative the doctors can be.

That's a bit like the policeman who doesn't really want to cite you for some small violation, but who has no choice because that is his job. The policeman tells you to argue the case in court, and to pressure your politicians to rewrite the

---

[59] You might think you're a careful person and you might feel you're doing sufficient "due diligence" by researching the companies, the websites, and the products they promote – maybe you even do a Google search for "(company name) fraud", and all you find are positive articles, so you feel reassured that the company or product is trustworthy.

But did you know there are companies – they call themselves "reputation management" companies – that charge sizeable sums of money to ensure that when people search for one of their clients, they only see good positive articles online. They'll even create a network of seemingly independent sites, all with some generic articles and also positive articles about their client. Needless to say, some of the people spending tens of thousands of dollars every month for reputation management services have deservedly bad reputations to start with. So it is very hard to really truly know who and what to trust.

Yes, I know, I'm saying, by obvious implication, "don't trust me". And I'm happy with that statement. That is why I'm never asking you to trust me "just because", and am supporting everything I say with what I hope to be links to credible sources.

Back to my point. Because doctors have seen so much that is untrue and false, they've developed an immediate rejection type response to most new information that doesn't appear in "trustworthy sources". But the conservativism of those trustworthy sources, while working in everyone's favor in normal times, is a problem in fast-moving fast-changing situations such as we are in at present with the virus. We all need to open our filters a crack and at least consider some of this stuff with a slightly open mind. Just because most alternate type medicine is nonsense doesn't mean it is all nonsense.

law. He's just the man in the middle, following rather than making policy. Or the policeman who personally thinks writing speeding tickets for 2 mph over the limit is crazy, but he's been given a quota he must fill to get good personal reviews every year.

Being compared to a policeman is an unglamorous description of a doctor, but many times it is a fair one. A family doctor is surprisingly limited and constrained in what he can and can't do, and much of the time, these constraints are strict and strange and have been enacted by politicians and regulators, for reasons that in truth are not always as valid and altruistic as they should be. Doctors might not tell you this directly, but the grim reality of the ever more obsessive scrutiny of their work and required documentation and reporting about what they do is increasingly constraining their ability to pro-actively think outside the box and help patients with new and sometimes experimental medicines to resolve new and difficult medical issues.

While in theory doctors can prescribe drugs for off-label use (we discuss this below, see the section "Off-Label Use" on page 357), their liability for off-label prescribing is higher than for normally approved use prescriptions. This leads to the next point.

The **second** reason is similar to the first. The other threat to a doctor being able to keep his job is that posed by the professional liability insurance he needs. Using a similar analogy to the policeman one, we all know that the biggest penalty, if we get a speeding ticket, is not the fine we pay to the court, but the hit on our insurance premium. We need, by law, insurance cover to take our vehicle onto the road. Our mortgagor requires us to have insurance on our house before they will lend us money. And a doctor needs his professional liability insurance – and needs to have a good record with low/no claims to keep his insurance cover – and therefore to be able to practice.

If he starts prescribing off-label medicines, then he is not only opening himself up to liability from his patient if the medicine doesn't work as hoped for,[60] but his insurance company will react very negatively too.

---

[60] While a patient might make any number of promises upfront to not sue, no matter what the outcome, and while the doctor might make extremely full disclosures of any risks involved, try telling that to the ambulance-chasing attorneys if things subsequently turn out negatively.

This is even more certain if the patient dies, and an action is brought by the patient's grieving family (who never promised not to sue), demanding compensation for their loved one's "wrongful" death due to "medical malpractice".

There are so many ways a non-standard course of treatment can be twisted and turned and made into seemingly medical malpractice.

The **third** reason is a practical one. Doctors are overworked and don't have the time to fully and fairly study the literature on every last long-shot possible cure for every different disease. Neither do they have the time, if they give a patient a non-standard treatment, to then closely monitor the patient to ensure no unexpected side-effects or responses to the non-standard treatment. Most medical practices are set up to work on a very scripted regulated basis, processing patients in the most efficient way possible, and conforming to industry "best practices" with little opportunity to break free of those constraints.

This isn't just because doctors are greedy (most are not) and wanting to make as much money as possible. Closely related to not having the time is the **fourth** reason - your medical insurance may not cover the cost of experimental treatments, and has dozens of complex requirements and restrictions on what they will cover, and how much of a doctor's time they'll accept in any given course of treatment for any given ailment. The doctors are being squeezed by both their liability insurance and your medical insurance into a narrow "safe ground" with little room for variance.

There is one more – the **fifth** – reason as well. It is one I've experienced myself, not as a doctor, but as a lowly travel agent. I owned a travel company for just over a decade and noticed an interesting thing. When a client came and asked for, eg, the lowest possible fare to fly to Europe; while I was keen to find them the very *best* fare possible, I was avoiding offering them the very *lowest* possible fare on the cheapest no-frills airline. This absolutely wasn't because I wanted to sell them a needlessly over-priced ticket and get a little more commission. It was because I knew that the lowest ticket, on the cheapest airline, came with a whole bunch of potential problems that might make life difficult.

For example, back in the happy days before "no change/no refund" policies became common, tickets with those types of restrictions would create problems if a person subsequently needed to change or cancel their travel. Sure, I'd tell the person upfront about the restrictions, but they'd unconsciously reject what I was saying and believe that, if such an issue arose, they'd be able to persuade me or the airline to make a special exception for them. These requests would almost never be granted by the airline. I knew that, but my clients did not (and when their request for a waiver of the rules was summarily refused by the airline, they would invariably blame me rather than the airline).

For further example, some charter airlines would have very low fares, but would only operate one flight a week. If you needed to change your departure or return, and even if your ticket rules would allow you to do so, you wouldn't have a choice of an earlier/later flight the same day, or even the next day. You had to wait a week, which of course could be terribly inconvenient and often ended up requiring the person to have to buy a last-minute one-way ticket on another airline (costing much more than the original roundtrip ticket – and, of course, they'd not even get a refund on the unused portion of their original restricted ticket).[61]

Now, here's the thing that applied to me, and which I suspect applies to many doctors as well. I knew that perhaps one person out of every 50 people I sold these restricted discounted tickets to would end up with a problem, which of course meant that I too would end up sharing that problem. If I told the person about that risk, they'd invariably say "A 2% chance of problems? That's fine, I'm willing to take the risk. The odds are in my favor, it will probably not happen to me."

The person saying that was indeed probably correct. A one in 50 chance of a problem is not a big risk to take.

But, and here's the point. For me, I was selling 100 or more tickets to Europe, every week. One chance in 50 meant that each individual traveler probably had no problems, but meant for me that I would end up with two nightmare problems, every week. I was more risk-averse than my passengers, because my risk exposure – even though involving the same event – was very different from theirs.

It is the same with doctors, only more so. The limit of the risk and "nightmare" that I had to endure was nothing more serious than an irate passenger blaming me for things that in truth were not my fault or liability,[62] and the extent of the reparations demanded was hopefully no more than refunding an airfare.

But for a doctor, he is risking malpractice suits, losing his insurance and/or his medical license to practice, public vilification in the media, and also seeing patients that he truly cares about suffering the consequences of bad medication choices, possibly even dying.

So we fully appreciate and understand why doctors sometimes seem to be closed-minded and opposed to medical experimentation.

But their low tolerance for risk does not mean that alternative approaches to curing a disease are automatically wrong for you, just like my unwillingness to book passengers on "risky" flights did not mean that what was bad for me would also be bad for my clients.

---

[61] Usually, the problem arose when the charter airline had to cancel a flight. Best case scenario, it might refund a small portion of the original fare, but it would never offer to re-book you, for free, on another airline to keep you more or less close to your original travel dates and times.

[62] And sadly also, things I was unable to resolve – travel agents don't set airline policy and only rarely can prevail upon airlines to vary their policies.

It also raises the interesting ethical/social issue – who should be in control of our healthcare? Politicians, administrators and regulators, and insurance companies? Doctors, either subject to or freed of the constraints detailed above? Or us, ourselves?

Surely, at the end of the day, we deserve the right to at the very least participate in a discussion about how our illnesses should be treated. My Californian friend couldn't even get a doctor to have that discussion, let alone open-mindedly consider the issues and possibly allow a non-official treatment regimen.

It is in the spirit of self-empowerment and allowing more fully-informed participation in what may literally be life and death decisions about you, yourself, that we provide this material now.

The Fallacies of Scientific Tests and Trials

Have you noticed how two different groups of people can take the same statistic and interpret it in opposite ways? For example, an economic statistic can simultaneously be claimed to be an excellent improvement, or a terrible underperformance.[63]

Economics is interesting because it makes a distinction between "macro-economics" – the broad impacts on a country as a whole – and "micro-economics" – things that impact on you and me personally and directly. That is why the country's economy might be booming, but your personal economy might be on life-support – for example, even though employment in general is rising, your employer just laid you off.

We need similar distinctions in other fields too, including the medical field. This is particularly so in the case of studies that are used to evaluate the efficacy and safety of possible new medical treatments. Almost without exception, all of these trials, while possibly showing a sufficient skew in the results and outcomes to either support or contradict the claim of a new medicine working well, will also show some people/patients who experienced completely the opposite. Understandably, the focus and finding of the trial is on what most patients experienced, but sometimes there is very helpful information to be gleaned by studying the other outcome.

---

[63] We see this in every election campaign, don't we. The incumbent quotes numbers to show wonderful the economy is, the aspiring other candidate uses the same data to "prove" how the economy has been woefully mismanaged. The numbers are the same, it is how they are interpreted that varies. This ability to selectively interpret data in many different ways is a theme running through much of the rest of this section.

The point we're building up to is that even the most negative study might show some grounds for hope for some patients. With the main purpose of most medical research being to find and enable new cures, shouldn't even negative and disappointing studies be further looked at to see if there is some possible added factor that determines if a patient is likely to have a positive or negative experience, and then adjust the treatment plan to allow for that?

It is interesting and significant, whether a trial is largely positive or negative, to understand why that is so, and to see if it is possible to further shift the results or adjust the treatment to improve the positive outcomes, and to understand which patients are most likely to safely secure the positive outcome. It can be equally valuable though to study the other part of the results – the negative/undesired outcomes, and learn from those too.

We've progressed to a point of understanding and risk-averse approach where we will let even a low level of severe side-effects prevent or at least marginalize the use of a new drug. That may or may not be appropriate – for example, if there is a disease that kills half of all people who acquire the disease, and if a treatment is proposed that would cure two-thirds of people with the disease, but condemn the other one-third to a painful death, should that treatment be allowed or not?

Happily, that's not a question that we need to answer here![64]

And now for the particular examples we have in mind. Let's look again at the "poster child" of bad science/bad result interpretation, hydroxychloroquine. We have to bring up, in particular, the bizarre hate that is being lavished on

---

[64] But if we were to answer that question, we'd probably say that rather than a blanket ban on the new drug, or a blanket approval, it should be left up to each patient and their physician to evaluate and decide. We know that some doctors are unscrupulous, and of course, most patients are not well-informed about medical issues, but when it comes to you and your health, who do you most trust? The doctor you're dealing with face-to-face, and yourself; or nameless faceless bureaucrats in Washington, DC, who have made "one size fits all" rules and regulations that don't have the flexibility to consider you and your specific case and situation?

We'd also point out that this question/dilemma is *not* a medical issue. It is a public health policy issue, and we all (should) have an equal voice in the formulation of such matters. And, most of all, it is both a public health policy issue in general, but also a very personal life and death decision for each patient individually.

At the risk of touching on a very contentious issue, we (and most other societies around the world) allow women to decide if they have an abortion or not. So why can't we also allow patients to make other major issues about their healthcare? Don't we have a similar "right to choose"? Isn't it a similar protected privacy issue?

And, for the many good people who are uncomfortable about abortion and opposed to it, hopefully they'll agree there's a huge difference between decisions involving the life of an unborn child and decisions involving only one's own life.

hydroxychloroquine (HCQ), and the unfair methods that have been deployed to "prove" the drug is either unhelpful or possibly even harmful.[65]

The situation is simple. Some doctors have claimed that for patients early in a Covid-19 infection, and with mild rather than severe symptoms, giving them a combination of HCQ and zinc (Zn) (and possibly azithromycin (AZ) too) has resulted in their patients' symptoms not getting worse, and instead seeing the patients quickly cured of their infection, without hospitalization, and without dying.

There are three key elements of this claim :

- Early in an infection
- Mild symptoms
- Combination of HCQ and Zn (and possibly AZ)

So, if you were a medical researcher, and wanted to do a formal "scientific" trial to confirm or rebut the efficacy of using HCQ in patients with Covid-19, what would you choose to do :

(a)   Test using HCQ and sometimes AZ but not Zn on patients with severe infections who have already been admitted to hospital

(b)   Test using HCQ but not zinc nor AZ on patients already in a hospital

(c)   Test using HCQ and Zn and possibly AZ on patients early in an infection with mild symptoms and not yet needing hospitalization

The correct answer is, of course, (c). Unsurprisingly, every trial that has tested that scenario has been strongly positive. The few negative-result trials have been either (a) or (b).

While it would be interesting to also understand if HCQ by itself works, or if it needs to be combined with Zn and/or AZ, and of course it would be great to know if the drug can also help patients with more severe doses of the virus, the first point is surely to prove or disprove the apparent value in the early treatment with HCQ + Zn (+ AZ) as has been claimed.

Now, let's say that for whatever reason you too did a test using the (a) or (b) scenario, and it shows that the HCQ has little or no effect. What do you then announce to the world?

(a)   HCQ is useless for all patients with Covid-19 infections

---

[65] HCQ has become the most vivid example of a drug getting an undeserved bad reputation, but many other drugs are also being totally ignored. They're not being criticized, they're just being ignored, even though other countries are using them with positive results – for example, ivermectin.

(b)   In the specific scenario you tested, HCQ did not have
         any positive effects, but the benefit of using HCQ in
         other scenarios and as has been claimed by the earlier
         studies can not be determined by your trial

We don't know why, but not only have most of the negative-outcome HCQ
trials been to test scenarios where there has been less compelling evidence that
HCQ would work, but when the results subsequently came back to show that, yes,
indeed HCQ did not work in those scenarios, somehow the results have been
misstated, by the popular press and by medical professionals too, as "proving"
that HCQ never works in any scenario.[66]

There is no rational ground for that at all. A test/trial can only ever report on
the results observed in the scenario being trialed. Extending and generalizing a
specific outcome of a specific test is a very dangerous and seldom substantiated
thing to do (and yes, both in terms of extending negative and positive results).

Hopefully, you understand this and why it is. I understand it too. But I do
not understand, for the life of me, why it is that people have run the "wrong" trials
and then come to the doubly wrong conclusions at the end of the trials.

---

[66] You might say "But, David, if HCQ doesn't help seriously ill patients, surely it also
doesn't help people with milder infections?". That's a fair question to have, but most
anti-viral drugs work best in the early stages of a virus attack.

Think of the virus infection like a leaky old boat. The more that water leaks into the
boat, the more it continues to leak and the faster the water floods in (more water
pressure as the boat settles into the water, and more holes get below the waterline as
the boat gets deeper and deeper into the water). Eventually, the water breaks over the
sides of the boat and then it rapidly completes its sinking.

Now think of HCQ (or any other anti-viral drug) as a bailer. When the first leak starts,
the bailer can easily handle all the water coming in, and there's no problem. But if you
don't start bailing right away, the leak slowly gets bigger, and the rate of water coming in
increases. Now, if you start using the bailer, you can barely keep up with the water. If
you wait a bit longer still before responding, more leaks start letting in more water, and
the bailer can no longer keep up with the rate of water flowing in. Eventually – if you
don't get to shore in time – the boat then has the water flooding over the sides and
nothing will save it.

The analogy with the virus is to think of the virus growth like the growing rate of water
coming into the boat, and HCQ like a moderate-sized bailer. In the early stages, HCQ
may be able to defeat the virus, before it gets established and reaches a
critical/sustainable level of infection. In the middle stages, HCQ might slow the
deterioration of symptoms to a noticeable degree (or might not). And in a late-stage,
almost nothing will make a difference.

Maybe if I was a doctor, I'd understand? No, I think not. This is universal logic and plain common sense. No amount of medical education changes the fact that these trials and their results are unhelpful.[67]

Now for a really big question : What else are medical researchers and the public policymakers who use their findings making similarly fundamental errors about?

One more point needs to be made. Conducting a medical trial is an extremely complicated process. There are a multitude of challenges – three in particular stick out. The **first** is that every person is different. They have different ages, body masses, lifestyles, existing ailments and conditions, and react to different drugs in different ways. How can you distill out of a range of results which factors are based on what variables, and how can you be sure there isn't an unknown "X factor" that is influencing your entire study?[68]

The **second** factor is to try and understand what would have happened if the same people had received (or not received) the same or different treatment? If three-quarters of your test subjects got better after taking a trial drug, that is great; but how do you know what percentage would have got better, anyway?[69]

All the accepted practices and procedures to try and resolve these issues can reduce the random "wild card" unknown factors, but don't eliminate them. The

---

[67] By all means, write to me and explain otherwise. I've no vested interest other than optimizing my own chances of surviving a Covid-19 infection. I'm seeking the truth, wherever and whatever it is.

[68] For example, Covid-19 testing on people in Laos, where only 3 people per million have contracted the virus, would probably give very different results to people selected in Luxembourg, where 11,861 people per million have contracted the virus. No-one knows why, but there's an X factor that is causing something.

There are ways to reduce unknown additional factors, but it is hard to know there isn't some subtle obscured bias that has managed to sneak into the trial.

[69] What you do is to have two halves to your trial, with as similar as possible groups of people in each. One half is taking the drug that is being tested, and the other half is not (and no-one knows which is which). Then you can say "we had 50 women in their forties, all of European background, all vegetarians, all slim, all with two children, in happy marriages and working in similar jobs, living in the same town, going to the same church, none lactose intolerant, none with high blood pressure, (and so on and so on in as much detail as possible to eliminate other factors that might impact on the outcome…..) in each group, and 30 of the women in one group experienced a positive outcome and only 20 of the women in the other group did – therefore this drug seems to improve the chance of a positive income by 50%".

only way to do that is with repeated trials with different samples of subjects in different locations, and with the largest possible groups of subjects.

If a number of tests/trials are performed by different researchers in different places and with slightly different scenarios, and some return positive and some return negative outcomes, one shouldn't abandon all further research. Instead, one should be encouraged by the positive tests, and excited to identify what the as-yet-unknown "X factor" is that makes some trials negative and others positive.

The **third** factor is in analyzing the results. Remember you already don't know exactly what caused the results, and you're not sure what the outcome would have been if the test element hadn't been added. But after those two variables, you now have the third one, which in its essence, is "do these results actually mean anything?".

For example, if you toss a coin four times, and it comes up heads every time, does that mean this is a magical coin that will always come up heads? Or is it just random chance? Is the next toss more likely to be heads again, or maybe tails to help even out the past numbers? You can guess both those answers fairly readily by using your general knowledge of statistics, sampling, and coins.[70]

But with an unknown test element, and uncertain other factors, you don't know what to expect, and while there are statistical methods to help you determine the confidence you should place in the results, and what the possible range of actual answers might be implied from the results you've received, even an apparently overwhelmingly and convincing seeming outcome might actually be statistically insignificant (like the coin-toss example) and likely to be random chance.[71]

---

[70] That points to another possible error – "confirmation bias". This is an insidious and subtle effect that can flow into and taint every element of a test/trial, starting with the way the trial is designed in the first place, and running through to the analysis of the results in the end.

Our "confirmation bias" from the coin tosses would depend on if we'd randomly pulled a coin out of our pocket, or had been playing a gambling game based on coin tosses in some shady gaming room. Our bias also extends to "knowing" intuitively that a coin will only land heads or tails, and "never" on its side. These are obvious examples of confirmation bias, and because they are obvious, they are less dangerous. It is the more subtle ones that we don't pick up on that can come back to haunt us, later.

[71] Test design and validation is an exceedingly complicated field. But here's a fascinating article, easily readable, about how one person "proved" the existence of ESP while simultaneously following what appeared to be all the best test design practices. https://getpocket.com/explore/item/daryl-bem-proved-esp-is-real or https://cov.cx/a1a34

(continued on next page)

There are other complicated issues too. What say, for example, you decide to conduct a trial to see if a new drug helps cure Covid-19 sufferers, and you decide you will monitor the test subjects for two whole months to see who survives and who dies. That seems to be very careful and cautious, and possibly even too much so. As time passes, there is a growing possibility of other semi-random events influencing a person's survival, and most Covid-19 people have either been cured or died in much less than two months. So, based on that possibility, the longer you keep checking survival rates, the more you allow new variable factors to intrude. But maybe this experimental drug miraculously extends everyone's life three months, but then its effect wears off, the virus comes back to life, and one day later, they are all dead. Your trial won't have registered that ultimate outcome.

So how long should the trial be?[72]

I could continue, but the point to focus on is simply that even the most apparently rigorous and perfect of tests may still be full of issues and unknowns. I'm not saying that meaningful testing and trial results are impossible, but I am saying they are much harder to get than first meets the eye. There are "best practices" that can address many of the issues I've mentioned above (and more issues I've glossed over), but testing and trials are an uneasy mix of art and science.

At another level, it is possible to surround an apparently robust theory or test analysis with such an impenetrable wall of babble and jargon as to cause all readers to "give up" on their analysis and simply accept the result, as ridiculous as it may be. This is most famously exemplified in the Sokal Hoax.
Seehttps://physics.nyu.edu/sokal/Chronicle_Jan_1_17.pdf or https://cov.cx/a1a35
We are NOT saying that all (or even any) of the many drug studies to do with Covid-19 treatments have been deliberately distorted, but we are saying that whether deliberate or accidental, it is possible that test weaknesses may have slipped into an analysis, undetected. There are already examples of some such studies that have even been "refereed" before publication in very esteemed journals (namely, The Lancet in Britain and NEJM in the US) which have subsequently been exposed as failing to meet even the most basic and rudimentary standards of test/analysis protocol.

[72] You might say "those other causes of death can easily be distinguished on the death certificates, so there's no danger of confusion". I'll disagree with that. Our authorities, in the US, are finding it an enormous struggle to accurately count true Covid-19 deaths at present, due to how death certificates are completed and the varying requirements for what is needed to qualify a death as being counted as a Covid-related death.
The most strident example of this was in Washington state, where gun-shot victims were being counted as Covid deaths for a while. See
https://www.freedomfoundation.com/washington/washington-health-officials-gunshot-victims-counted-as-covid-19-deaths/ or https://cov.cx/a1a36

To close this part, I need to state that I am not saying HCQ has yet been proven to always, guaranteed for sure, help people beat their Covid-19 infections. I doubt that level of certainty will ever come about.

But I am nailing my colors to the mast and saying that the trials (at least that I'm aware of) claiming to prove it doesn't work and never works have not been targeted at the use-cases HCQ is being advocated for, and so their results, while possibly accurate for the scenarios they researched, tell us nothing at all about if HCQ might help in other circumstances.[73]

In round figures, in mid-December, every day sees another 200,000+ people in the US will become infected with Covid-19, and 2,000 of those people will die. This is a national disaster of the gravest of proportions. Why are we not scrambling every possible resource to solve the problem?

We are spending many trillions of dollars to try and compensate people for the harm caused by the virus to our national economy and to people directly, and we're on the verge of spending many trillions of dollars more for another round of compensations. How about spending some small percentage of this on positively researching potential cures?

Shouldn't the medical experts be giving the highest possible priority to finding how and when HCQ might save lives, rather than dismissing it on the thinnest of excuses? This strange disconnect is all the more astonishing because it isn't as though there are other, better, and formally approved treatments that could be taken instead.[74]

---

[73] See https://c19study.com/ or https://cov.cx/a1a24 and the (as of 17 Dec 2020) 205 studies about HCQ they review.

[74] There are other unproven treatments. The thing that strikes us is how the "medical establishment" reacts so extraordinarily negatively to all such possibilities. Rather than saying "Wow, those preliminary results are really promising, let's rush to research it further to see if it checks out" there's an overwhelming rejection, saying "You haven't proven this already to the nth degree with multiple trials involving thousands of people over many years, so we're not interested in hearing what you've got to say".

That is sometimes accompanied by an ad hominem attack – "You can't be trusted, because you have a vested interest in the outcome and success of this". But if having a vested interest is to be a disqualifier, what about all the Big Pharma companies? Why are we investing billions of dollars to rush through the production of untested vaccines, while refusing to listen to "Small Pharma" and their under-funded early results of promising new drugs?

The most recent example is this hit-piece/hate-piece about another possible product that might help people who get the virus more quickly recover.[75] Ignore the people and personalities involved – we need to focus on the reality of the potential promise of the product.[76]

Ultimately, the issue right now, is "What right does someone else have to forbid me from choosing my preferred course of treatment?".

The Truth Changes

Here is another important introductory comment. The truth changes. By this we mean three things :

First, we are still discovering new things about the virus – how it is transmitted, what it does, possible cures and treatment plans, and so on.

Second, the virus itself changes. It mutates. There have been hundreds of minor changes to the virus already, most having very little impact, but there have also been more impactful and significant changes too.

Third, the infection – the global pandemic – is still raging all around us. The numbers of cases and survivors/deaths change every day, and so too does the analysis and interpretation of those numbers.

Even in this document, you might notice where we refer to a number somewhere (for example, total US cases) but elsewhere in the document, we use a different number for the same thing.

This is unavoidable because, as we write and update the document, we don't update every occurrence of every number, and as long as the change isn't material and important to our statements and interpretations, and as long as there is a general sense of the number applying at a certain point in time, we let some of the older versions of numbers slip through the system.

Because the truth is indeed changing daily, you need to consider this when reading any material about the virus. If you're reading material that was written back in March and April, there is a good chance that it needs to be revisited and possibly very much rewritten and changed now, with different facts, percentages, timings, and conclusions.

---

[75] See https://www.axios.com/trump-covid-oleandrin-9896f570-6cd8-4919-af3a-65ebad113d41.html or https://cov.cx/a1a37

[76] The actual 18-page research paper (not peer-reviewed) showing the promise of oleandrin is here :
https://www.biorxiv.org/content/10.1101/2020.07.15.203489v1.full.pdf or
https://cov.cx/a1a38

This is regrettably and particularly the case because much of the early analysis necessarily focused on data from China. Up until April, China's disclosed virus numbers represented the largest part of the world's total and so seemed to be a great source for analysis and interpretation.[77]

Unfortunately, there are two problems with that. The **first** is the Chinese data is widely believed to be unreliable. It has been suggested that China has hugely understated both their total cases and also their total deaths. It would be risky to make major policy decisions based on any numbers from China.[78]

Secondly, there are extraordinary regional differences in numbers, both in terms of the number of cases per million people, and in terms of the number of deaths and mortality rate.[79] For reasons that are currently not at all well understood, some countries have been very fortunate, with extremely low rates of cases and deaths. Other countries have been very unfortunate with extremely high rates. Even more puzzling are cases where similar seeming countries, geographically close to each other, are at the opposite extremes of the spectrum.

---

[77] My, how times have changed. We in the US alone, although with four times fewer people than China, are now reporting more cases in a single day than China has acknowledged, in total, right from the very start of the virus onset.

[78] It is interesting to remember the horror and amazement which those of us monitoring China's official numbers in February felt – up to a maximum of about 3,500 new cases a day – numbers which seemed apocalyptical and impossible to countenance. But now, India is reporting over 90,000 cases in a single day – India is having more new cases every day than China has reported in total – and the 90,000 cases a day barely rates a mention in the (non-Indian!) press. And we in the US are leaving every other country in the world behind us, with up to 250,000 new cases every day.

[79] For example, looking at this site https://www.worldometers.info/coronavirus/ or https://cov.cx/w-c on 17 December, we see there are 20 countries with total infection rates greater than 40,000 per million people, and 62 countries with total infection rates less than 1,000 per million people. Similarly, the case fatality rate (the percent of total cases who die) ranges enormously, and some countries with what you might think are primitive healthcare systems have much lower CFRs than countries with sophisticated healthcare systems (such as, ahem, the US and UK).

I'll concede that different countries have different ways of counting cases and deaths, different approaches to testing, and all sorts of other differences too. That might explain the difference between the US and Cameroon, but is less likely to explain the huge difference between the US and Canada, or between different countries in the EU such as Germany and France. There are some mysterious unknown factors also present. We should be moving heaven and earth to identify these and then use them to our advantage.

Because we don't know why there are such huge changes, it is risky to rely too much on any data from other countries, because there are these mysterious unknown factors that greatly change from each country to each other country.

The Truth is Not Absolute, Facts are Seldom Certain

Our western Judeo-Christian society values truth and morals as absolutes. Promises should be enforceable and inviolable, and right and wrong are universal concepts.

While people can hopefully perceive some issues are more nuanced – which is of course why there are multiple political parties and viewpoints; some things, particularly "scientific" things, are thought to be absolutes and incapable of multiple different interpretations. Facts, after all, are surely right or wrong. Two plus two always equals four. Water is always liquid, and fire is always hot.

But these are gross over-simplifications,[80] particularly in the context of something that deceptively seems simple – public health management. You might think it is simple – a person is either healthy or sick. They either have this disease or that disease. They either survive or die.

None of those seemingly black and white issues are indeed absolutes. As you know yourself, being healthy or sick is a continuum with many mid-points. Some days you feel "a bit off-color", other days you feel definitely unwell but still get out of bed after hitting the snooze button on the alarm a couple of times, and sometimes you are so unwell you moan, groan, turn off the alarm, and stay in bed all day.

As for having this or that disease, that too is surprisingly variable, particularly in terms of how each disease affects you, its severity, and its possible interaction with other medical conditions you have. Even a single disease might actually not be a single disease, but a collection of several different strains of a similar/related virus or bacteria. Something as simple as a "sore throat" can be caused by several different bacteria (or might be a symptom of something much darker, like

---

[80] Even the 2 + 2 = 4 assumption is a simplification, but that's not something we'll dive into here! It can also be subject to computer errors (if not represented as integer type values – also not something to go into here).

Water can also be a solid, a super-cooled (solid) liquid, or a gas. Some flames burn very coolly because they require almost as much heat to evaporate the liquid they're burning as they generate in heat.

cancer) and those several different bacteria may vary in terms of whether they will be eliminated by various different antibiotics.[81]

Some diseases mimic other diseases, and some diseases (using the word in its broadest sense) have mysterious and puzzling root causes that are still subject to conjecture.

Even the most extreme measure of healthcare – does the patient live or die – is also nuanced. We discuss this in the section "Your Risk of Dying" which starts on page 148.

Beyond the examples of debatable and possibly miscategorized causes of death, there is also the issue that living is not an absolute outcome either. There is more to living than simply breathing (especially if only doing so while connected to a mechanical ventilator and sedated). What is the quality of life that the "recovered" patient now experiences? Have they made a full or only partial recovery? Will their future life expectancy be the same as if they had not been ill, or will they die prematurely, albeit years/decades in the future?[82]

---

[81] We'd also point to the fascinating story of how our understanding of what causes stomach ulcers has evolved. For the longest time, they were thought to be caused by stress. An obscure doctor in western Australia dared to think otherwise, and was ridiculed for doing so by "the experts". But he persisted in his research and even infected himself to prove his theory, and eventually came up with conclusive proof that stomach ulcers are caused by bacteria. He and his partner-researcher ended up winning the Nobel Prize for medicine.

So much for "all experts agree that .....". Most advancements in medical science start with a need to rebut the implacable deadening of open-minded inquiry and experimentation caused by the "all experts agree that ...." statement.

See, for example, https://www.discovermagazine.com/health/the-doctor-who-drank-infectious-broth-gave-himself-an-ulcer-and-solved-a-medical-mystery or https://cov.cx/a1a39

[82] Yes, there are point scales to measure degrees of severity of illness and degrees of recovery as well. But they are very subjective – just think when a doctor last asked you "On a scale of 1 – 10, how would you rate the pain you are feeling at present?". When I'm asked that question, I have no idea where in the scale any pain should be placed, and I also suspect that whatever my rating might be will be several points higher or lower than the next person with the same pain.

Facts Are Meaningless, Interpretation is Key

This brings us to another important concept. We also urge you to beware of accurate but misleading or irrelevant facts.[83] The most obvious example of this is the often-quoted claim that "The US has almost twice as many virus deaths as any other country". On the face of it, this is sort of true. In mid-December, the US had 317,000 deaths. The next largest death count is in Brazil, with 185,000.[84] [85]

But this is a meaningless number. Of course the US will have a very large number of deaths because it is the third-largest country in the world. The largest

---

[83] An example of this happened to me, almost 40 years ago. I was doing a major research project for a retailer in a small New Zealand city, and part of that involved surveying both their shoppers and the shoppers of competing stores in the town. We had interviewers outside the exits to all relevant stores, asking questions of people as they left. One of the other stores objected, claiming that the people leaving their store were "their" customers and that their customers' opinions were a trade secret that we were trying to steal. A nonsense claim, of course, but the last thing we and our client wanted was a major argument and possibly a court case in a small town where you needed to cooperate positively in the community.

I asked my senior partner what we should do? We needed the data. He said, "Offer to give the other store a complete copy of all the survey data we get, both from their store and other stores". I marveled "Doesn't that mean we're giving them a free copy of what we are charging our client many thousands of dollars for? That doesn't seem fair. What will our client think?" The older wiser partner replied "The raw data is meaningless and has no value. Anyone can collect data. What we are charging for is how we analyze the data, and the recommendations we derive from its interpretation. The other retailer won't know what to do with the data."

He was correct. We uncovered interesting differences in perceptions and attitudes between the different stores, and the client retailer made successful changes as a result. The other complaining store made no changes at all, even though we saw issues and opportunities for them too in the data we gave them.

The moral of the story is that raw data, by itself, is useless. The magic of its meaning lies in how you interpret it. The data might be absolute (but usually isn't). Its interpretation is almost always subjective.

[84] In case you wondered, there is then another large drop in death numbers to India, with 145,000 deaths, and then Mexico with 116,000, Italy with 67,000, and so on.

[85] Remember also our point above that the truth changes. Countries often swap places on these lists and can shift from way below average numbers to way above average, or vice versa. Between 14 Aug and 17 December, India went from fourth place to second place, and then back to third place. Many other countries have changed their rankings, too. This will of course continue into the future, just as it has in the past.

country, China, is widely thought to have massively undercounted its case and death rates as a matter of national policy, and the second-largest country, India, while way behind the US, is experiencing steadily increasing rates of daily deaths, some days exceeding the number in the US.

The meaningful measure in this case is not total deaths, but deaths as a percentage of total population. When we shift to that measure, the US goes from being the worst-performing country to a more modestly placed ninth position on the list in mid-November. That's nothing to be proud of, for sure, but it is also very much different from claiming that we are the worst in the world.

There's another interesting measure as well – the "Case Fatality Rate" or the percentage of people who get the disease and then die.

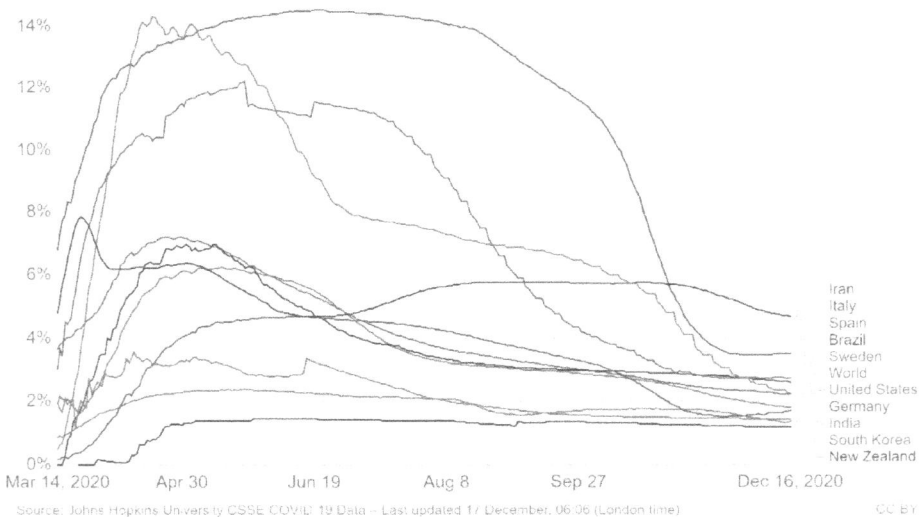

Figure 2 Case Fatality Rates by Country

As this chart shows above,[86] the US is slightly lower than the world average when it comes to this measure. That's a very good thing, and miles away from the opening statement "The US is the worst country in the world for Covid-19

---

[86] Taken from this page, you can visit it for the current updated data and additional data from other countries https://ourworldindata.org/mortality-risk-covid#the-case-fatality-rate or https://cov.cx/a1a40

deaths". You can also see the way that different countries have changed their relative rankings over time.

So here's the thing. While "numbers never lie"[87] they can paint very different pictures of an underlying situation at different times. As the chart above shows, the relative positions of different countries shifts from time to time. Conclusions made in March – while perhaps valid then – are very different from the conclusions you'd draw in April, and neither set of conclusions helps you guess for what will happen in May and June.

It isn't just time that impacts on these numbers. You need to question and consider what the number is measuring and think about other related measures that might be more helpful and relevant, and whether other measures might be impacting on the numbers you are measuring in subtle ways you've not yet factored into your analysis.

Even if the numbers are correct, they can be displayed in deceptive ways. A classic "trick" is to show a graph where the origin (the bottom left-hand corner) is not zero. This exaggerates changes in numbers – this is a trick beloved of politicians who use this trickery to exaggerate either their accomplishments or to denigrate the problems of their opponents.

---

[87] That's a totally wrong statement, and obviously made by someone who never heard the aphorism "There are lies, damn lies, and then there are statistics"!

Big Change

Little Change

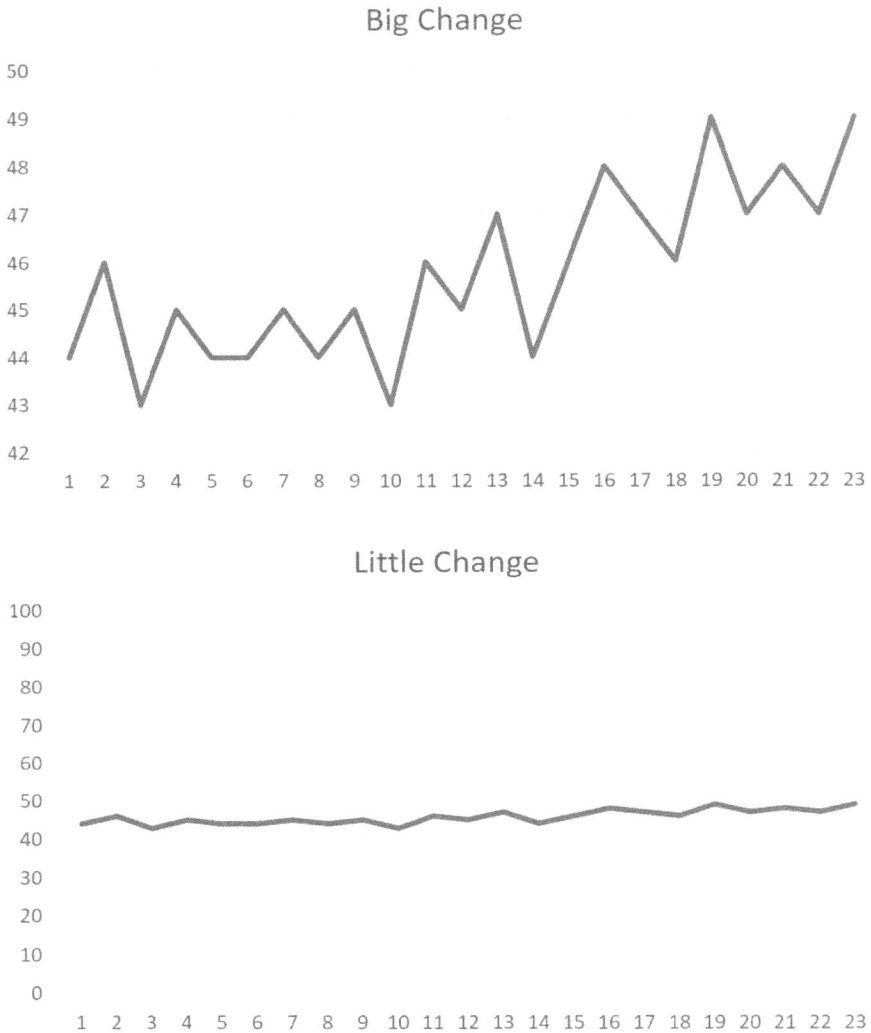

Figure 3 A big or small change in values?

The two charts above use the same data, perhaps it might be showing the percentage of people who support a political party, or could be anything else at all. The numbers are identical, but the top chart, with a narrow range of values, suggests a big shift, whereas the bottom chart, with space on the chart for all possible values from 0 to 100, suggests the difference is trivial.

This also brings up another issue that we touched on above. Whenever analyzing multiple data events (most commonly a time series) how far back do you go for your data series? It is possible to selectively pick a starting point when the value at that time is either unusually low or unusually high, making the overall trend and change in data from that point through to the endpoint (which is usually the most current data but also might be selectively chosen) look either good or bad.

Longer time series indeed tend to show trends more clearly, but if you make a time series too lengthy, other factors may have occurred during the time series that impact on the data you're tracking. For example, with airfares, you could track data for a short time – the last nine months – and you'd see a plunge in pricing. You could track airfares from say 1 January 2002 through to 31 Dec 2019 and show that air prices had massively increased. But do you see the deception there? 1 Jan 2002 had airfares very low, in the aftermath of the 9/11/2001 terror attacks in the US. You could track airfares all the way back to say 1975 and show how the average airfare has either dropped or stayed the same, but that ignores the major event in 1979 – airline deregulation, which resulted in plunging airfares for a decade or so. And you also then have the confounding effects of inflation, jet fuel prices, new airplanes being developed with lower operating costs, and a need to compare the varying cost of airfares with other transportation modes, and so on.

So short data series can be deceptive, but so too can long data series. Basically, in either skilled (deliberately deceptive) or inept (accidentally deceptive) hands you can make most data series tell very different stories based on how you choose them and interpret them.

Another display tool that needs to be understood is whether numbers are shown with a linear or logarithmic scale. For example, look at these two charts of the same data series. One looks very alarming, the other looks very reassuring.

Do you notice how it is that the two lines are so totally different, even though the underlying numbers are identical?

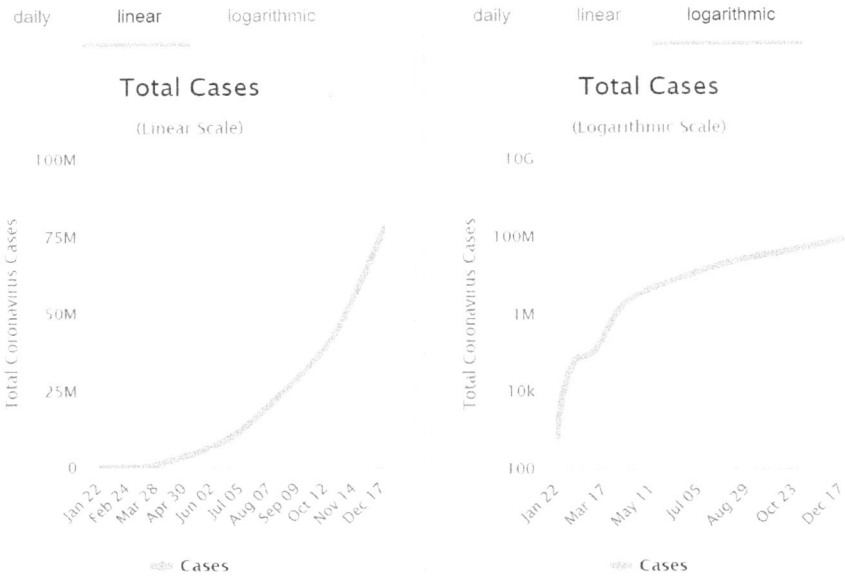

Figure 4 Showing the same data very differently

As you can see in the fine print on each image, the left image has a linear scale on both axes, and the right image has a logarithmic scale on the vertical axis. The linear scale is the most commonly used one in most situations, where each unit of measure relates to the same number of items being reported – in this case, each horizontal line is 5 million greater than the one below it. But see in the logarithmic scale, how each unit of measure is increasing – each line is ten times greater than the line below it?

There are sometimes valid reasons to show things with an exponential/logarithmic scale, sometimes on one axis, sometimes even on both axes, but the way they then show data is very different from the same data on a linear scale. You need to not only perceive which type of scale is being used but also be able to make a value judgment as to if it is relevant and fair or not.[88]

Other distortions can apply to showing data as well, maybe deliberately and maybe inadvertently. For example, look at this chart showing the change of Rt

---

[88] An example of an appropriate use of a log scale would be measuring different sound levels, because we hear sounds logarithmically, and indeed the typical measure of sound – Bels and decibels – is a logarithmic measure.

values (we explain this measure in our chapter "4. How the Number of Infections Increased So Quickly", starting on page 50, below) over time in Hawaii.[89]

Figure 5 Numbers with different meanings

On the face of it, this seems like a very fair presentation of the data. 1.0 is the point where infection rates either increase (if the value goes above 1.0) or decrease (if the value is less than 1.0). The vertical scale (ie the y-axis) is equally spaced, the same space between each 0.2 of value.

But, here's the thing. The meaning and impact of each unit on the y-axis is not the same. For example, a value of +1 unit (ie 2) means "doubling" but a value of -0.5 units(ie 0.5) means "halving". A value of 1.9 means "almost doubling" but a value of 0.1 means "reducing ten-fold".

In this case, perhaps the y-axis scale should not be linear.

One more thing – and I'll try to make it the last thing before we turn to the "real" meat of the book.

Many of the issues and actions involve **subjective values as well as objective science**. "This is an effective cure" or "that doesn't work" usually are not absolute truths, even though they are stated as such. Almost every "effective cure" works less than 100% of the time, and may have side-effects and risks associated with its deployment.

Another element of effectiveness is unavoidably cost and resource consumption. How much cost are we prepared to accept to cure a person of something? $1 million? $1 billion? Or? Will we pay more to cure a new-born babe than we would to cure an 85-year-old? Will we pay more to cure the

---

[89] See https://rt.live/us/HI or https://cov.cx/a1a41

President[90] or Elon Musk than we would to cure a convicted murderer or a homeless person?

These are awkward issues that most people consciously or unconsciously avoid examining, but need to be considered as part of any evaluation and which lie uncomfortably concealed beneath the surface of blanket statements.

Similar but opposite comments apply to the statement "that doesn't work". Now, for sure, some things will never work, like taking a sip of sugar water as a hoped-for cure for cancer,[91] but many things rejected as cures are rejected not because they don't work, but because they don't work often enough, or because they are accompanied by too high a level of side-effects, or because they are too experimental and have not yet been proven to work, or because they are impossibly expensive.

There's a mile of difference between "this never works" and "this does work sometimes but not always and carries severe risks of causing other problems", and so on. Furthermore, if you're just looking for something to salve a sore throat, your willingness to take a risky experimental drug is rightly very low, but what say you're in the final stages of cancer and with a very short life expectancy

---

[90] Well, we now know the answer to that question, don't we! President Trump got VIP treatment and a barrage of experimental, expensive, and scarce drugs such as the rest of us could never hope to get.

[91] Well, even that *might* sometimes work. The placebo effect is very real. And how to explain the loyal following and supporters of homeopathy, which involves taking substances that have been so diluted that there is no longer any active ingredient at all remaining in the medicine – not even a single molecule. Homeopathy supporters even acknowledge this but claim that the past presence of the chemical in less dilute portions of the medicine has somehow changed the state of the now completely diluted water.

That sounds like a ridiculous and laughable unscientific piece of nonsense. But so too have any number of "folk medicines" where unlikely mixtures of plant and animal life are claimed to cure all manner of evils. The interesting thing is that many of medicine's most exciting breakthroughs have been by examining and understanding what the active ingredients are in such folk remedies. So – who knows – let's not yet dismiss homeopathy entirely (but yes, feel free to be very cautious about it, too!). We discuss homeopathy further in the chapter on medicines, supplements, etc.

The homeopathic example points to another mystery of life and medicine – no matter how much we surround ourselves with science, there is still an enormous amount we don't know about life, diseases, and treatments, and many modern treatments and medicines have evolved out of folk-remedies that were at one time popular, then ridiculed by people preferring "science" over folklore, only to be subsequently shown to actually contain some ingredient that truly does influence a specific disease.

and very low quality of life at present. What would you say then to a drug that has a 50% chance of curing you but a 50% chance of hastening your end?

Medical professionals often talk "in shorthand" and make absolute statements because their time is short and the matter is complex, and they fairly perceive that their patient wouldn't want or comprehend a two-hour lecture on the complexity of issues underpinning the recommendation/finding they are offering up. You need to be aware that while their shorthand "bottom-line" comments may be appropriate, they also may not be complete, and the reality of the matter might be much more complicated than the single short absolute statement implies.

One of the life lessons I hold dear is that the more certain an expert is of something, the less credible he is. Even the basic laws of physics end up, in the ultimate quantum sub-particle levels, changing from simple certainties, equations, and laws that we learned in high school to matters of variable chance and imprecision. True experts, as they learn more about their field, come to understand not how simple the underlying truths are, but how complex they are.

Beware of "experts" who speak only in absolutes.

We could continue, but we're already way too far into the book, and possibly haven't even started what you primarily came here to read! But this section is important – you need to view every element of this issue as being comprised of shades of gray rather than being absolutely either black or white.

If you can't perceive the grays, you need to ask someone to identify them for you, because they are ever-present and make interpretation of data and decision-making based on such interpretations difficult rather than easy.

You also need to understand that even "hard facts" are not necessarily either hard or factual, and the representations of those facts can be deliberately or accidentally very distorting.

Can I close the introduction with one last and important point. I absolutely do not wish this document to be an extended critique of the medical profession or researchers or anything/anything else. That would be wrong at so many levels.

But I equally strongly wish to encourage you (and medical professionals) to look behind the façade of certainty and perceive the imprecision, the unknowns, and the range of potential possibilities hidden behind it.

If this lengthy preamble has helped you to look at all data, on all topics, with a more open and questioning mind, then the book has already served a noble purpose.

2. Have the Sacrifices We've Made So Far Been Worth It?

This is a controversial question, but one we surely all wonder about, and one the politicians answer in very different ways. Have we adopted the correct balance of virus-limiting controls, sufficient to be effective, while inflicting only the minimum amount of damage to our lives, our jobs, and to the nation's economy as a whole? Or have we done too much, or too little?

These are impossibly difficult issues because we don't know five essential things :

- We don't know how many actual cases and deaths have occurred as a consequence of the virus (please don't start disagreeing with that statement yet – I'll explain shortly)
- We don't know what would have happened if we had more (or less) restrictions
- It is even difficult to know exactly what the cost (social, economic, and by any/all other relevant measures) has been of what we've done so far
- It is hard to understand and compare the differences between our numbers and those of other countries – some major unknown factors seem to be at work
- I don't think anyone can even accurately and succinctly state exactly what our controls are or were, or what the compliance level with them has been, and they've regularly changed in any event

Let's start with the third point. What has been the cost of the virus and our response to it?

We should remind ourselves of some of the things that have changed since March. Some changes are hopefully temporary, others might be longer-lasting, and, of course, for businesses that have closed, some are tragically permanent.[92]

- *Retail Shopping*

For some time, retailers have been struggling. It has been common to blame online shopping for making things harder for traditional "bricks and mortar" stores. While there can be no denying that many retailers have found life more difficult, and the rise of online shopping is obvious to us all (Hello, Amazon!); in reality, online sales had only reached about 11.5% of total sales in the first quarter of 2020, which on the face of it doesn't seem like an uncontrollable monster that threatens all retailing, everywhere.

However, the second quarter simultaneously saw total retail sales drop while online sales increased, and as you can see, the share of online sales rapidly increased in the April-June and July-September quarters. We expect to see a further significant increase in the fourth quarter. This trend can be seen here:[93]

---

[92] This interesting article in the Wall St Journal includes the observation that ten years of consumer adoption of e-commerce was compressed into three months. Many of the social changes forced upon us are likely to be lasting. See https://www.wsj.com/articles/four-reasons-the-stay-at-home-economy-is-here-to-stay-11605934806 or https://cov.cx/a1a42

[93] Taken from https://www.census.gov/retail/mrts/www/data/pdf/ec_current.pdf or https://cov.cx/a1a43

Estimated Quarterly U.S. Retail E-commerce Sales as a Percent of Total Quarterly Retail Sales:
1st Quarter 2011 – 3rd Quarter 2020

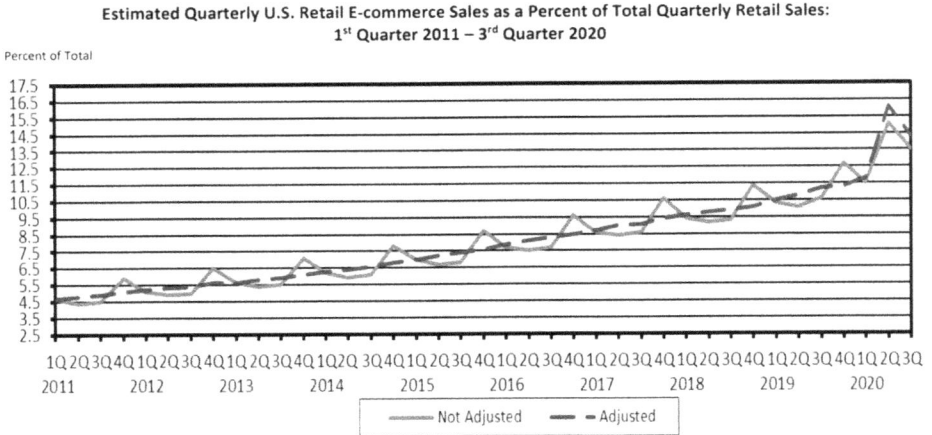

Figure 6 Online share of US retail sales

In the first quarter of 2020, these statistics show $1.204 trillion in traditional retail sales and $160 billion in online sales. In the second quarter, traditional retail sales dropped, and in the third quarter, traditional retail sales had recovered and slightly risen above the first quarter, to $1.259 trillion. Online sales increased to $210 billion.

It seems surprising that a brief drop in traditional retail sales could be so impactful, and perhaps that is due to an uneven impact on sales. Some retailers never closed (supermarkets for example), others tried to shift to curbside pickup or delivery, others closed completely and a few experienced a surge in sales – Costco in particular. Perhaps I'm not the only person who currently thinks it is better to make occasional bulk shopping runs than several-times-a-week minor "topping up" trips to a local supermarket. Instead of buying one or two cans of beans or soup at a time, as needed, and from a local store, I buy a carton of them from Costco, and so on.

We also don't know what will happen when things return back to "normal". It is possible that many new people have been introduced to buying many new things online (or in bulk from Costco and similar outlets) and they may never return to regular retail purchases.

The bottom-line has yet to be determined, but one report in June projected 20,000 – 25,000 retail stores will close this year.[94]

---

[94] See https://www.foxbusiness.com/markets/future-malls-coronavirus-25000-stores-close or https://cov.cx/a1a44

In addition to the general impact on general retailing, there seems to have been a greater impact on large indoor shopping malls. They've been struggling for several years already, and one report in August suggests a quarter of all malls will close within the next five years (in addition to the malls that have closed over the last while).[95] Not all of this can be blamed on Covid-19, but surely it has had a measurable impact on retailing, and perhaps for stores that have been struggling to survive, it has been "the last straw" that has hastened their end.

It isn't just retail shopping, by the way. It is also retail services – you've probably noticed the ever-fewer number of banks that have anything more than a lobby with a few ATMs, or perhaps a couple of tellers, but no-one to talk to about general banking needs.

Many other professional service type businesses have been quietly transitioning to consolidated operation centers that have no public access, the virus has hastened that trend. An obscured second part of that issue is that when operation centers are separated from the markets they serve, it makes little difference if they are ten or ten thousand miles away, encouraging the concept of more off-shoring of services.[96]

We also wonder if we're noticing another trend – businesses are using the virus as an excuse to cut back on customer service functions. If you've needed to call a customer service line for any reason, there's a measurable chance you've been told to expect a longer wait than normal due to the virus.[97] We don't believe that excuse and think it is more a case of businesses opportunistically trying to turn a challenge into a benefit.

---

[95] See https://www.cnbc.com/2020/08/27/25percent-of-us-malls-are-set-to-shut-within-5-years-what-comes-next.html or https://cov.cx/a1a45

[96] To give two examples of unexpected offshoring, the first is that when you next go to your local fast-food drive-through, there's a chance that the voice coming out of the speaker wanting to take your order isn't coming from a person inside the restaurant, but from someone in a call center, possibly in a totally different country.

The other example – you go to a hospital and need an X-ray. The radiographer who "reads" that X-ray might not be in the room next to the X-ray machine. He might be in India – the X-ray is digitally sent through the internet to an off-shore radiographer, and their analysis is sent back the same way.

[97] Most infamously, I tried to call Google Fi support on their 800 number, and was told "Due to the virus, we are not offering phone support at present". That's appalling. The virus doesn't travel down phone lines, and surely Google of all companies would be able to allow their support reps to work from home, the same way so many other companies do (and have been doing for years).

• *Restaurants and Bars*

If you're like me, you struggle to understand how a few dollars worth of food ends up costing $25 when cooked and served to you in a restaurant, and how a couple of dollars of alcohol costs you $10 to drink in a bar. Based on those numbers, restaurants and bars seem like some of the most potentially profitable businesses out there.

The truth is that most restaurants and many bars struggle to do much more than barely break even, have high failure rates, and the owners and managers of those that remain in business work very long hours for very low return.[98]

The outright closure orders imposed on restaurants and bars in many states of course were very harmful to these businesses. And the subsequent requirement to reduce the number of people allowed in at one time with partially restricted re-openings does not solve the problem.

From the cost analysis in the footnote above, food and labor costs are about 60% - 70% of gross income, all other costs are 25% - 35%, and profit is about 5%. If a restaurant can now only service half as many people, that means the "all other costs" percentage close to doubles because most of those costs are fixed, whether the restaurant serves one person or one hundred. The 5% profit can not now absorb another 25% - 35% of costs.

Unsurprisingly, many restaurants and bars have already closed, and many more will in the future.[99] Those that stay open will need to increase their prices or come up with imaginative new ways to earn additional income.

While not quite the same thing, Starbucks and other types of coffee shops are also suffering. Starbucks, which built its success on the concept of creating European-style "meeting place" type coffee shops, is permanently closing up to

---

[98] I'll not make this a lengthy treatise on the economics of restaurants and bars, but the short answer is that particularly in restaurants, the highest cost is labor. You know yourself from cooking at home how much time goes into buying food, preparing it and cooking a meal, serving it, and then cleaning up and doing the dishes afterward. Food and labor costs alone represent 60% - 70% of your meal price, and then rent is another 8% - 10%. Other overheads – utilities, repairs and maintenance, depreciation and capital equipment purchases, advertising, and so on, take up most of the rest, leaving maybe 5% for profit – sometimes (rarely) more, often less.

[99] Here's an interesting albeit slightly confusing report on a survey done by Yelp for the six months through the end of August, showing the proportions of various types of businesses it lists that have closed, either temporarily or permanently. Food businesses and other general retailers were hit the most, professional service providers the least. https://www.cnbc.com/2020/09/16/yelp-data-shows-60percent-of-business-closures-due-to-the-coronavirus-pandemic-are-now-permanent.html or https://cov.cx/a1a46

400 of its US stores this year[100] and shifting away from that style of store, with future emphasis on drive-through and to-go type mini-stores instead. We expect other independent coffee stores are similarly impacted.

- *Office Environments*

It is hard to know exactly what the net effect might end up being with office workplaces. The emptying of many offices and working from home trend has resulted in, depending on who you listen to, either a positive or negative impact on people and their work/life balances, and similarly, an uncertain impact on productivity.[101]

We expect that to start with, everyone worked harder – but inefficiently – as companies rushed to adapt to remote work. Then people stopped making special efforts, but work processes became more efficient, so perhaps there were periods when productivity was up, and other times when it was down, and if we had to guess, perhaps overall, things are more or less a wash. Certainly, things are not as impactful for office-type businesses as they are for restaurants and bars.

There have been various surveys and reports about what the actual impacts have been in the earlier stages of remote working, but we think due to the somewhat changing nature of remote work back then, they should all be viewed with care, rather than accepted as absolute truth today. But this mid-May Gallup poll seems to suggest that in general terms, considerably more people enjoy remote working than dislike it.[102]

---

[100] See https://www.cnn.com/2020/06/10/business/starbucks-closing-400-stores/index.html or https://cov.cx/a1a47 It will be sad to see them close. I'm sure I'm not the only one with memories of internet-driven "blind dates" at Starbucks stores in the past.

[101] Perhaps the least commented on aspect of working from home is that in many cases, not only did the parents start working from home, but their children were home too due to school closures. The initial chaos of developing new "office" work routines at home was made much more complex by having one's children present, with no school work being given to them, and impacting on everything too.

It may well be that in the future, with the children either busy doing school work remotely rather than being unoccupied, or the children back in school, working from home will become even more popular for parents.

[102] See https://news.gallup.com/poll/311375/reviewing-remote-work-covid.aspx or https://cov.cx/a1a48 A subsequent Gallup poll in September/October showed that people have been returning to their offices. Of the remote workers, two-thirds want to continue working remotely and one-third would like to be back in their former office

(continued on next page)

It seems clear, whether a success or not, remote working, at a greater level than before the virus, will become more common.[103] This June article is even more positive, and claims 98% of employees would like to be able to work from home at least some of the time.[104]

Here is an interesting chart showing average office occupancy this year, as measured by swipe cards for building access.[105]

OCCUPANCY OVER TIME — MARCH 5 TO DECEMBER 16

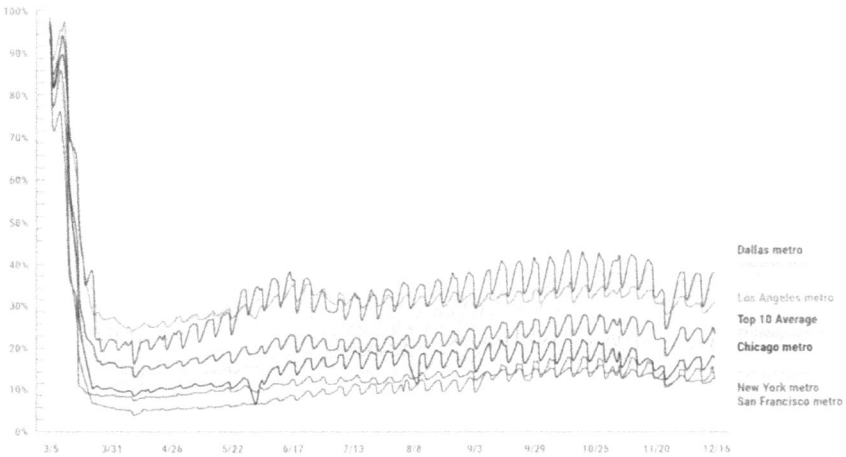

Figure 7 Office occupancy levels since March

What we find particularly interesting is to match these numbers with the numbers shown in Figure 8 US Air Travel compared to 2019 on page 61, below. It might seem reasonable to expect some sort of general correspondence in

---

environment. See https://news.gallup.com/poll/321800/covid-remote-work-update.aspx or https://cov.cx/a1a49

[103] Here's a vague and pompous declaration to that effect
https://www.ey.com/en_be/covid-19/why-remote-working-will-be-the-new-normal-even-after-covid-19 or https://cov.cx/a1a50

[104] See https://www.weforum.org/agenda/2020/06/coronavirus-covid19-remote-working-office-employees-employers or https://cov.cx/a1a51

[105] See https://www.kastle.com/city-by-city-views-of-americas-office-use/ or https://cov.cx/a1c21 for the most recent data.

numbers, but as can clearly be seen, there has been a much greater recovery in air travel numbers than there has been in office attendance levels.

What will this reduction in office staff numbers do to the need for office space in expensive high-rise buildings? In some cases, greater distancing between staff members might use up the office space freed by fewer people working in the office, although in general there is usually six feet or more between people in most offices already. On balance, we guess that companies may require about the same or slightly less office space than before.

This shift to remote work (whether all the time or perhaps a mix of some days at home and some days in the office) will mean fewer people in the center of cities, which will weaken downtown retailing and restaurants/bars even more. It will harm commercial property owners.[106] It will impact on public transport services[107] – reduced ridership will mean fewer operating buses, and/or greater losses and higher fares, and ridership will reduce further because people will see driving in their car as safer and also easier with less rush-hour commute traffic. Plus fewer riders will probably mean a reduced frequency of services, encouraging still more people to shift to their cars.

- *Live Entertainment*

I was watching video footage of the "Last Night at the Proms" in London just before writing this section. The "Last Night at the Proms" is an annual event and the last in a series of casual classical concerts held in London's Royal Albert Hall every summer. Normally the last night event is full of literally standing room only attendees (the Hall has a normal capacity of 5,272 people), an orchestra of 300 players, and a huge choir. This year, it had 65 musicians, a handful of singers, and no attendees, and was performed purely to be broadcast on the BBC.[108]

Most other concert and theater events have just been canceled entirely.

---

[106] This will be a long-term trend rather than a sudden sharp shift, because companies with multi-year leases may not be easily able to immediately reduce the space they lease, and even when renewing, some companies will prefer "too much" space but keeping their present location and layout and everything rather than the hassle and costs of moving.

[107] See https://ny.curbed.com/2020/3/24/21192454/coronavirus-nyc-transportation-subway-citi-bike-covid-19 or https://cov.cx/a1a52

[108] The Proms have been held every year since 1895, without interruption, until 2020. https://en.wikipedia.org/wiki/The_Proms or https://cov.cx/a1a53

Also in London, the always-every-show-still-sold-out musical, Phantom of the Opera, after being temporarily closed as part of Britain's social gathering restrictions, announced it would formally close in late July because the producers couldn't see how they'd ever be able to produce it profitably in the future with social distancing restricting the number of people who could be in the theater for each performance.[109]

The same is true of all other forms of live public entertainment. These businesses have been built on a model and expectation of certain sized audiences, and if they can't get those sized audiences they're either going to have to close down or downsize their productions. This applies to both live entertainment and also to movie theaters, although the new style of low-density deluxe seating type theaters probably will be more likely to re-open, and sooner, than the traditional high-density theaters. But will there still be new first-run popular movies for the remaining theaters to screen?

Movie studios are now – very reluctantly – experimenting with releasing major new movies direct to premium streaming channels, and there have even been some attempts at reviving drive-in movie theaters, albeit with no real success. Sony said in September it won't release any blockbuster movies to theaters until after the pandemic is over.[110] Other studios are delaying releases of such eagerly awaited movies as the latest in the James Bond, Indiana Jones, and Mission Impossible franchises.[111]

- *Sports*

Sporting events are another form of live entertainment, and they are such a key part of our society they deserve a separate mention.

---

[109] See https://www.vulture.com/2020/07/phantom-of-the-opera-closes-on-west-end-amid-coivd-19.html or https://cov.cx/a1a54

[110] See https://www.cbr.com/sony-covid-19-no-major-movies-in-theaters/ or https://cov.cx/a1a55

[111] See https://en.wikipedia.org/wiki/List_of_films_impacted_by_the_COVID-19_pandemic or https://cov.cx/a1a56 There were rumors in October that possibly Apple might buy the rights to the James Bond movie and take it direct to streaming, but MGM and Apple were unable to agree upon a price – with MGM allegedly wanting $600 million and Apple offering perhaps $400 million. https://variety.com/2020/film/news/james-bond-no-time-to-die-netflix-apple-1234814809/ or https://cov.cx/a1a57 The movie, which was due to be released initially in April 2020, has now been twice delayed and currently is set to be released, in theaters, in April 2021.

The possibly saving grace for professional sports is that for quite some time, their revenue has come less from the live crowds in stadiums and more from television broadcast rights and advertising.[112]

Even though most of us choose to watch sports on television, there has always been the opportunity to go to a game, and there's been the "buzz" of the crowd adding to the involvement when passively watching at home or in a bar somewhere. There's been some sort of abstract "sense of place" when watching a "home game" in the local stadium that always feels more special, even more special than watching a home team play an away game.

But what, now? Watching teams sequestered inside "bubbles" play games in almost empty stadiums – even worse, if they add computer-generated images and soundtracks of cheering crowds, as has been suggested – is a sad sight and not nearly as engaging as watching "the real thing". We wonder also what the teams and stadiums are doing without the ticket sales each match, and how engaged the public as a whole will remain when a match changes from a social event that company groups attend for fun, and other people go as a family outing or for a date, to something one can only watch on television (and probably not even in a "sport's bar" due to it being closed or allowing only reduced occupancy).

At a more personal level, seeing our children and grandchildren deprived of their chances to enjoy "little league" type games feels like a sad loss of part of life's growing up rituals (for them) and of parenting (for us).

- *Education*

It is perplexing and regrettable that our schools were very slow to embrace "distance learning". Companies switched to Zoom and other video technologies in a matter of days. My daughter's high school closed in March and for a couple of months did nothing at all, before sending some offline work to her and other students in the last month or so of the school year, work which required only a couple of hours a day to do, even though she had a good load of Honors and AP classes.[113]

Things are going better for her and most other children in the new school year, with more effective use of video technologies to recreate classroom-type experiences, but inexplicably, her school days now start later and finish earlier,

---

[112] This article says Major League Baseball typically gets only 25% of its income from stadium ticket sales. https://www.startribune.com/schafer-how-major-league-teams-can-still-make-money-in-front-of-empty-stands/571676282/ or https://cov.cx/a1a58

[113] She and all her peers were then given "A" passes for the year in all their subjects, no matter how well or poorly they were doing prior to the collapse in education in March.

with no lessons at all scheduled on Wednesdays. But why did it take so long to transition to remote learning?

While it varies from school district to school district, many parents are left with the distinct feeling that their children are being shortchanged by their schools at present. And talking about shortchanging, how about people at colleges – sometimes paying $50,000 or more per year of education, and then finding themselves being fed the equivalent of a series of "Great Courses" programs?

A depressed level of learning for a while is perhaps acceptable at early levels of education, but by the time young adults get to tertiary levels and need to acquire specific job-related skills before starting work in their chosen field, their lives are on hold – even if the fees are not.[114] [115]

- ### *Travel – Business and Leisure*

Air travel plunged in March, dropping to about 5% of 2019 numbers in April, and has been slowly inching up since then. In mid-December, it is at about 33% (1/3rd) of last year.[116]

---

[114] A humanities/liberal arts graduate can probably proceed into the workplace with a bit less of a thorough grounding in their chosen subjects, but what about an accountant. "Oh, sorry, I missed that section on tax law in my training". Or a doctor. "I think you might have a tropical disease, but unfortunately they didn't teach us that subject because of the virus." Or an architect. "Here are the plans for your new home, except for the bedrooms. We didn't cover how to design bedrooms."

[115] There's another aspect of schooling that is currently being lost – the social element. While, as an anxious father, at one level I'm sort of glad that my high-school daughter is not being surrounded by teenage boys all the time, realistically I feel it is not a good thing that she is missing out on the traditional evolution and maturing of developing relationships with the opposite sex, and fear that when these restrictions are lifted, things might happen more quickly and more impactfully than otherwise might have been the case.

[116] See https://www.tsa.gov/coronavirus/passenger-throughput or https://cov.cx/tsa-c - a very useful counting of people going through TSA checkpoints every day

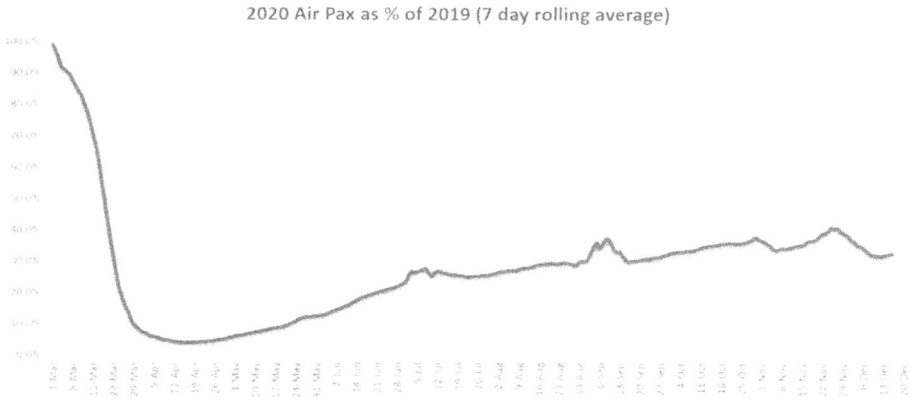

2020 Air Pax as % of 2019 (7 day rolling average)

Figure 8 US Air Travel compared to 2019

Other types of travel have been impacted to greater or lesser extents, and in general it is fair to say that the air travel trends probably reflect much of the broader travel market.

Of interest is this survey in early November, showing the impact of the virus on people's past, present, and future travel plans.

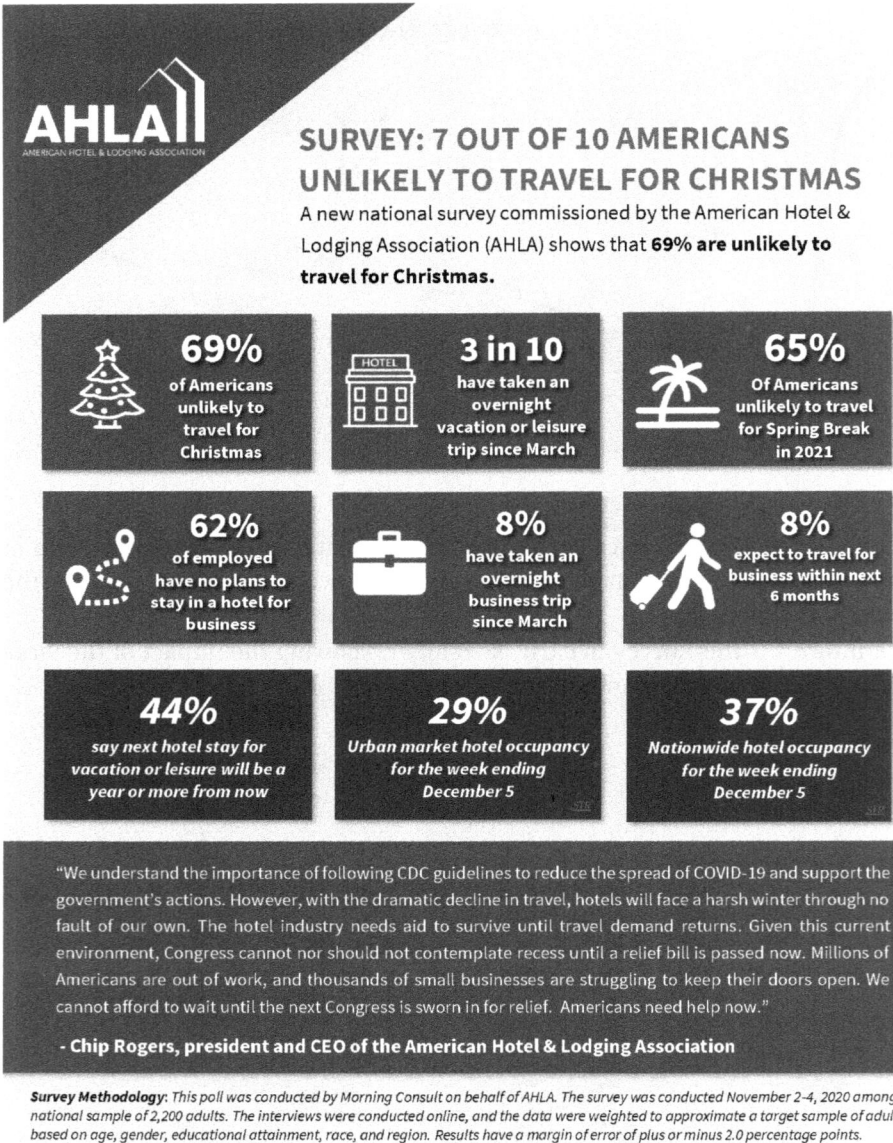

SURVEY: 7 OUT OF 10 AMERICANS UNLIKELY TO TRAVEL FOR CHRISTMAS

A new national survey commissioned by the American Hotel & Lodging Association (AHLA) shows that **69% are unlikely to travel for Christmas.**

69% of Americans unlikely to travel for Christmas

3 in 10 have taken an overnight vacation or leisure trip since March

65% Of Americans unlikely to travel for Spring Break in 2021

62% of employed have no plans to stay in a hotel for business

8% have taken an overnight business trip since March

8% expect to travel for business within next 6 months

44% say next hotel stay for vacation or leisure will be a year or more from now

29% Urban market hotel occupancy for the week ending December 5

37% Nationwide hotel occupancy for the week ending December 5

"We understand the importance of following CDC guidelines to reduce the spread of COVID-19 and support the government's actions. However, with the dramatic decline in travel, hotels will face a harsh winter through no fault of our own. The hotel industry needs aid to survive until travel demand returns. Given this current environment, Congress cannot nor should not contemplate recess until a relief bill is passed now. Millions of Americans are out of work, and thousands of small businesses are struggling to keep their doors open. We cannot afford to wait until the next Congress is sworn in for relief. Americans need help now."

- Chip Rogers, president and CEO of the American Hotel & Lodging Association

Survey Methodology: This poll was conducted by Morning Consult on behalf of AHLA. The survey was conducted November 2-4, 2020 among a national sample of 2,200 adults. The interviews were conducted online, and the data were weighted to approximate a target sample of adults based on age, gender, educational attainment, race, and region. Results have a margin of error of plus or minus 2.0 percentage points.

Figure 9 Past, present, future travel plans

One of the big worries is that the halt to business travel is demonstrating to companies that business travel is not as essential and unavoidable as it has held to have been.

The obscured truth is that few corporate travelers enjoy traveling around the country and the world on a regular "one week in two" type of basis. Well, some of us went through an early phase of enjoying it, a period of being entranced by frequent flier miles and upgrades, but then disillusionment sets in, and other than a select number of "grand tours" showing the corporate flag to special customers and at special events and industry gatherings, we all cut back our travel as much as we can, and pass those duties on to newer more junior team members.

Not only is corporate travel stressful, and not only does it eat massively into personal time, but it is very time and cost-inefficient.[117] [118]

Video-conferencing, with zero travel time and zero travel cost, is massively better for most people and most purposes.[119]

The future will of course see some continued corporate travel, but probably less than before. Instead of monthly visits to clients "just because", there might be quarterly visits or coordinated meetings scheduled around industry trade shows and conventions. There's a paywalled Wall St Journal article that quotes

---

[117] Even a relatively short 2 – 3 hour flight takes up 5 or more hours from start to finish – driving to an airport, checking in and waiting for the flight, the flight itself, deplaning, collecting bags, getting a rental car, or somehow then going to one's meeting, then the same in reverse at the end of a trip.

Plus the cost. Assume $400 for a roundtrip airfare, then $100 for other transport and parking, maybe meals, and who knows what else.

Add it all up and you're looking at the high side of $500 in above-the-line costs, and a full day out of the office, in return for which you get one or possibly two meetings – perhaps two productive hours out of a 10 – 12 hour grueling day. All of that could be done, for free, from your desk, with a normal day's schedule and six hours left over for everything else.

Don't forget – that's a close to best-case scenario assuming a short two-hour flight. If you're going coast to coast, you have entire days of travel and nothing else, and you need to add hotel costs (and greater personal life disruption at home) to the equation as well.

[118] Amazon reported that it has saved $1 billion in travel costs during the six months of its second and third quarters of 2020, see https://skift.com/2020/10/30/amazons-1-billion-corporate-travel-shutdown-reinforces-a-bleak-2020/ or https://cov.cx/a1a59

[119] The travel industry is desperate to obscure these truths. See, for example, this article that hails the wonder and magic of corporate travel. https://www.bbc.com/worklife/article/20200731-how-coronavirus-will-change-business-travel or https://cov.cx/a1a60 As a former corporate traveler and travel agent, I disagree with its claims of the irreplaceable value of corporate travel.

an "industry expert" as believing one-third to one-half of corporate travel might go away for an extended time.[120]

The effect of that on the travel industry will be disproportionately large. Corporate travelers are the ones who buy the most expensive airfares, hotel rooms, rental cars, and restaurant meals.[121]

Cruise ship voyages have currently stopped entirely for the US market. Of course the cruise lines are gaspingly desperate to get their expensive ships back into service again, and occasionally they try in various parts of the world, but we're not sure how they'll manage to successfully come up with a changed product that allows for social distancing but also relaxed fun and indulgence on board, plus the ability to enjoy port calls without creating new risks of infections during port stops.[122]

There's also the challenge for the cruise lines, the same as restaurants, sports stadiums, hotels, and airlines – can they be profitable if they operate their ships at reduced levels of passengers?

- *Car Sales (and Other Durable Goods)*

The impacts of the virus closures have spread to just about every other type of trade as well. For example, new car sales dropped by about one-third during

---

[120] See, if you can, https://www.wsj.com/articles/what-travel-will-look-like-after-coronavirus-11596026858 or https://cov.cx/a1a61

[121] A lot of businesses might have a profit model like, for example, "We need to average $100 per customer. We will charge business travelers $150 because they are happy paying that, and we will then charge leisure passengers $50 because that is all they are prepared to pay, but on average we still get the $100 we need." If they then lose most of their $150 paying customers, they need to start charging their leisure customers closer to the $100 average, and with leisure customers being price sensitive, they stop buying the product, meaning that if the company charges the necessary rate, it won't get enough customers, and if it charges the rate the market will stand, it won't get enough revenue. That's a terrible lose-lose with no obvious solution.

[122] The risk of becoming infected during a port call is a huge concern. Cruise lines can do some things to improve the bio-safety on board the ship, but most of us go on cruises as much to enjoy port visits as we do to enjoy the ship itself. The current thinking is that passengers will only be allowed to go on official cruise arranged port tours, and will be required to stay with the group, and not break away to see or do their own thing at all. That will greatly reduce an essential part of most cruise experiences.

the second quarter.[123]   The impact of this slump is even more severe because many auto-manufacturers introduced various incentives to try and encourage sales, meaning they were making less profit on the cars they did sell.

Although there has been some recovery in sales volumes in July, a 10% increase in July compared to last year's July figure in no way makes up for three months of 33% decreases.

But even if every car that wasn't sold in the second quarter ends up being sold in the third or fourth quarter, that doesn't mean the auto-manufacturers have caught up on their sales.   They have suffered three – six months of extended ownership of the tardy buyers' older cars, and now the tardy buyers are starting the clock on their next however many years of car ownership 3 – 6 months later than they otherwise would.

It is the same with any other durable goods.   The 3 – 6 months of longer ownership of current products will ripple through the next upgrade cycle too, and so on.

- *Apartment Living*

There's been a marked shift away from apartment living, whether as rentals or as condominiums, and a preference for free-standing single-family dwellings. This has selectively boosted the residential property market in many parts of the country.

This shift in preference is easy to understand.   It is bad enough to be experiencing second hand your neighbor's cooking smells and smoking choices, but when you start to risk also experiencing your neighbor's virus infection too, apartment living loses a lot of its appeal.

And those high-rise apartments with great views?   How do you feel at squeezing into an elevator now?   Or, if there is enforced distancing in elevators, how do you enjoy the five-minute waits (or longer) for your turn to get into an elevator?[124]

---

[123] See https://www.wsj.com/articles/car-sales-fell-in-the-second-quarter-despite-deals-and-covid-19-stimulus-11593621053 or https://cov.cx/a1a62

[124] We can understand how there can be a (hopefully orderly) line of people waiting on the ground floor to take the elevator up to their apartment, but what happens when you want to go down from your apartment to the ground floor, and every time an elevator stops at your floor, it is already full of the reduced quota number of people allowed in it at one time? That seems like an uncontrollable wait unless the building owner reprograms the elevator controls to a totally different logic for answering button press calls for service.

How widespread this trend will become and what it will mean to the property market is anyone's guess at present, but we'll wager that whatever it means, it won't be good for any of us.

- ## *The Multiplier Effect – ie, Everything Else*

I could continue through many more business types and elements of our normal lives, but I think you get the point already. I'll add one final point though – talking about the multiplier effect.

The multiplier effect refers to the flow-on impacts. For example, what happens if an airline stops flying one of its daily flights into your airport? That means a pilot, a few flight attendants, a baggage handler or two, and an airport gate agent or two might lose their jobs. Say, six jobs are lost.

But those six people no longer go out to eat at restaurants and bars, because they can't afford to. So maybe a server loses their job at a restaurant. And now those seven people no longer spend as much money on clothing – they're staying at home every day. That means someone in a local clothing store might be laid off (and maybe someone in a clothing factory). Those people now cut back on something else (or perhaps better to say "cut back on everything else"!), causing more job losses, and then all these people travel less, meaning the airline cuts back on another flight, which starts the next round of the multiplier effect, and so on.

The point I'm making is simple. Even unexpected and unrelated parts of our economy suffer when there are broad hits to broad parts of the economy.

So, considering just these preceding illustrative elements of our lives that have been harmed, most people will agree that the impacts have been enormous, and in some cases, even if the virus should miraculously vanish tomorrow, things might never return to the old "normal". We've opened a Pandora's Box of new possibilities, we've challenged conventional wisdom about the unavoidable need for certain things, and our futures will change. We can hope the changes might be for the better, but we can be certain that changes there will be.

- ## *The Economy as a Whole*

To perhaps everyone's surprise, the economy has been extraordinarily robust, at least by common measurements. The Dow, NASDAQ, S&P500, and NYSE indices are all up so far this year (as of 17 December).

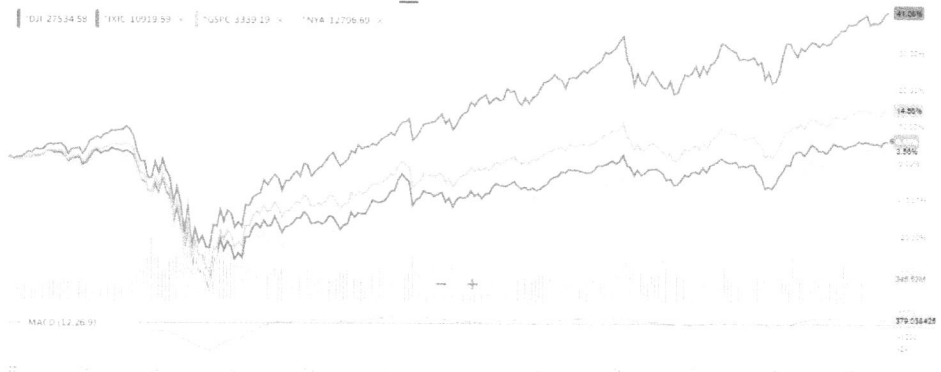

Figure 10 Major market indices for 2020

How about GDP?[125]

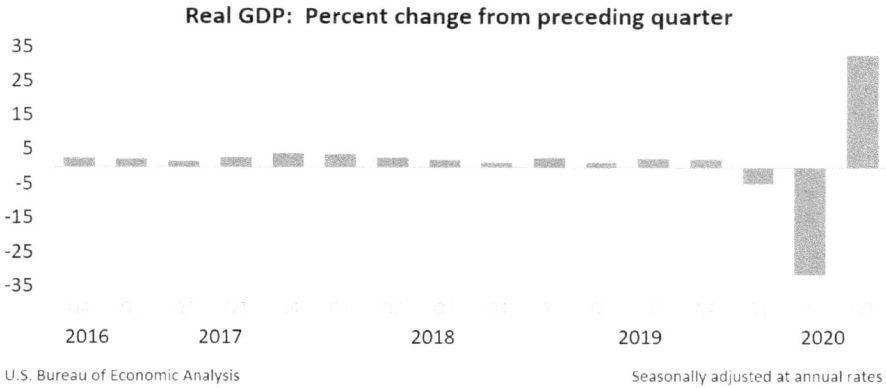

Figure 11 US quarterly GDP changes

As you can see in this chart, after steady rises since 2016, the GDP faltered in the first quarter, when the virus first started to make itself felt, then plunged a terrible 31.4% in the second quarter, before then rising a massive 33.1% in the third quarter, almost making up all the losses of the first two quarters.

_____

[125] See https://www.bea.gov/data/gdp/gross-domestic-product or https://cov.cx/a1f96

Employment numbers are not quite so positive, with a 6.5% seasonally adjusted unemployment rate at the end of November.[126]

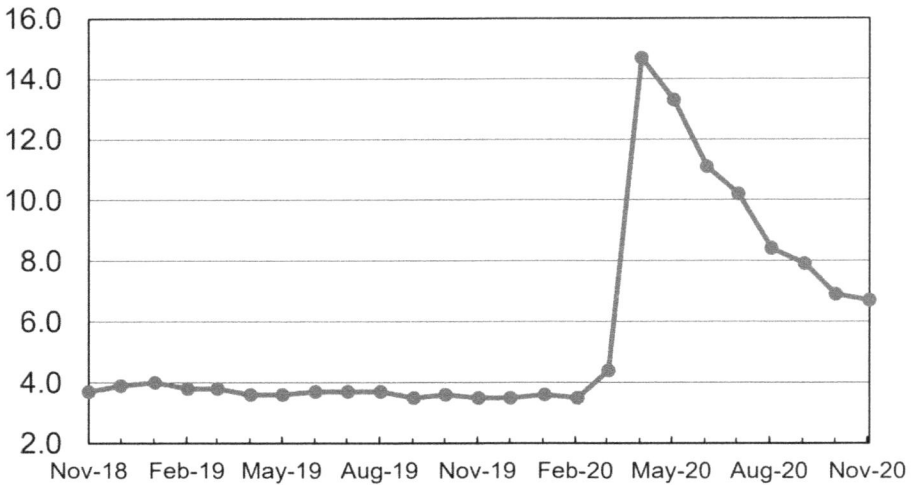

Figure 12 Monthly seasonally adjusted unemployment

But even this could be very much worse than it is. Although we see harm to our economy every which way, these three very direct measures – the stock market, GDP, and unemployment – all show much less harm than might have been guessed.

Does that mean we dodged a bullet, or does it mean the "silent economy" is hurting more than the obvious economy, or does it mean that the economy has some inertia that has kept it going, although if that inertia gets used up, might the economy now be more vulnerable to additional shocks and with the new "wave" of virus cases as we approach winter?

We don't know, and as we said at the start of this chapter, the problem with assessing the wisdom of our strategies to date is we can't know for sure what happened as a result of them.

After I wrote this section and came back to edit it, I realized there was a huge assumption that needed to be examined at the very start, and due to this being an assumption rather than clearly stated and agreed to, is perhaps where and how the disagreement or misunderstanding first occurred.

---

[126] See https://www.bls.gov/news.release/pdf/empsit.pdf or https://cov.cx/a1a63

What Were and Are Our Goals?

What exactly was (and still is) the reason for the various restrictions we've imposed on ourselves? What are our goals (and time frame for achieving them)?

Was it to eliminate the virus entirely and get the country back to normal? Was it to reduce the virus spread to a "safe" level (and if so, what exactly is the "safe" level)?

Was it to "flatten the curve"? This was the concept that if we allowed the rate of new infections to grow without limit, the hospital system would quickly become overloaded and would crash, with a much higher rate of deaths due to lack of care.

The problem with the concept of flattening the curve is that many of the visual representations were misleading, such as, for example, this example :[127]

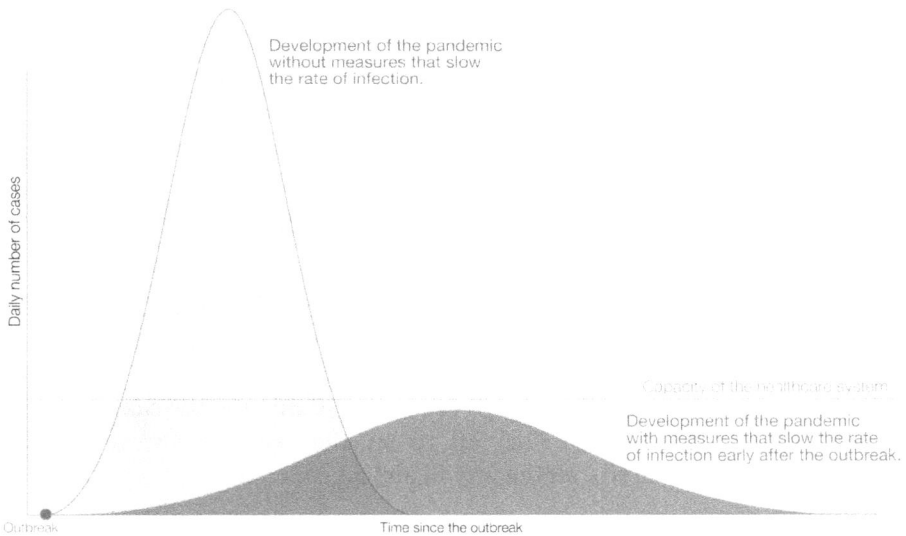

Figure 13 A false depiction of flattening the curve

---

[127] I'm not linking to its source because I don't want to unfairly cite one of the hundreds of examples of this.

The falsity in this chart is that the area under the purple curve (representing total cases) is very much smaller than the area under the yellow curve. In theory, the curve flattening should still show equal areas.[128]

When presented with a chart like the one above, of course there was enthusiasm for flattening the curve. But when one sees a more realistic drawing of what it means to flatten the curve, the appeal is much less strong :[129]

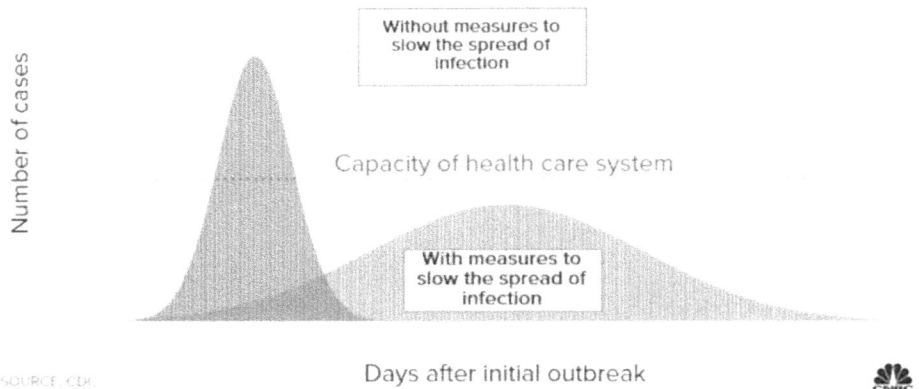

Figure 14 A fairer flattened curve

As you can now more clearly see, the flattened curve probably now has just as much area underneath it as the tall one, and it isn't quite such an appealing concept.

However, the thing about any type of curve flattening is the same – look at the right side of the curves. They all go up, then reverse direction and go smoothly and steadily down, all the way to almost zero.

---

[128] It is also true that there were sensible hopes that as a positive outcome of flattening the curve and buying us time, new treatments would be developed, a vaccine created, and so on. But the simple equivalency of these simple charts remains misleading.

[129] Taken from this generally very sensible article https://www.drjohnm.org/2020/05/can-we-discuss-flatten-the-curve-in-covid19-my-eight-assertions/ or https://cov.cx/a1a64

But look at the curve of US new daily cases as of 17 December 2020 :[130]

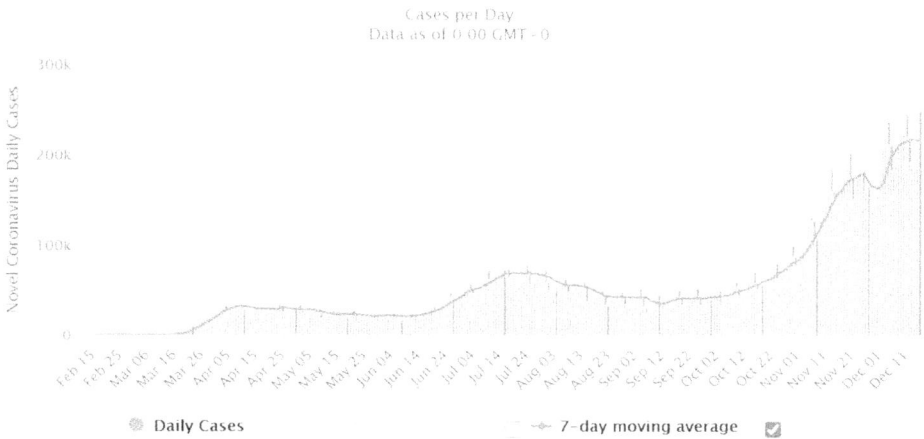

Figure 15 US Daily new Covid cases

Our curve might have flattened, way back in April. But it never massively dropped. It dropped a bit, then went up again, then down, and now up again. Worse, we're being told to expect continued rises in cases again as we go into winter.[131] As you see above, the new case rates now are very much higher than when President Trump first declared an emergency on March 13 – the rate of new cases on March 13 was so low it barely even appears on the above chart.

That, to me, is the biggest frustration. Although never clearly expressed, there has always been some vague sort of promise that shortly after flattening the curve, we would in some ill-defined way "beat the virus" and things would then return to normal. We've been promised many different dates for when normalcy might have returned, and while most states have pretended that normalcy is back and relaxed their social distancing requirements, the reality is things have become very much worse, not better, over the months since the 13 March emergency declaration.

During the initial emergency period, we were being told it would take two weeks to flatten the curve, and one week into those two weeks, Dr Fauci was saying that the two weeks would have to lengthen to "at least going to be several

[130] See https://www.worldometers.info/coronavirus/country/us/ or https://cov.cx/w-us

[131] See, for example, https://covid19.healthdata.org/united-states-of-america?view=infections-testing&tab=trend&test=infections or https://cov.cx/a1a65

weeks".[132] Those earlier hopes and promises now all seem impossibly naive and unreal when we look at the actual numbers that have followed in the eight months subsequently.

But, to look at the positive, we did flatten the curve after a fashion. At the beginning of April, new case numbers stopped shooting up, and didn't start again until mid-June, by which time we had better-prepared hospitals and infrastructure. This is just as well because the new rise starting in October threatens to test every element of our healthcare infrastructure if we don't get it quickly restrained.

Maybe our goal – albeit unstated – was to buy us time to find a cure or vaccine? We've indeed improved at treating the disease, and it seems that during the last six months, researchers have been using the time productively and getting us much closer to a vaccine, and in mid-November there are a handful of vaccine candidates moving toward the end of accelerated Phase 3 trials and expecting to be requesting FDA approval in the foreseeable future.

But, if the objective was merely to buy us time, let's also consider the cost of that purchase. As of mid-December, the US has suffered 295,000 deaths, and many of the 15.5+ million people in total who have had infections have ongoing debilitating conditions.

Shouldn't our goal have been not just to flatten the curve, but to do so as quickly as possible, and to get numbers to reduce as quickly as possible *and then to stay low subsequently*? That isn't an impossible goal, and the US is far from the only failure in that respect.

It is important to appreciate how things change over time.

Look for example at our neighbor to the north (Canada), which in mid-September had a proud chart to boast of :[133]

---

[132] See https://www.nbcnews.com/politics/donald-trump/fauci-predicts-americans-will-likely-need-stay-home-least-several-n1164701 or https://cov.cx/a1f90

[133] See https://www.worldometers.info/coronavirus/country/canada/ or https://cov.cx/w-ca

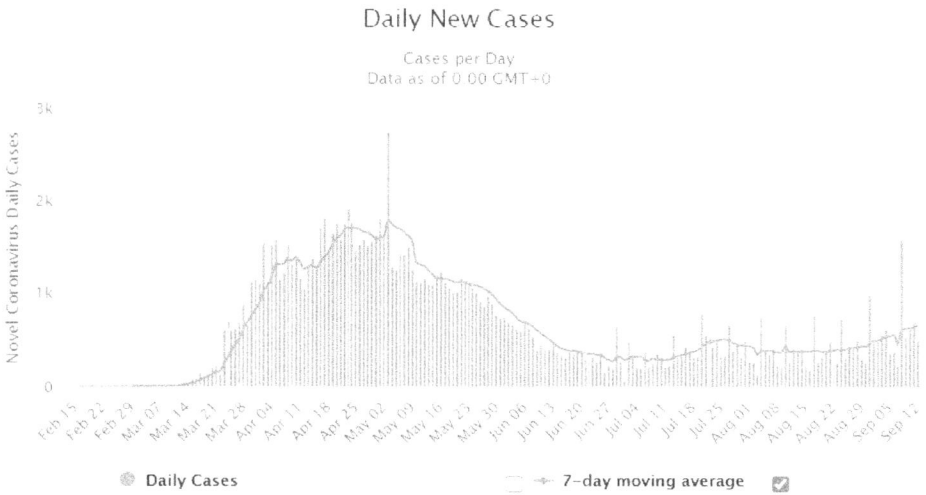

Figure 16 Daily new cases in Canada through mid-Sept

Canada had the same rise into April, but then instead of plateauing then rising again, they reduced numbers down back to March levels.

But you always need to beware of when a time series starts and stops. Let's make that chart more up to date and show it through mid-December.

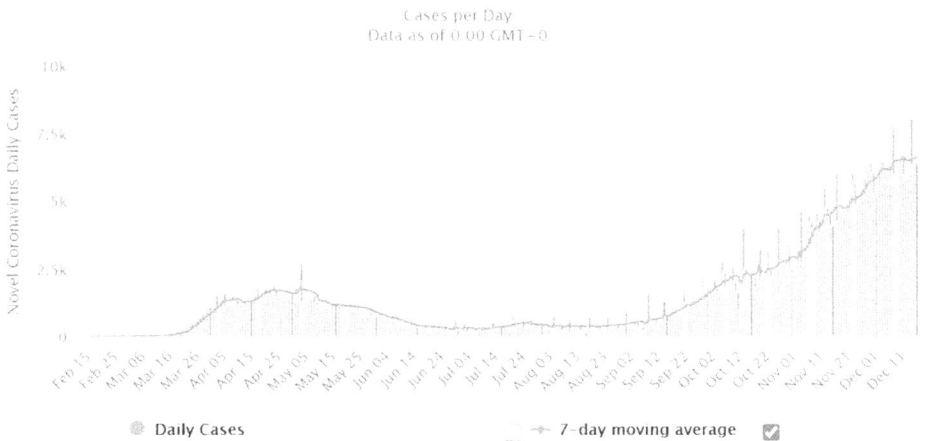

Figure 17 Daily new cases in Canada through 17 December 2020

Not quite such a success now. Many other countries are experiencing similar climbs in virus numbers again.[134]

Comparing the US with Other Countries

People who say we should have had (and still should have) more controls point to the 17.6 million virus cases and 317,000 deaths we have suffered, and observe that internationally, we have the third-highest rate of virus cases per head of population among major countries and the sixth-highest rate of deaths (as of mid-December).[135]

Ranking	Cases		Deaths	
	Country	Per Million	Country	Per Million
1	Czech Rep	51,963	Belgium	1,508
2	Belgium	51,204	Peru	1,097
3	USA	47,238	Italy	1,022

---

[134] And, in almost all cases, for the same reason. After implementing controls to limit the spread of the virus, these countries then relaxed their controls, with the entirely predictable outcome that the virus numbers started to grow again.

Strangely, the controls that such countries had in place back in March and April, and which obviously worked back then, have seldom been brought back again – are we becoming hardened to the impact of the virus?

[135] I've arbitrarily decided that these stats should not include minor countries. Tiny countries with less than a few million people can have a single outbreak of a few dozen cases and shoot up the tables due to something that might be a one-off "anomaly". That is easily explained. The more subjective part is at what size does a country become "major". For no particular reason, I chose the number 10 million.

But if I'd chosen 5 million instead, the US ranking would stay unchanged for both cases and deaths. The largest of the small countries with more cases is Luxembourg, with a mere 631,000 people. The largest of the small countries with more deaths is Bosnia and Herzegovina, with 3.3 million people.

The data for these two tables is taken from https://www.worldometers.info/coronavirus/ or https://cov.cx/w-c

4	Spain	36,898	Spain	1,005
5	France	35,349	UK	920
6	Netherlands	33,639	USA	888
7	Portugal	32,607	Argentina	882
8	Argentina	32,393	France	862
9	Brazil	31,341	Mexico	856
10	Sweden	30,097	Czech Rep	852
World Average		8,848		202

Figure 18 US ranked with other major countries (8 Dec 2020 data)

There is no denying the appalling nature of those numbers, and no denying that the US is among the worst-performing countries.

If we were to rank the US against even the smallest of countries, it could be said that it is fair to look not at the aggregate rating for the entire US, but to match our individual states against smaller countries.

Ranking	Cases		Deaths	
	Country or State	Per Million	Country or State	Per Million
1	North Dakota	110,133	New Jersey	1,977
2	South Dakota	98,386	New York	1,810
3	Andorra	92,629	Massachusetts	1,607
4	Iowa	78,851	Belgium	1,508

5	Nebraska	73,719	Connecticut	1,470
6	Wisconsin	71,868	San Marino	1,443
7	Utah	68,613	Louisiana	1,438
8	Montana	65,620	Rhode Island	1,401
9	Wyoming	64,751	North Dakota	1,396
10	Minnesota	64,493	Mississippi	1,358
World Average		*8848*		*202*

Figure 19 US states ranked with all countries (8 Dec 2020 data)

If it weren't for the micro-state of Andorra (with a population of only 77,319), US states would have all ten positions on the top case rate list, and if it weren't for even smaller San Marino (pop 33,962) our states would have nine of the ten positions on the top death rate list.

So, however we measure it, the US numbers are extremely bad. But the reason(s) for our poor results are not as simple as they might seem.

Some strange factors are influencing these numbers that no-one understands. Some countries where you'd expect very high rates of infection – densely populated countries with poor healthcare systems, such as much of Africa and Asia/Middle East – would seem to be prime breeding grounds for the virus. But no major country in Asia/Middle East even has half the cases per million that the US does (the most severely affected country is Iraq with a rate of 9,942 cases per million) and the same is true for deaths as well – Iran's death count, while the highest in Asia at 339 per million, is still only about half that of the US.

Those numbers seem very mild in comparison to the US, and the very worst-affected countries. Look at some of the least affected countries – Vietnam with a case rate of 14 per million, and a death rate of 0.4/million. Taiwan has 30 and 0.3 for its numbers. Thailand has 59 and 0.9. How is this possible?

Africa is similarly puzzling. South Africa is the worst-affected African nation (13,782 cases and 376 deaths per million) but it is a puzzling outlier. Lesotho, totally contained within the South African borders, has rates of 1000 and 20. Namibia, Zimbabwe, and Mozambique share South Africa's northern border, and their rates are 5,974/60, 730/20, and 518/4.[136] What is the mystery factor that kicks in on South Africa's border?[137]

There is some mystery factor (maybe several) that is making the spread of the virus very uneven. So while some part of the poor outcome in the US may be due to bad controls, some part may also be due to these mystery factors. [138]

If we match the US to Canada and Mexico, we see

---

[136] All these numbers are as of 8 December.

[137] A physician wondered if this might be due to higher rates of mask-wearing in Asia and less travel in Africa. We're not sure about either of those explanations. Many of the highly infected European countries report reasonably high compliance rates for mask-wearing. This site gives some data on mask-wearing by country, for example, this page on Belgium (the worst country for deaths and second-worst for cases) : https://covid19.healthdata.org/belgium?view=infections-testing&tab=trend&test=infections or https://cov.cx/a1f97 . Belgium has a higher mask-wearing rate than Vietnam (among the very best countries) – see https://covid19.healthdata.org/viet-nam?view=mask-use&tab=trend or https://cov.cx/a1f98 .

As for Africa and travel, it only takes one person and one case to "seed" a new viral outbreak, and most African countries have cross-border travel, local travel, and at least until March/April, international flights too. Plus, a hallmark of many African countries is dense urban centers – what one would assume to be rich breeding grounds for respiratory viral infections. A third of low scoring Mozambique residents live in urban areas, and even if we ignore all the rural inhabitants and therefore triple Mozambique's infection rates, at 1,554/12 they are still stunningly low and less than 1/30th of the US numbers.

[138] There is a theory that is becoming increasingly possible that one of the mystery factors might be the varying policy, country by country, to vaccinating people with the BCG anti-tuberculosis vaccine. Some correlations suggest the BCG shot also gives some level of protection against Covid-19 as well. But even if this is indeed a factor, there are probably other factors, too.

Another possible factor may be hydroxychloroquine use. A rather confusing website, https://hcqtrial.com or https://cov.cx/a1a66 contrasts mortality rates in countries where HCQ use is widespread or little used and suggests the clear difference might be due to HCQ use.

Still another factor that is now being given more credence is ivermectin and its potential value as a prophylactic/protective medicine. Ivermectin is often broadly prescribed as protection against various water parasites, particularly in Africa – countries with some of the very lowest virus rates.

Country	Cases/million	Deaths/million
Canada	11,324	340
USA	47,238	888
Mexico	9,128	850

Figure 20 US stats compared to Canada and Mexico (8 Dec data)

It is an oversimplification, but perhaps acceptable to say that the US and Canada are somewhat similar nations in many respects. How is it that Canada has less than ¼ the number of cases, and less than half the deaths per million people? Is it just because the Canadians are better at social distancing and mask-wearing?

Our conclusion, from all the above numbers, and even after allowing for "X factors" is that the US has been significantly more affected than most other nations by the virus.[139] So, from that point of view, perhaps we should have had firmer controls (yes, I hear you if you're shouting "No!" at me right now – we'll come to your point of view soon enough).

How Accurate Are the Numbers?

This is a question that, on the face of it, wouldn't even seem to need to be asked.

We can measure our virus experience in several different ways of course. How many people have been infected with the virus and how many people have died are the two obvious major factors, and perhaps the easiest to establish. Beyond that, many other measures could be used as well, if the data was easily obtained – the cost of providing healthcare, the number of days off work, the number of

---

[139] One more issue needs to be kept in mind. It is dangerous to draw too many conclusions from these types of statistics currently, because the virus is still active in all countries. Countries are going up and down the "most affected" lists daily, and some of the initially worst countries are now way down the list, while some of the countries now at the top were nowhere prominent at all a month or two ago.

In the case of the US, it fairly quickly rose to near the top of both the case rate and death rate lists, and has stayed near the top consistently, but maybe in the future, more countries will pass it and push it down the list.

years of otherwise expected healthy lives that had been lost per person who died, and so on into many different measurements.

We touch on these issues throughout this book, and the sad situation is that we don't accurately know how many people have been infected by the virus, nor do we know how many people have died.

The imprecision on counting deaths seems especially strange. A person is either alive or dead, right? It is very hard to mistake one of those two states for the other! That is true, but the problem comes in determining what caused a person to die. We discuss this in the section "Your Risk of Dying" on page 148, below.

What about the imprecision to do with counting how many people have the virus – surely that becomes easier to do than attributing causes of death? Well, yes, in some cases, this is very easy. A person goes to the doctor saying they feel unwell. They display the classic symptoms of the coronavirus, they are given a test for the virus, and the test comes back positive. Count them in the list of people infected with the virus, right?

Yes, that seems straightforward and simple. But how about a person who has no symptoms of the virus and feels perfectly fine, and is given a random test for the virus which comes up positive. The virus tests can be a bit unreliable (see our section on Testing, below on page 179, and how the count of false positives can greatly exceed the count of true positives, even with testing that is 99%+ accurate). If a person has no symptoms and doesn't feel unwell, should they be counted as having the virus?

The official answer, to date, has been that yes, they are considered to have the virus. You could argue the sense of that – like the classic question "if a tree falls in a forest and no-one hears it fall, does it make any noise", there's a fair question to be asked – if a person has no symptoms and doesn't feel unwell, and it is only because of an unreliable test that we think they might have the virus, should we count that as a case or not?[140]

How many cases that we're counting at present are of "truly sick" people and how many are of "asymptomatic" people? The CDC currently says 40% of all counted cases are of asymptomatic people.

---

[140] Even this question is more complex than it might seem. It appears that it is not uncommon for some virus-caused illnesses to be asymptomatic. Perhaps the best known of these would be HSV-2. So maybe it is correct to fairly count asymptomatic cases, but we would like asymptomatic cases to at least be double-tested to validate the diagnosis.

They also say that 75% of asymptomatic people can still infect other people. So from the perspective of helping the virus spread, asymptomatic people need to be considered in some form.

But if you wanted to say "if you don't feel sick, you don't count as an impactful virus sufferer because you don't require any medicine or healthcare support, you don't take time off work, and you have no risk of dying" then you could reduce the official count of virus cases by almost 50%.

On the other hand (and it seems there's often "another hand" that needs to be considered), if we only know about asymptomatic cases from random testing, and if we're only testing a very small percentage of the population, does that mean that maybe there are many other asymptomatic cases that we don't know about, in addition to those we do know about? Yes, that seems like a reasonable assumption.

So we have a death rate that may be too high (or possibly slightly low) and a case count that might be twice as high as can be justified by some approaches, or twice as low, due to not testing everyone. Ugh!

Some people have stronger opinions still and claim that most/all of the numbers about this virus are a lie. We don't understand their reasoning, particularly when it is placed alongside credible reports of hospitals – and morgues – full to overflowing with Covid patients, all around the world. If this is all a lie, it has been orchestrated on an extraordinarily massive scale, internationally. But otherwise sensible and sincere people, including many doctors, maintain this to be the case – see the video referenced in this footnote, below.[141] We were particularly surprised to see several doctors from Belgium, which in mid-December leads the entire world with the worst death rate, making these claims straight to the camera. We don't understand such claims but feel it necessary to at least acknowledge their presence.

The Need for Clever and Consistent Controls

There is another way we can rate our response. Never mind if it has been successful or not, has it been well planned?

There are two key elements – which sadly have both been largely missing – in any effective response to the virus outbreak.

---

[141] It is available on this Facebook page, assuming it hasn't been taken down. https://www.facebook.com/fiona.hine.7/videos/10164697404790441 or https://cov.cx/a1f94 . I urge you also to read the fact-checking rebuttal to the claims being made and to view all the claims being made in the video through the lens of the claims which are clearly wrong.

The **first** is to be "clever" - to have appropriate and targeted controls, rather than blanket controls for everyone and everything, no matter what the relative risks are. The adage of working smarter, not harder, applies in this context the same as it does in most other contexts.

The **second** is to have a simple consistent set of controls that are easily understood and equally adopted across the entire country.

These two requirements might seem to be contradictory. But they are both important and can co-exist. For example, the targeted controls don't necessarily mean "regionally targeted" – they can mean "type of business or activity targeted" as well.

The requirement for appropriate and targeted controls has been totally overlooked, being replaced by blanket impositions. And when states, counties, and cities did try and make exceptions, the exceptions were for strange reasons that seemed to relate more to the political power of various groups than for any epidemiological reason. This was obvious when states started closing down and allowing exceptions for some types of business but not others (and equally obvious with the curious sequence of removing controls too).

It doesn't encourage public confidence and cooperation when there are seemingly inconsistent policies and strange loopholes in what can and can't be done.[142] Compliance is best done with comprehension and cooperation rather than mandated by rules and penalties.

The bewildering range of different controls in every state – and often varying by county and even city too[143] – and made worse by adjustments and loosening

---

[142] See, for example, https://www.inc.com/gabrielle-bienasz-mariyam-khaja/covid-rules-regulations.html or https://cov.cx/a1a67 and https://www.bloomberg.com/opinion/articles/2020-04-16/coronavirus-protests-dumb-lockdown-rules-erode-public-trust or https://cov.cx/a1a68 - can we particularly point to how in MI you can buy drywall at Home Depot, but not paint (at the same Home Depot). Why is it safe to buy drywall but not paint?

There's something very wrong with our public health officials and leadership when they create beyond-stupid policies like that. How can we trust or respect anything they say when they tell us "drywall good; paint bad"?

[143] A great example of problems with such rules is in my own state of Washington. My county announced it would close all its public parks – lovely sprawling open outdoor spaces with few people and lots of space between them – an unnecessary and unfortunate decision. Of all the things to leave open, surely low-density open-air parks would feature highly. Happily – but confusingly – the city I live in said it would keep its parks open. So now we have parks, sometimes within a mile or two of each other, that are variously open or shut. I'd never even known, in my 35 years in WA, which were county or local parks. But now I need to.

or tightening of restrictions - is that even the most conscientious of us don't accurately understand what we can and can't do, and how those restrictions vary as we travel within our local area.

Do you know what restrictions apply to you? For example, do you have to wear masks outdoors? Indoors? Can you meet in groups with other people? If so, of what size? Are there different restrictions for meeting with other people indoors or outdoors? Are there time limits? Are there different restrictions for different activities? Do you have to socially distance? If so, are there exceptions? Are restaurants allowed to open with all their previous capacity? Half? A quarter?

What "level" of restrictions is your state/county/city in currently? What is required to move it up or down a level? For that matter, do you even know how well your local area is doing compared to other areas in your state, and how well your state is doing compared to other states?

We could continue with this "Covid Quiz" but you get the point already, I'm sure. No-one really knows what is being done or why or what will happen next.

As for even and consistent adoption and enforcement, some sheriffs are refusing to enforce their county or state laws – an alarming constitutional situation which few have commented on sufficiently.[144] There is even one sheriff who refuses to allow his deputies and other staff to wear masks.[145] That must put his deputies in an awkward position – how can they arrest a person for not wearing a mask when they aren't wearing a mask themselves? Should they be arresting each other?

There's another problem as well. The virus attacks us through our weakest links. So if a person goes to another jurisdiction where there is little or no restriction on "normal" activities, they might become infected with the virus, and

---

[144] See https://www.tmj4.com/news/coronavirus/these-wisconsin-sheriffs-say-they-wont-enforce-gov-tony-evers-statewide-mask-order or https://cov.cx/a1a69 (and many more examples in many other states too). There have been other cases of sheriffs and their departments "looking the other way" in other situations, of course, and even of publicly and totally refusing to enforce laws (for example, some firearms laws). I'm reminded of what the police officer tells me when handing me a speeding ticket – "We don't make the laws, we just enforce them, if you want to contest this citation, take it up with the judge and your elected representatives".
It makes me wonder if the opposite can apply too – if sheriffs are free to choose which laws they enforce, are they therefore also free to invent new laws, too? Isn't that the same sort of thing? Is "frontier justice" still appropriate in the 21st century?

[145] See https://www.npr.org/sections/coronavirus-live-updates/2020/08/12/901756223/florida-sheriff-orders-deputies-and-staff-not-to-wear-face-masks or https://cov.cx/a1a70

then when they return home, they bring the virus back with them and potentially infect people in their home area.

We know how the Tenth Amendment to the US Constitution[146] gives the states sweeping autonomy in many things, but this makes it very difficult to create a consistent national policy. We know there have been exceptions granted to this requirement in the past, and the first section of the Fourteenth Amendment[147] and the Commerce Clause of the Constitution[148] have between them given "cover" to activist judges to annul individual state rights pretty much whenever they choose.

We also know that some states have taken very different views on how to respond to the virus than other states – ND and SD in particular have never required masks to be worn.[149]

This is an issue that calls out desperately for a more consistent approach.[150] [151]

---

[146] The powers not delegated to the United States by the Constitution, nor prohibited by it to the States, are reserved to the States respectively, or to the people.

[147] The "equal protection" part at the end of Section 1, which in its entirety reads :

All persons born or naturalized in the United States and subject to the jurisdiction thereof, are citizens of the United States and of the State wherein they reside. No State shall make or enforce any law which shall abridge the privileges or immunities of citizens of the United States; nor shall any State deprive any person of life, liberty, or property, without due process of law; nor deny to any person within its jurisdiction the equal protection of the laws.

[148] Article 1, Section 8, Clause 3 :

The Congress shall have power to regulate Commerce with foreign Nations, and among the several States, and with the Indian Tribes

[149] Partially as a result of that, partially because of allowing the Sturgis motorbike rally to proceed, and perhaps partially "just because", ND and SD are now the two states with the highest infection rates – 71,261 and 62,625 cases per million respectively. The national average is 31,078 cases per million.

[150] For what it is worth, there are problems in other countries comprising multiple semi-independent regions. Britain has to accept different policies in Scotland, England, Wales, and Northern Ireland. Canada's provinces have responded differently and with enormously different rates of success.

[151] The federal government, with the support of the courts, has succeeded in eroding many of the state privileges under the guise of interstate commerce, or by linking

(continued on next page)

What Worked and Didn't Work

So, what – if anything – has helped us reduce our cases? Perhaps this heading should also be "what we used and didn't use".

We haven't done well on testing. President Trump likes to say we've done more testing than any other country in the world, and that's sort of right, but it is also sort of wrong.

It is sort of right because, by simply counting the tests administered, it seems the US has administered almost 158 million tests (as of 7 November). Only one country is claiming more tests – China, with 160 million tests.[152]

But the most relevant measure of everything, including testing, is not absolute numbers. It is numbers per so many people.[153] When we switch to that measure, the US drops from second place to **20th place**. That is the most meaningful measure, and that is the one President Trump should be using.

We have administered 475,000 tests for every million people so far.

It is very important to realize that there is a lot of difference between saying "we have administered the equivalent of 475,000 tests for every million people" and "we have tested 475,000 out of every million people".

We have actually tested very many less than 475,000 people per million because many people get two or three or more tests. If you get a positive test, you probably get another test to confirm the positive test, then another two tests to confirm you are free of the disease too. Some people are being tested every day or two.

This is shown in the numbers for the countries with the highest numbers of tests per million. In the tiny Faeroe Islands, there have been 3.2 million tests per million people – what looks to be every person being tested three times. Nine other countries also have more tests than population (Gibraltar, Andorra, Luxembourg, Bermuda, UAE, Monaco, Iceland, Bahrain, and Denmark).

"voluntary" compliance with federal requirements to eligibility for federal funding. Why has the federal govt been able to do this for all manner of things but shown no interest or willingness to do the same now for virus response measures?

[152] Like many statistics to do with China, this is a strange number, in the sense that it has not changed in the last ten weeks. Is China no longer testing anyone? We're sure they are.

[153] Some places use numbers per million, some use numbers per hundred thousand, or per some other quantity. It doesn't particularly matter what the "per quantity" is, as long as it is consistently used, and of course, it is easy to convert as between per million and (eg) per hundred thousand (just divide or multiply by 10).

Just because you don't have the virus today doesn't mean you mightn't catch it tomorrow. A test is only a snapshot at that instant in time, and quickly becomes an irrelevant bit of history, rather than a lasting guarantee of future safety. So testing people multiple times makes sense.

If we'd done more testing – and (something that doesn't appear in that simple test count statistic) – if we'd got test results back sooner, we'd have found more infected people sooner and (in theory) been able to ask them to isolate before they infected other people. That would have greatly reduced our case numbers.

The other part of testing is the tracing of people that an infected person has possibly passed the infection on to. That's a very "painless" procedure, and almost completely non-disruptive. It doesn't really impact on most of us, most of the time at all, and doesn't require us to socially distance, stop working, or anything else.[154] That makes it is a very desirable activity, and we have scored extremely poorly in that respect. I know people who have "officially" had the virus and haven't had any contact with any contact tracing people at all.

As for the other elements of what has worked and not worked, it becomes fairly hypothetical to know which things made the biggest difference. But it is fair to say that most of the outdoor social distancing rules were of very little value, and outdoor mask-wearing even less valuable again. And while the authorities have been slow to walk this particular claim back, it now seems the initial eager exhortations to compulsively wash our hands all the time were not necessary, either.[155] We discuss this further in our chapter "10. How to Avoid Infection – In General" starting on page 214.

On the other hand, most of the indoor social distancing rules and mask-wearing requirements are probably important and beneficial, and deserve greater emphasis.

Do We Know if Anything Worked?

Some people believe that every part of our virus response was unnecessary, or if not unnecessary, too extreme and well into the realm of vanishing returns.

---

[154] Don't misunderstand, please! We still need to do those things, but in terms of getting better control of the virus, tracing is something we can do that is easier than tightening up on mask-wearing and social distancing.

[155] Almost no-one is thought to have caught the disease after touching an infected surface and then transferring some virus particles to the mouth, nose, or eyes. This was "health theater" (a bit like many of the meaningless "security theater" controls at airports these days) and perhaps intended to "give us something to do" and make us feel more in control of things.

They say we should never have closed anything, and that mask-wearing is unnecessary.

More nuanced versions of those broad statements suggest we should have only limited restrictions to the most at-risk sectors of our community, and be more selective at the restrictions we've placed on businesses.

We certainly agree that our "one size fits all" approach has been poorly designed, and the contradictions and loopholes in terms of what types of business can be open or must close, and the different degrees of limits between states (and even between cities or counties within a state) have not only been confusing but have weakened the credibility of the underlying claims that such restrictions are necessary.

Younger people are indeed at very low levels of risk of dying from a Covid infection. But they're at equal (or at least very similar) risk of contracting a Covid infection, and they then pose an equal (or similar) risk of passing infections on to other people who might be at higher risk. It is not possible to segregate high-risk and low-risk people and keep each group away from the other.

We also agree that there has to be a balance between the benefit of protecting people from the virus and the cost/harm of the protection. Where does one set the compromise point?

We're not going to argue these issues in this book. We acknowledge the existence of these issues and opinions, and in general terms relating to how entire states and countries have developed their public health responses, some of these points are credible and relevant. But the main focus of this book is on you and what you should do, more than what the country as a whole should be doing. However, there is of course a link between what the country is doing and what we are doing, individually, and if it is wrong at a national level to impose some restrictions, it may be wrong at a personal level too.

Can we prove – to their satisfaction and ours – that any of what we've done has actually worked? I think we can.

Let's start by looking at this chart of US new cases – it is slightly different to the ones you are probably more familiar with)[156] :

---

[156] Taken from https://covid19.healthdata.org/united-states-of-america?view=infections-testing&tab=trend&test=infections or https://cov.cx/a1a65

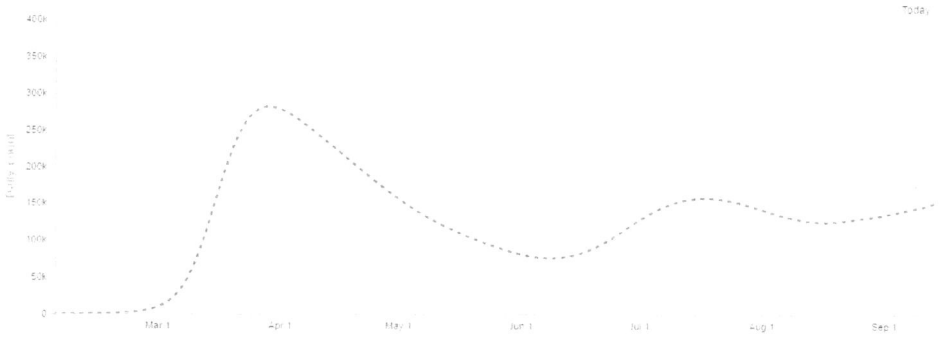

Figure 21 *Daily US new cases (adjusted)*

If you've been following the virus spread in the country, you will notice two interesting things about this chart compared to the common charts usually shown, such as this one[157] :

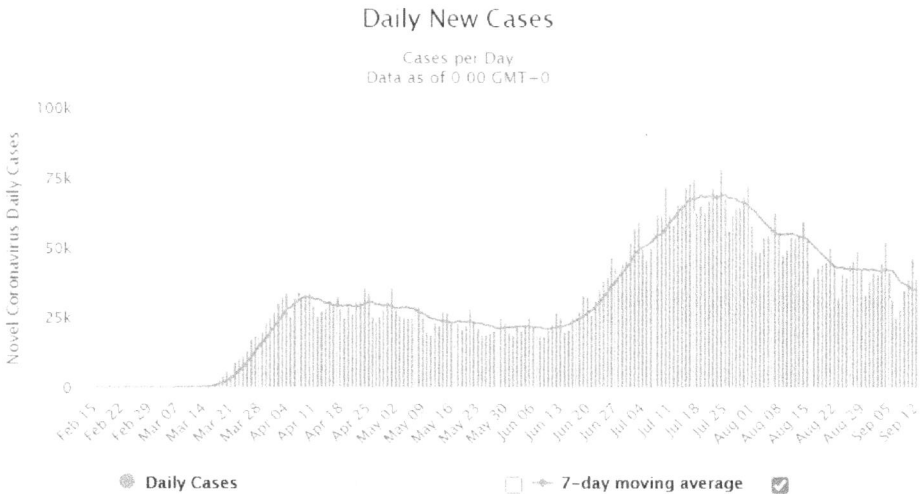

Figure 22 *Daily US new cases (raw)*

The two obvious differences are that in the first chart, the second bump is not as high as the first, and that in the first chart, the first bump goes up higher than 250,000 new cases a day.

---

[157] See https://www.worldometers.info/coronavirus/country/us/ or https://cov.cx/w-us

To explain, the second chart shows the number of **officially confirmed** new cases every day. The first chart shows the number of **estimated** cases and adjusts for factors such as the number of tests we do each day, with the assumption being that if we test more people, we find more asymptomatic cases.

The second chart doesn't make that adjustment, and with the expectation of "If you test more, you find more cases", it could be said that part of the reason for the second rise in cases is simply due to a rise in the number of daily tests conducted, as shown here :[158]

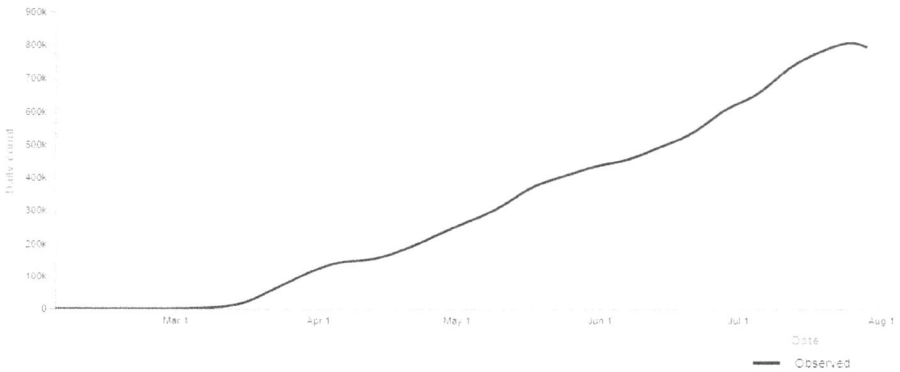

· *Figure 23 US Daily testing rate*

Both of the two "daily new case" charts have their value and use. The second chart with "raw" data tells us about the cases we know about, and by implication, these cases are more likely to be impactful on the healthcare system, and on people's lives.

The first – adjusted - chart is perhaps more interesting because it tries to guess what is happening "beneath the surface".

The adjusted chart in particular shows us several things that we can think about and try to match with how we've responded to the virus outbreak.

---

[158] See https://covid19.healthdata.org/united-states-of-america?view=infections-testing&tab=trend&test=tests or https://cov.cx/a1a65 – although we took this chart in mid-September, it strangely doesn't have data subsequent to late July.

First, you see the truly astonishing rise in daily cases until late March. Something happened at some time in mid-late March[159] to stop that rise, otherwise it would have continued to skyrocket into April.

Could it be because on 13 March President Trump declared a national emergency? Well, not entirely – his declaration was mainly about administrative issues and funding. But perhaps his actions encouraged the states to join in because from then through the end of the month, almost all the states issued various orders mandating some types of social distancing and closures of restaurants and bars and other activities.

We'll also mention we note the changes in case rates sometimes seem to precede the imposition and removal of restrictions. It is almost like there is some type of unconscious collective wisdom that senses either the need or absence of need for restrictions, causing us to adjust our behaviors without the official prompting.

So maybe those measures did indeed work and stopped the virus growth. Not only did they stop the virus growth, but they caused new case numbers to start shrinking every day, until about the beginning of June. Here's an example of what we mean[160] :

Figure 24 Rt rate for new cases in WA state

You can see how the rate of new cases was already declining before the shelter order being announced – indeed, almost immediately after the shelter order was

---

[159] Generally, virus symptoms appear four or five days after infection, and probably people get tested a day or two after that, so whatever you see in the chart more or less reflects changes in external factors 5 and more days previously.

[160] Taken from https://rt.live/us/WA or https://cov.cx/a1a71

announced, case rates stopped dropping every day and started increasing again!
The removal of the shelter order didn't result in an immediate runaway of new
cases again, and indeed, case rates dropped for a while again. The IHME site
shows data on mask use and an empirical measure for social distancing too, but
it is hard to match those up against the chart above.[161]

Moving on from the state closures in March, starting from about mid-May,
states started to re-open again and relax their social distancing controls. So we
see the rate of decline start to flatten out and then more sharply turn to a rise
again in June.

Beyond that, it is interesting to see a see-sawing effect. Things get bad, people
become more careful, things improve, people become more careless.

Alas, while it was easy to track when states first issued their shut-down orders,
and moderately easy to track when they started to relax them again, since that
point, it has become extremely difficult to track what is happening. Many states
seem to be deciding things on a separate county by county level, and some cities
have made their own decisions too, and there is a morass of "Stage 1/2/3/4" types
of restrictions and other variations of what is being allowed, but in general, and
as hinted by the chart above, things have been getting less and less restrictive.

It is hard to know how much of the increase and decrease in daily case rates
is actually due to regulations and how much is due to some sort of innate group-
sense of what is happening.

Here are three more charts that give interesting oblique measurements of
how we're responding to the virus :[162]

---

[161] See https://covid19.healthdata.org/united-states-of-
america/washington?view=mask-use&tab=trend or https://cov.cx/a1a72

[162] See https://covid19.healthdata.org/united-states-of-america?view=mask-
use&tab=trend or https://cov.cx/a1a73

Mask Use

Social Distancing

Daily New Case Rates

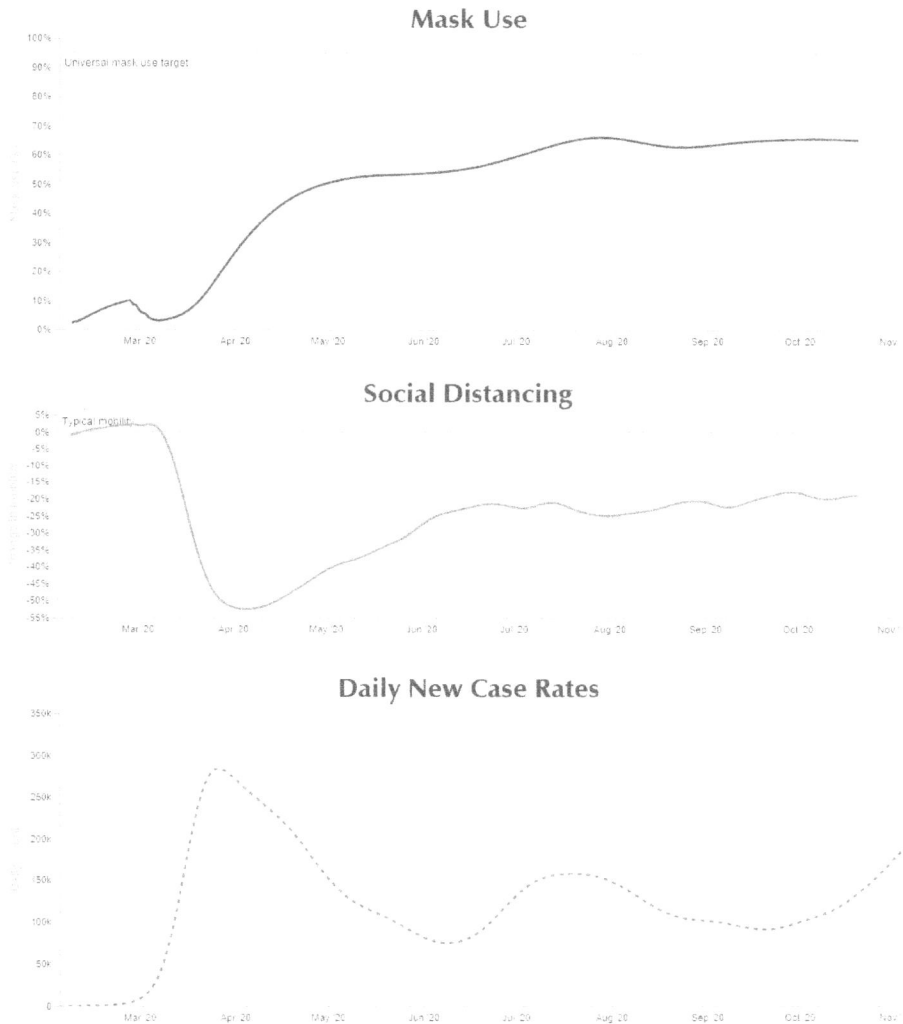

Figure 25 Mask use and social distancing in the US

Can you see any correlations between the two "behavioral" charts and the estimated infection chart at the bottom? There does seem to be some type of link between the very imperfect measuring of social distancing and new case rates, but it is hard to say anything specific.

Keep in mind that in the first chart – mask use – the higher the line goes, the more mask-wearing there is, and so the harder it is for the virus to spread. But it is the opposite in the second chart. The lower the line, the less contact we have with others, and the less we move around, and so, in that chart, the lower the line, the harder it is for the virus to spread.

It might be possible to weakly match up the first two charts to the third chart – for example, in mid-July, virus case numbers started to decline until mid-August, and we see that mask usage had been rising until the start of August then declined, and we also see that social distancing reduced in mid-July for a couple of weeks before rising again in August.

These measures are very inexact, and a case could also be made that it is necessary not to examine the US as an entirety, but to break it down state by state. As you know, some states had early peaks in virus cases then declined (like New York, for example) and other cases had later peaks (like Arizona). Here's a chart showing this, with New York and Arizona highlighted :[163]

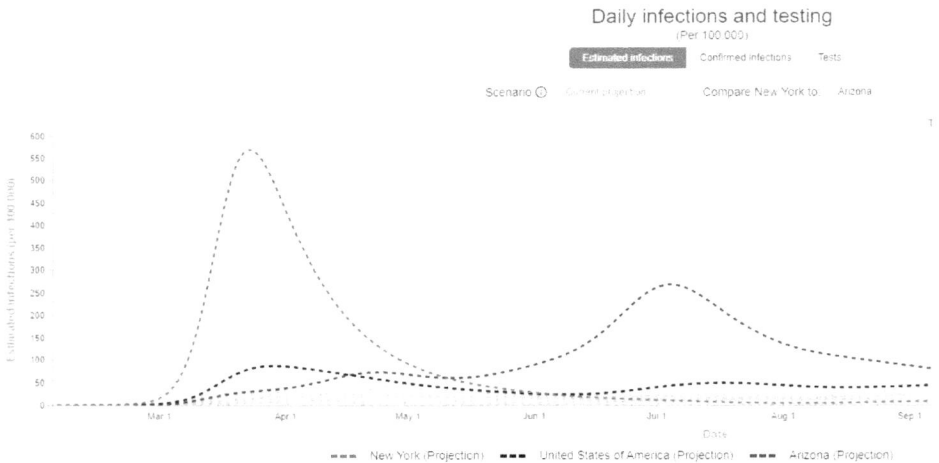

Figure 26 Comparing NY and AZ infection rates

You can probably vaguely see other gray lines on the chart as well – those are all the other states, and the black line is the resulting total for the entire US.

Some people would say we should drill down even further, to specific regions, and that is generally sensible (although it also makes things 50 times more complex for a book such as ours!). In the case of New York, you know there were extreme problems in the city of New York, but most of upstate New York was not

---

[163] See https://covid19.healthdata.org/united-states-of-america/new-york?view=infections-testing&tab=compare&test=infections or https://cov.cx/a1a74

nearly so strongly impacted by the virus back in the terrible days of late March and early April.

We're not going to do that, because this entire discussion is somewhat tangential to the main topic of the book,[164] although by understanding what has and has not worked in the past, we get strong pointers as to what we should do in the future.

At this point, I hope you'll agree that it seems there is a measurable impact on virus cases, depending on how we socially distance and wear masks. Hopefully, you'll also acknowledge that some forms of controls and social distancing are probably more beneficial than others.

To close off this section, let's look back at what people who disagree with the controls we've had in place say and put them in several contexts.

Usually, these people will also claim that the virus case numbers and death counts are greatly overstated. We discuss those claims in the preceding section "How Accurate Are the Numbers?", back on page 78, and elsewhere in the book too.

Yes, there are amazing imprecisions in terms of how we've been counting both cases and deaths, but we don't believe there has been any sort of orchestrated campaign or "conspiracy" to overstate the numbers. We put this more down to bungling, inefficiencies, and over-stressed systems failing. If it were to be a conspiracy, it would have to be worldwide, not just in the US, and that is unlikely. We also believe that there are significant scenarios where the numbers might be undercounted as well as overcounted, and perhaps the two – the overcounting and the undercounting – might more or less balance each other out.

If we accept the numbers as being kinda sorta close to reality, it is abundantly clear that the virus is extremely serious. In the space of nine months, it has become the third most common cause of death in the US – only heart disease and cancer are greater killers. Worse than that, it is becoming increasingly common, daily, for Covid deaths to be higher than either heart disease or cancer.[165]

---

[164] The purpose of the book is to help *you* decide what *you* should do. But we talk about these general issues so that you understand the broader concepts and can better than pick and choose what you do and how you do it, personally.

[165] Heart disease runs about 655,381 deaths a year or 1,796 a day. Cancer runs about 599,274 deaths a year or 1,642 a day. These numbers vary from year to year and from source to source, but are around these sorts of levels. We have now had some days with over 2,500 deaths in a single day from Covid – almost 50% higher than either of these two other causes, and the seven-day moving average has been higher than the heart disease 1,796 number consistently since 3 December through 8 December.

The key point, which naysayers[166] overlook, is that whether these numbers are true or not, what we don't know is *how much worse the numbers would have been* without the controls in place. That is the big and unavoidable gap in their argument. Even if their contention of the Covid statistics being inflated is correct, we don't know and can only guess at what would have happened if the controls had not been in place.

If you agree with me on those points, that is great, but it still leaves one other point unaddressed. Has it all been worth it? Let's see if we can answer that question, too.[167]

Comparing Costs and Benefits

This is the really big question, isn't it. We've sort of shown that in some way, to some extent, the sacrifices we've made have paid off in terms of fewer cases and fewer deaths. Maybe not as many as we hoped for, and probably with less effectiveness than in many other countries, but every saved life is a small achievement.

Can we say exactly how many fewer cases and deaths? As we said just a few paragraphs above, no, we can't. It is very hard to guess accurately at what would have happened if we'd acted differently. But let's have a try (and keep in mind these are guesses).

Here's a copy of the graph we saw earlier (Figure 21 Daily US new cases (adjusted).) :

---

[166] This word is not meant in any pejorative or offensive manner at all. A lot of good and sincere people, and a lot of well-credentialed people, sincerely believe the country has made grave mistakes with the controls that have been imposed on us.

[167] I don't expect you to believe me when I tell you this, but at this point, as I start to write this section, I really don't know what the answer will be. I truly have no preconceived notion. I'll simply look at the facts as best we can determine them and let the conclusions emerge as may become apparent. I hope you're similarly open-minded.

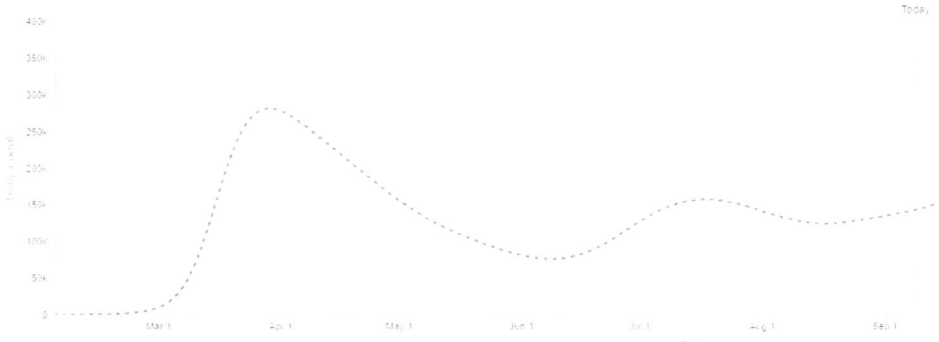

What would have happened if we did nothing in March? It seems almost certain that the daily new case count would have continued to rise. We'd be at half a million cases a day by early April, at a million cases a day by mid-April, and perhaps things would stabilize at about 5 million cases a day by the end of April – or maybe not, maybe they'll continue to double at least once more every week. [168] Basically, pick any numbers you like, and whatever scenario you choose, the disastrous nature of this increase is obvious. (See "4. How the Number of Infections Increased So Quickly" on page 50 for a refresher on exponential growth.)

With this uncontrolled scenario, even if things stabilized with "only" 5 million new cases a day, by the middle of May, we'd have about half the country infected, and so we'd be getting close to herd immunity (assuming it exists). That means, in theory, cases would start dropping off, and sometime in June, we'd be past the

---

[168] Someone will validly point out that surely, at some point, people would wise up and start reacting and responding to the virus without the need for a legislative mandate. As I observed a page or two back, this actually appears to be a phenomenon – maybe it truly is "the wisdom of crowds". The biggest influence of all on infection numbers, at least in the US, doesn't seem to be external government controls, but rather some sort of hard-to-measure group sense of concern and response.

Should we rely on the "wisdom of crowds", such as has largely been done in Sweden? I'll answer with a definite "maybe". To support my "maybe" I point to the Sturgis motorcycle rally, August 7-16, when 462,182 motorbikers all descended upon the small town of Sturgis SD for a week of partying, most of it with no social distancing. Where was the sense in that? Some studies are suggesting that one event has been responsible for over 260,000 new Covid cases, and a healthcare cost in excess of $12 billion. And ND & SD, in their entirety, with no mandated mask-wearing, have the highest infection rates in the entire country.

The other point is that the whole thought exercise we're talking about is "if no-one does anything". Social distancing is social distancing, whether it is voluntary or government-mandated.

herd immunity point – cases would continue, because people from other countries would bring new infections in, but new outbreaks would not be large and would die out on their own. Life would be – sort of – back to normal by the end of June.

However, let's think about what would have been happening in April and May. Remember the panic in March about ventilator shortages, ICU congestion, shortage of needed drugs and resources, and of course, the lack of masks and other PPE for health-care workers?

What would have happened if, instead of actual case numbers leveling out in April and then slowly declining (and the actual underlying case numbers steeply dropping), everything had continued to relentlessly double and double and double, every five or so days?

We'd run out of hospital beds, staff, ventilators, medications, and PPE. The healthcare system would collapse. It wouldn't just be Covid patients dying. People with most types of treatable illnesses needing hospitalization would be unable to get care and would die.

Think of the most terrible scenario you can think of, and then keep on thinking some more. Remember also the scare with toilet paper shortages? And the scare about meat shortages – even now in October, it seems the cost of meat is still more than 50% up on what it was in February.

Instead of shortages, there'd be outages. Instead of some workers absent in some meatpacking plants, we'd be talking most workers out of work in most meatpacking plants. Plus there'd be a shortage of truck drivers who transport the cattle to the plants, and who then take the processed beef to the supermarkets. And the same for every other category of food and consumable product, and every other part of the distribution industry.

If you think the Black Lives Matter rioting earlier this year has been bad, imagine how much worse it would be if the rioters were also starving and needing food, rather than just "wanting" flatscreen televisions.

You can choose to create your own projection as to what might have happened, but keep in mind what was happening, and what the future seemed to be threatening until we managed to stop the rise in cases in early April.

So, what did we achieve? Three things. **First**, we prevented the system from failing, all-over, everywhere. In doing so, we allowed our healthcare system to continue to work as best it can, and so, **second**, we kept the death rate as low as practical, and without much "collateral damage" from other neglected urgent-care cases.

Third, we bought ourselves some time. Time to ramp up hospital capacities and regrow inventories of supplies. Time to come up with better care plans for infected patients, and time to get closer to a vaccine. We can see a difference in death rates already – although be careful how you compare deaths and cases.

It might be better to compare adjusted cases to actual deaths rather than raw cases. Because we've been detecting more cases, the average degree of severity per case has been reducing, as much because we are finding more people who are only mildly sick, as because of new treatment regimes.

Here's a comparison of adjusted cases and actual deaths – I shifted the timeline to more closely match each day's deaths with the time the case was first registered :[169]

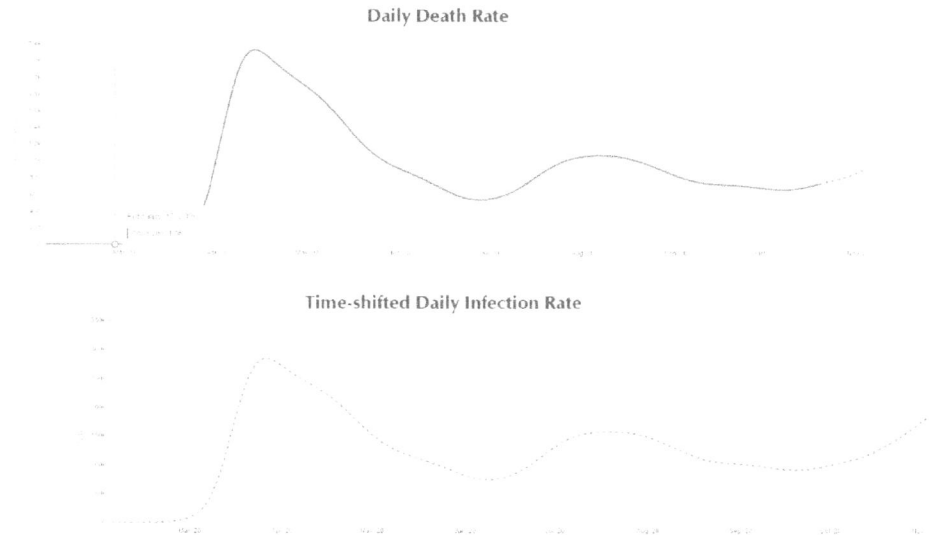

Daily Death Rate

Time-shifted Daily Infection Rate

Figure 27 US deaths (top) and new cases (bottom)

These numbers are reasonably closely linked, aren't they.

Conclusions, if Possible

So, where does that leave us? It is time to start trying to wrap all this up.

On the one hand, we're all getting a bit frustrated and "stir crazy". When can we do normal things, normally? When can we simply go to a restaurant, enjoy a cocktail or three, have a great meal, and enjoy some good company; and do all of

---

[169] Again, data from this site https://covid19.healthdata.org/united-states-of-america?view=infections-testing&tab=trend&test=infections or https://cov.cx/a1a65

that free of fear and consequence? When will the virus be less present in our lives than it has been over the last some months?

By these measures, we're no better off today than we were in March, and if we look at actual rates of cases, we're very much worse off – the virus is much more active now than it was then. But if we'd done nothing, things would be very much worse.

There are some improvements, even if somewhat obscured. We are better equipped to manage cases now than we were six months ago. We're six months closer to a vaccine. We continue to identify new possible drugs to treat cases, reducing their severity and increasing survival rates (even though none of these new possible drugs have yet been officially acknowledged or approved). And, most of all, for six months, our healthcare system has continued functioning at close to a normal level of service, for most of us, for most of our needs. We've spared ourselves from a disaster that few of us can fully comprehend.

So we have some benefits from the time we have bought. But how much has it cost us to buy those benefits?

That's a hard number to guess at, and even harder to visualize.[170] A new word has silently entered our everyday language – trillion. That's a thousand billion. A number so hard to comprehend, that maybe it helps to look at it. Look at all those zeroes :

1,000,000,000,000.

You can have fun with a number like that. For example, say you have a trillion dollars and invest it at 5%. At the same time you stand on a street corner, and every second of every day (there are 86,400 seconds in a day) you give someone $1,000. That's $86,400,000 you give away, every day. How long does it take to give away the entire trillion dollars? The short answer is that you're getting $137 million every day in interest, and only giving away $86 million. You literally can't give the money away fast enough.

Say you had $1 trillion in $100 bills. How high a stack would that be? As high as the Empire State Building? As high as Mt Everest? Actually, a huge amount higher. Mt Everest is 5.5 miles high. Your stack of bills is 125 times higher than

---

[170] I guess I'm showing my age. I remember, as a young lad in intermediate school, having the headmaster come into the classroom and, apropos of nothing, regale us for ten minutes on the subject of how unthinkably vast the number one million was. Being a millionaire meant someone with unimaginable wealth. It wasn't until 1987 that Forbes started publishing its list of billionaires. That list grew to feature 2,200 people in 2018 but has dropped to 2,095 in 2020. The wealthiest billionaire is Jeff Bezos, now worth a reduced $113 billion. But that is still 113,000 times more money than what a millionaire has.

that – 680 miles high. The International Space Station is only 220 miles up. Most of us have never even seen a one-inch stack of $100 bills.

Say you asked for $1 trillion in ransom after kidnapping someone. How could you get paid? At a gold price of $1930/troy ounce, that would buy almost 36 million pounds. You'd need 450 semi-trailer trucks, each with an 80,000 maximum weight load of gold, to haul your ransom away.

Maybe you decide to get it in bitcoins instead. In total, there can only be a maximum of 21 million bitcoins, due to how it works. Today they are worth $12,895 each. Your $1 trillion could buy up every bitcoin that can ever exist, and you'd still have $730 billion unspent.

As I said, you can have fun with that sort of number, can't you.

Now to talk about the government's spending, and we need to switch from talking about "just" one trillion to now talking about many trillions. We know the federal government has authorized about $5 trillion in relief payments due to the financial harm of the virus shut-down on us all. That's the equivalent of $15,000 for every person in the US. How much of "your" $15,000 have you seen? I've not seen the first penny of mine.

We also know there are many other expenditures, at state level, and the Federal Reserve is doing things that presumably have costs associated with them too.

But that's just half the equation. That is government spending. How much extra has this all cost you, directly? There are invisible costs such as loss of quality of life for half a year (and counting). Maybe you've also had some uncompensated loss of earnings. Maybe there have been major disruptions in your life. And for sure, there's plenty of justifiable worry, for us all, about the future.

The economy as a whole has proven remarkably resilient, but is it really as strong as the indexes suggest? Most of the S&P 500 strength has been because of movements in just half a dozen high tech stocks. Take that out, and much of the rest of the S&P stocks have been falling. Extend the virus problems much longer, and sooner or later, the economy is going to realize what has been happening to it and may disintegrate entirely.

My sense is many businesses have been struggling to stay open, and have done so only in the hope that this will all soon pass. But as the expectation of a fast fix starts to fade, and as businesses exhaust all their cash reserves and fail to see any light at the end of the tunnel, very soon now they'll start to close. For sure, if there's no hope for a fast turnaround at the end of the year, retailers who are currently grimly holding on in the hope of a good Christmas season will close their doors late on 24 December, re-open for a "going out of business sale" on 26 December, and be gone by 31 December.

The same is true of many other businesses. Restaurants and bars of course are all hoping for a great "holiday season". Movie theaters are now so desperate for business, any business at all, that the AMC chain is now allowing people to hire their own theater for as little as $99.[171] That's not a viable strategy, but at least it helps keep the lights on for now. If something wonderful doesn't happen very soon, we'll be facing not so much a "second wave" of virus cases, but a second wave of business closures.

What will happen when governments of all types face up to the falling tax revenues that are happening and will happen?

Let's hope the economy will be more robust and self-healing than it might seem to be.

For want of a better number, say that the virus outbreak has cost the nation, in some form or another, $10 trillion, so far, and more with every extra passing day.[172]

Is it worth $10 trillion to keep our life more or less normal for six months? That's an impossible to answer question.

But phrase it differently. If we guess that if we'd not done anything, then one of the early projections, predicting 2.2 million deaths by about now,[173] would have come to pass, is it worth $10 trillion to save 2 million lives?[174]

Here we have a question that can be answered. The current federal guidelines are that a life is worth $10 million. The two million lives we saved with the $10 trillion represent a cost of $5 million per life. So that is good value for money – we're spending $5 million to save a life valued at $10 million.[175]

---

[171] See https://www.msn.com/en-us/money/companies/you-can-now-rent-a-private-amc-theater-for-just-99/ar-BB1a8aXw or https://cov.cx/a1a75

[172] This site shows $5 trillion spent, and a total of $11.6 trillion authorized to be spent, at the federal level alone. So going from $5 trillion spent federally to a total of $10 trillion doesn't seem an impossible reach. But pick a number, any number, and do your own sums. https://www.covidmoneytracker.org/ or https://cov.cx/a1a76

[173] See https://www.businessinsider.com/coronavirus-uk-report-projects-2-million-deaths-without-action-2020-3 or https://cov.cx/a1a77

[174] I'd actually put the total potential extra deaths as way higher than 2 million. But we can run with that as a conservative "low number" for the sake of this thought experiment.

[175] My numbers have been wild and wooly – both lives saved and the costs for saving them. Here's a totally different set of calculations for both lives saved and costs (and

(continued on next page)

A related question is "Can we afford $10 trillion to save two million lives?". But that's probably not a question we should ask, because think about what would have happened if we did nothing and the virus took over the entire country. There'd truly be massive social disruption, massive economic loss, and unthinkable consequences every which way. The $10 trillion didn't just save two million lives. It also saved our entire society and social system, which otherwise was at risk.

So, did we do the right thing? I'm not going to say yes we did, because even though things are very much better than they could be, they are also very much worse than they could have been and should have been. Our responses to the virus have been crude, confusing, and inconsistent. There is nothing we can be proud of when we look back at the last six months.

But "did we do the right thing" wasn't the question we opened this chapter with, was it. The question is "Have the sacrifices we've made so far been worth it". My answer to that is a bit like how I view the ridiculously inflated cost of buying a bottle of water at Disneyland on a hot day. When you're parched, you don't begrudge the dollar or two for a bottle of water. It is worth a couple of bucks for a bottle of lovely cool water. But when you see the same bottle of water for sale at a store right outside the gates for half or quarter the price, was the Disney price good value? Absolutely not.

So, worth it? The alternative would have been beyond bad. What we did was necessary. But we surely could have done things very much better. Maybe our response hasn't been perfect, but it has been better than no response would have been.

---

over a very different time period); but amazingly, it comes up with a very similar cost per life saved. They estimate $6 million, compared to my $5 million estimate. See https://news.yahoo.com/169-bn-29-000-lives-013740202.html or https://cov.cx/a1a78

3. When Will the Virus Finally Go Away?

This is a question many of us wonder, every day, in a semi-despairing and impatient manner. We are all keen to return to our normal lives. As you surely agree, while wearing a mask might be beneficial, it is not pleasant. We've been living with an ever-present concern that so many elements of our normal lives and routines now have an element of danger to them, with the potential of coming down with a severe case of the virus, for too many months.

The good news is there are truly hundreds of various research projects and clinical trials underway at present, at various stages of progress.[176] Hopefully, some of these might eventually come up with some solutions to allow us to get free of the terrible hold the virus has on our lives at present.

So, when will it finally go away? The answer to this question is not one you'll like. It is unlikely the virus will disappear, completely, any time soon.[177] It is

---

[176] This is a great site that updates regularly and lists details of all the research and trials it can uncover. See : https://racetoacure.stanford.edu/ or https://cov.cx/a1a79

[177] See, for example, this article :
https://www.independent.co.uk/news/uk/politics/coronavirus-uk-pandemic-end-vaccine-flu-ongoing-mark-walport-a9683246.html or https://cov.cx/a1a80 . WHO are, in my opinion, way too optimistic when they say the pandemic might last another two years, based on, of all ridiculous reasons, the Spanish 'flu two-year outbreak after World War 1. The two outbreaks have nothing in common, and the two viruses also have

(continued on next page)

incredibly difficult to completely eradicate any type of disease – only two have ever been successfully eradicated – smallpox, and rinderpest.[178] Other diseases are hoped to eventually be eradicated, but not yet.[179]

The problem with Covid-19, and all other infectious diseases, is that as long as there is a single small occurrence of the virus, anywhere at all; in our modern connected world it is entirely foreseeable that an infected person from that region will fly to somewhere far away, and start introducing it to the rest of the world, and the next thing you know, we'll be back to the position we find ourselves in now.

An example of that was recently shown to us by New Zealand. The small island nation had entirely eliminated the virus, and shut down its borders to keep it out. As a result, for 102 days, there were no new infections anywhere in the country. But on the 103rd day, a newly infected person was discovered. Strangely, no-one knows, even now, two months later, how/where the person became infected.

Because the country had relaxed all its social distancing controls, in the short time between the man becoming infected and his infection being discovered and the almost instantaneous re-introduction of social distancing requirements, there ended up being a cluster of over 110 new cases of people with the virus. Until the virus is <u>totally eradicated everywhere</u>, if the world lets its guard down, then the virus can (and will!) rush back without warning and get firmly established, the same as it already has.[180]

So, for the foreseeable future, until a distant time when maybe we'll eradicate the virus causing Covid-19, what is the best we can hope for? If we completely return to normal, the virus will return and catch us unawares, exactly like happened in New Zealand, and whereas NZ was still on a high standby alert,

---

nothing in common. It is ridiculous to try and draw lessons from Spanish 'flu and apply them to Covid-19. See https://www.the-sun.com/news/1350542/coronavirus-pandemic-another-two-years-who/ or https://cov.cx/a1a81 Making it more ridiculous is the article even includes contradictory statements by WHO's emergencies chief.

[178] You've probably not heard of rinderpest. There's a reason why – it is a disease that primarily affects cattle, and doesn't affect people at all.

[179] See https://asm.org/Articles/2020/March/Disease-Eradication-What-Does-It-Take-to-Wipe-out or https://cov.cx/a1a82

[180] It isn't just New Zealand. There are other examples of countries and regions having ostensibly become free (we're not sure we agree they were ever truly free) from the virus, but then after relaxing their controls and restrictions, the virus comes back even worse than before.

anticipating the virus might somehow get back into the country; that is probably not a sustainable basis for the entire world, all the time.

There are essentially four possible ways to reduce the threat of the virus down to something minimal which we can live with, in something close to normalcy. Each poses a different timeline.

Vaccination

If a long-lasting and highly effective vaccine is developed, that would be tremendously liberating. We could simply be vaccinated, and then relax and live normal lives, free of fear if/when there are fresh outbreaks of the virus.

As we discuss below in the section on Herd Immunity (see page 216) the other benefit of being vaccinated is that if enough people are vaccinated, herd immunity means that future virus outbreaks among the unvaccinated die out rather than grow larger and larger.

The current situation with vaccinations has become more promising during November. In total there around 100 different vaccines are going through the various stages of development (numbers seem to vary in different sources) and 42 more going through three phases of trials. In early November, two of these reported positive early results (being made by Pfizer and Moderna), a third made a similar release in mid-November (AstraZeneca). We hope those results will be confirmed with the balance of their testing, but nothing is yet guaranteed.

The current most likely to soon succeed vaccine candidates are not expected to give 100% protection to 100% of everyone who is vaccinated – indeed, it is very rare for any vaccine to be 100% effective, all the time, for everyone. The FDA reduced its requirement for effectiveness down to "anything better than 50%" as part of what I think was an ill-advised way of accelerating vaccine development and approval; happily, the current vaccine candidates all claim effectiveness levels above 90%.

We should define these terms.

• *How Are Vaccines Measured?*

We're now talking about vaccines that don't work all the time, something that few of us have ever stopped to think about. We get a tetanus shot, and we expect that means we'll 100% not be at risk of tetanus – and that's actually a reasonable expectation - the tetanus vaccine is about as close to 100% effective as any vaccine ever gets.

On the other hand, most people sort of vaguely sense, without knowing the numbers, that the annual 'flu shot doesn't work for everyone. It improves our odds but doesn't guarantee us immunity from the 'flu that season.

This brings us to two terms that are often used interchangeably, but which mean slightly different things.

Efficacy is a measure of how well something works in perfect conditions.

Effectiveness is how well a measure works in the real world.

Why is there a difference?[181] In the case of vaccines for Covid-19, there are various points of "imperfection" that might reduce the real-world effectiveness below the perfect-world efficacy. For example, maybe the vaccine being administered is stale rather than perfectly fresh, or perhaps the temperature control of the vaccine while being shipped and stored was not perfect. Maybe the time difference between the two injections was not exactly the optimum time period.

In the case of a vaccine, hopefully there's not a large difference between the two measures, and unless there's a need to specify which term is being used, we'll continue to use the two interchangeably.

The other interesting point is how are the various Covid vaccines having their efficacy/effectiveness measured? This is a point of vital interest to understand, of course. What does it mean when a drug company says their vaccine is 90% effective?

In simplest terms, it means that 90% fewer people got the virus after being vaccinated compared to people who weren't vaccinated.[182] For example, if there were two equal-sized groups, and in the vaccinated group, 10 people came down with the virus, and in the unvaccinated group, 100 people came down with the virus, then the effectiveness is calculated as being)

$$VE = \frac{(NU) - (NV)}{(NU)}$$

Where VE is vaccine efficacy or efficiency, NU is the number of virus cases among unvaccinated people and NV is the number of virus cases among vaccinated people.

In our example, this calculates out to be 0.9 or 90% effective.

---

[181] A classic example of the difference between the two measures is with contraceptives. A condom has almost 100% efficacy, but only 85% effectiveness. https://www.plannedparenthood.org/learn/birth-control/condom/how-effective-are-condoms or https://cov.cx/a1a83

[182] This is an easy to follow explanation if you'd like to see it in some more detail https://www.cdc.gov/csels/dsepd/ss1978/lesson3/section6.html or https://cov.cx/a1a84

That is a relatively easy thing to understand, but it is surprisingly meaningless by itself. Yes, the effectiveness claims being quoted in November by the now three different vaccine companies are meaningless.

We need to know how statistically significant this number is. For example, you can toss a coin twice, and it comes up heads both times – does that mean this coin will always come up heads? You'd not really know after two tosses, but after 2,000 tosses, you'd have a better idea, wouldn't you.

In statistics, it is common to talk about a "confidence interval". This is where you say "95% of all results will be between this number and this other number". What is the confidence interval for the vaccine effectiveness? Are we 95% certain that the vaccine will work somewhere between, perhaps 80% and 95% of the time, or are we 95% certain that the vaccine will work somewhere between 25% and 99% of the time?

Clearly, the narrower the confidence interval we have, the more likely the cited effectiveness percent is going to be correct. But the drug companies haven't given us that number yet.

I can guess, however, by looking at the data they have disclosed, and using the Reporting Odds Ratio (ROR) formula and its associated formula for determining the confidence interval.[183] A quick guess[184] suggests that the confidence interval probably ranges from about 80% to 95% for a claimed 90% effectiveness, based on the apparent numbers of cases reported in both the trial and control groups in the various Phase 3 trials that have been conducted.

There are some other points of uncertainty as well. There may not yet be sufficient results to be able to make meaningful claims about effectiveness for specific population sub-groups (such as the over 70 year-olds, or people with specific comorbidities).

We don't know how the trials are measuring things like mild cases of the virus compared to severe cases. Or, for the people in both groups who do get the virus, how long their respective hospitalizations are, and how many in each group die.

We point this out not to suggest there are dark secrets currently being withheld. We expect and hope the FDA will be searching out these questions and their answers as part of their approval procedure. But we'd really like to know the information ourselves.

------

[183] The ROR is also easy to understand, but working out the confidence interval gets a bit more "interesting". See https://allaboutpharmacovigilance.org/43-reporting-odds-ratio-ror/ or https://cov.cx/a1a85 for a great explanation.

[184] For our purposes, a quick guess is good enough, and remember that statistics are always somewhat vague and never as exact as the calculated numbers imply.

We have written to Pfizer, BioNTech, Moderna, and AstraZeneca, asking them for more information. We'll add any information we receive back to future updates to the book and will maintain a page on our website with updates too.[185]

- *Vaccine Issues*

It goes without saying that there are billions of dollars in profits available to the first company to get a vaccine approved. The stakes have been magnified further because it has also become a matter of national pride for countries and their leaders to claim first place in this race, and having a vaccine then gives a country national and diplomatic leverage when it comes to deciding which other countries it will share the vaccine with.[186]

The largest drug companies, all around the world, are competing against each other in a race to be the first to come up with an approved vaccine, with the prize being the billions of dollars in vaccine sales. In a case where the US FDA has said "the first vaccine to give us 50% effectiveness will be accepted and approved", there was a credible fear that drug companies would focus on the fastest quickest 50% solution, rather than work on a possibly slower and more complicated development of a 60% or 70% or 95% effective vaccine.

Happily, however, while some of the vaccines being trialed do seem to have only low effectiveness rates, the two most promising vaccines at present both are suggesting very high effectiveness – possibly as high as 95%. The more traditional types of vaccines seem likely to be less effective than ideal, but these two new vaccine candidates both use a new process of "mRNA" that seems to work much better than other approaches, although mRNA vaccines have yet to be proven in any other applications, elsewhere, so they are all entirely new and with more potential unknowns lurking in the background.

Low vaccine effectiveness would mess up the herd immunity equation. If we need 60% immunity for herd immunity to kick in, and if vaccines are only 50% effective, then herd immunity is impossible to achieve.[187]

---

[185] See https://thecovidsurvivalguide.com/vaccine-information or https://cov.cx/c-vi

[186] This BBC article about the vaccine development is headed "Coronavirus vaccine : Short cuts and allegations of dirty tricks in race to be first" – see https://www.bbc.com/news/world-53864069 or https://cov.cx/a1a86

[187] Because if everyone is vaccinated, and only half get immunity, that means we have a 50% level of immunity but need 60% for herd immunity to be effective.

On the other hand, that's a bit of an over-simplification. As well as vaccine-derived immunity, there is also immunity as a result of having had the virus and recovered from

(continued on next page)

It would be nice to focus all the pharmaceutical companies on a higher goal right from the start; but happily, it seems the two mRNA vaccines will resolve this challenge.[188]

The trials that are being run at present are taking longer than any of us wish but ideally should take longer still (the FDA has agreed that a normal six-month trial period can be compressed to only two months). They also provide weak rather than certain evidence of a vaccine's efficacy. This is because the trials

---

it. Different studies come up with different levels of recovered virus sufferers. Maybe recovered sufferers have stronger immunity? We don't really know for sure.

The reason for different findings from different studies is the added complexity of evaluating symptomless cases. How many are there is a question that needs to be answered but by definition can only be guessed at. The other always present problem is being able to find truly representative random population samples that can be used to estimate the overall spread of recovered and now immune people, either from symptomatic or symptomless infections.

This also implies the assumption that recovering from the virus gives one immunity. On that point, the best one can say is that the immunity from having had the disease might be only short-lived, the same as may be true of vaccines. It also may not be conferred to every person who had the virus.

[188] So if 50% is too low, what percentage would be acceptable? It might seem like this is a totally theoretical question with no scientific answer, but there is a calculable minimum percentage needed.

Assuming our goal is to achieve herd immunity through vaccination – a worthy goal we must have – there are two factors to point us to the necessary vaccine effectiveness. What percentage of the population needs to be immune for herd immunity to kick in, and what percentage of the population will agree to be vaccinated.

Let's accept the often-stated requirement for herd immunity as being "at least 60% immunity" and call that 65%. The harder question is what percentage of people will agree to be vaccinated? Surveys have shown widely varying numbers. Only about half the population gets a 'flu shot each year, but we expect more people will take a Covid-19 shot. On the other hand, if they have to have a double shot, three weeks apart, and if due to special ultra-cold refrigeration storage requirements, the shots won't be offered everywhere, unlike 'flu shots, the hassle factor rises and that will reduce total numbers. But, for want of a better number, let's say 75% of people are vaccinated.

That means a vaccine would need to be 87% effective to generate a 65% herd immunity level. You can adjust the numbers and create your own scenario any way you like, but the simple math is unavoidable – you can't get 60%+ herd immunity, even with everyone being vaccinated, if the vaccine is only 50% effective. The minimum effectiveness goal should never have been set so low.

There's of course another entirely different perspective as well. If you get vaccinated, you want it to work and protect you, don't you! So from that perspective, the closer to 100% the better.

essentially comprise a group of people who are vaccinated and another group of similar people who are not vaccinated, then they are monitored for several months to see how many people in each group end up getting infected by the Covid virus. In theory, with enough people and enough time, the random variations will be reduced and the trial results will become meaningful.

Frustratingly, there is a very simple way we could massively increase the data we get from the trials – through a process known as "challenge trials". Currently, if, by the end of the trial monitoring period, the test subjects have not been infected by the virus, there is no way of knowing if that was due to luck, washing hands, wearing masks, etc, or due to the vaccine working and preventing a potential infection. That is a terrible point of imprecision, and all that can be said is "statistically we would expect this number of people to have got the virus and in reality, this (smaller) number of people were infected, so we think the virus might be working".

Over an extended period, and with tens or ideally hundreds of thousands of trial subjects, that vagueness reduces, but we don't have that time or those people. We're talking about rushed trials with many fewer trial subjects (some tens of thousands, half of which are probably taking a placebo). The data from a shorter trial with fewer people is of course less accurate.

With a challenge trial, *volunteers* – this is important to keep in mind, the challenge trial participants would all be volunteers – are deliberately exposed to the virus to see if the vaccine prevents an infection from taking hold of them or not. This is a very valuable data point and can be quickly obtained. Get 100 volunteers, vaccinate them, give the vaccine a week or however long is needed for it to settle into the volunteers, then in some way create a scenario where there is a very high likelihood they'll catch the virus. Wait another week or so after that exposure, and then test to see who has the virus. That's an invaluable and clear test result in as little as two weeks and requires a much smaller group of subjects, rather than taking many months with a massive group of subjects and getting a fuzzier result.

Sure, the trial should continue beyond that point to ensure no surprises in terms of reactions to the vaccine and other issues/complications, and to also check the longevity of the vaccine protection, but almost immediately, within a couple of weeks, there would be an excellent set of data indicating if the rest of the trial was worth continuing or not.

Some people have protested, saying it is unethical to deliberately infect people with the virus. Certainly, it would be ultra-unethical to do this by force, and equally unethical not to tell the subjects what was being done to them and give them the choice to participate or not. But these are good-hearted people lining up to *volunteer* to be exposed to the virus because they know that every day, worldwide, another half-million people get the virus and another 10,000 people die – it is an extremely urgent problem to solve, and these good people are willing to risk their own health to help.

Isn't it instead unethical to refuse to allow these people to speed up progress to a vaccine? 10,000 or more people are dying every day. If 100 volunteers could cut a couple of months off a vaccine development program, that might represent over half a million saved lives.

Instead, the appropriate US Agency, the National Institute for Allergies and Infectious Diseases says it is "studying the issue", and an article in August said they will probably reach a decision on whether to allow such challenge trials toward the end of this year (it is now November and no decision yet).

Why do they have to study the issue? Isn't this something they've studied endlessly for decades in the past? Why, if they need to study the specifics of a Covid challenge trial, will it take so long to come up with an answer? Can't all the people who need to sign-off on the concept all meet together, in a room or on Zoom, and sort it all out in the course of a single meeting lasting less than a day?[189] It isn't rocket science.

Alternatively, why don't the drug companies do challenge trials in countries that are more accepting of the concept? (We believe some of this might quietly be occurring.)

Meantime, two months and more after that August article, and with no decision from NIAID yet, instead of saving half a million lives, that number of lives have been lost due to their prevarication and inactivity.[190]

The other point of uncertainty is how long a vaccine will protect. Unlike some vaccines that give almost lifetime protection, it seems a realistic expectation might be for a Covid vaccine to protect for only a year or possibly two, and the worst case (far from improbable) could mean as short as three months of protection.

The length of protection depends on both the vaccine and how our body "remembers" what the vaccine has "taught" it in terms of how to respond to the virus, and also on the virus itself. If the virus mutates into a new form, the new form might not be one the immunity created by a vaccine recognizes. This is part of the problem in developing a vaccine for the common cold – the coronavirus that causes the cold keeps mutating. It is also a reason why we need annual 'flu shots because each year's predominant strain of the influenza virus is usually

---

[189] Of course, the truth is that "study the issue" means "do nothing and hope the issue goes away". We pay these people six-figure salaries – surely we should expect something better than doing nothing from them in return.

[190] See https://news.yahoo.com/us-developing-coronavirus-strain-human-220417655.html or https://cov.cx/a1a87

sufficiently different from the previous year as to need a different vaccine to combat it.

How long will it be until the virus causing Covid-19 mutates to a form that requires a new vaccine? No-one yet knows, although in mid-November, there was speculation that a new strain of the virus, first found in mink in Denmark, might be one which current vaccine candidates will not protect against.[191]

Russia has already claimed to have developed a vaccine, which it terms "Sputnik 5", and China is now testing a vaccine candidate on "real people" as well as on test volunteers. Very little is known about either of these vaccines, however, in terms of their effectiveness; indeed, Russia released its vaccine *before* it had even undergone the third phase of the traditional three-phase trialing process.[192] [193]

In the US we have been regaled with varying promises – a vaccine in November, a vaccine by the end of the year, a vaccine early in the new year. We now understand that on Friday 20 November, Pfizer has formally applied for an Emergency Use Authorization for their vaccine, and we believe Moderna will be doing the same within a week or so.

On 23 November, AstraZeneca announced its vaccine study findings, also claiming an over 90% efficacy rate, and anticipating a fast approval too.

The FDA is meeting on 10 December to consider the Pfizer application, and a week later to consider the Moderna application.

What will this mean in terms of you and me? When will the vaccine be available in sufficient quantity for us to be vaccinated, to bring the virus under control in our communities, and in the world as a whole?

It seems probable that we'll start to see mass vaccinations becoming available in the early part of the second quarter next year. This brings us to another point.

- *Who Will Get the Vaccine First?*

Even once a vaccine is approved, it will take an unknown number of months before most of us can go somewhere and get vaccinated. There are likely to be

---

[191] See https://www.theguardian.com/environment/2020/nov/04/denmark-announces-cull-of-15-million-mink-over-covid-mutation-fears or https://cov.cx/a1a88

[192] Slightly amusingly, shortly after Pfizer broke the news of its vaccine candidate initially showing 90% efficacy, Russia then announced its vaccine was showing 92% efficacy.

[193] See https://www.bbc.com/news/world-asia-china-53917315 or https://cov.cx/a1a89

complicated processes for distributing the vaccine, and also complicated processes for deciding who gets it first and who gets it last.[194]

There is already a lot of jockeying for priority positions for the vaccine, both at an international level and also within each country. WHO is trying to convene and coordinate an international distribution program, but the largest countries in the world are not joining that program (including the US), deciding their first loyalty is to get the vaccine to their own citizens, not to nobly sacrifice their citizens while allowing other people elsewhere in the world to get the virus first.

Several different countries have already signed up some of the most likely seeming vaccine candidate manufacturers and obtained commitments for priority shipping of products if approved. The US is going one better than many other countries and is actually buying up vaccine supplies now, in the hope that if one of the vaccine candidates they've bought a bulk supply of is then approved, we'll be that much further ahead of the eight-ball and can instantly start distributing the supplies that have already been manufactured and shipped to staging locations.

Assuming that demand outstrips supply, some counter-intuitive decisions need to be made about who gets vaccinations first. But the assumption about demand outstripping supply is also a bit uncertain. It is far from clear how many Americans would wish to be vaccinated. Studies seem to show about half the population is wanting to be vaccinated, perhaps another quarter is not sure, and the remaining quarter is opposed.[195]

A survey in late Aug/early Sept asking the slightly different question "Would you get a Covid-19 vaccine before the election if it was free and FDA approved" showed more caution than earlier surveys. It is not clear if this is an evolving negative attitude in general, or a specific concern about rushing a vaccine out there too soon :[196]

---

[194] This is an interesting article about some of the issues involved with how the vaccine is likely to be stored, distributed, and then allocated and dispensed :
https://www.usatoday.com/story/news/health/2020/09/06/covid-vaccine-complex-distribution-supply-chain-follow-approval/5712053002/ or https://cov.cx/a1a90

[195] See, for example, this survey in June
https://www.sciencemag.org/news/2020/06/just-50-americans-plan-get-covid-19-vaccine-here-s-how-win-over-rest or https://cov.cx/a1a91 and this survey about six weeks later https://news.gallup.com/poll/317018/one-three-americans-not-covid-vaccine.aspx or https://cov.cx/a1a92

[196] See https://www.axios.com/covid-vaccine-election-f267a641-a19f-43e0-80a0-87c8e6eb303f.html or https://cov.cx/a1a93   It is slightly amusing to note that Republicans are less trusting of a Republican administration and Democrats!

Yes   No

	Yes	No
Total	42%	54%
Democrats	50	46
Independents	41	56
Republicans	36	60

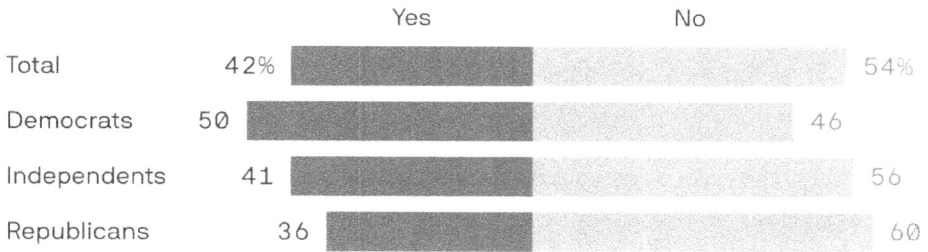

Figure 28 Attitudes to a pre-election vaccine release

It is interesting to compare US attitudes with those of other countries, too. Here's a recent study that shows the US to be one of the more skeptical countries when it comes to the vaccine.[197]

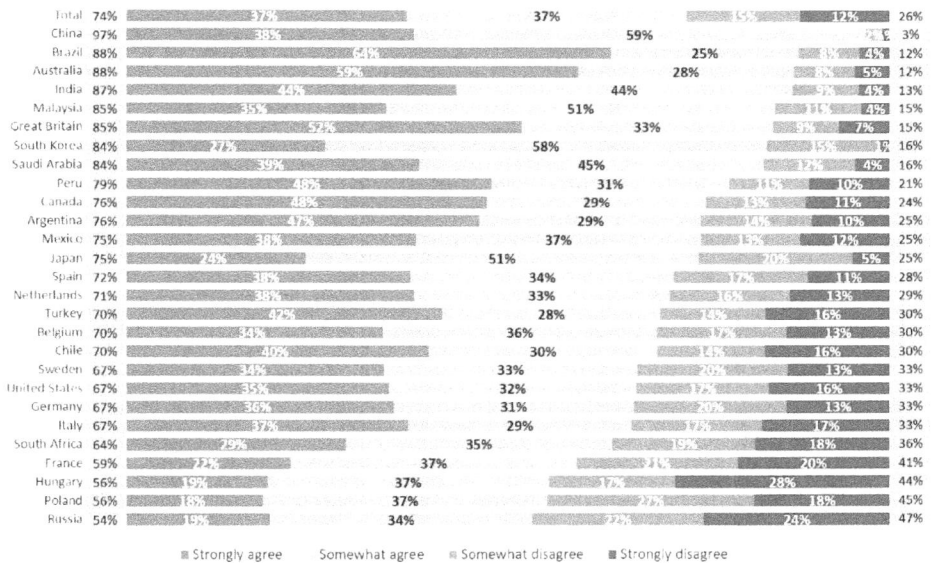

Country	Total	Somewhat agree		Strongly disagree	No
Total	74%	37%		12%	26%
China	97%	59%			3%
Brazil	88%	25%		4%	12%
Australia	88%	28%		5%	12%
India	87%	44%		4%	13%
Malaysia	85%	51%		4%	15%
Great Britain	85%	33%		7%	15%
South Korea	84%	58%			16%
Saudi Arabia	84%	45%		4%	16%
Peru	79%	31%		10%	21%
Canada	76%	29%		11%	24%
Argentina	76%	29%		10%	25%
Mexico	75%	37%		12%	25%
Japan	75%	51%		5%	25%
Spain	72%	34%		11%	28%
Netherlands	71%	33%		13%	29%
Turkey	70%	28%		16%	30%
Belgium	70%	36%		13%	30%
Chile	70%	30%		16%	30%
Sweden	67%	33%		13%	33%
United States	67%	32%		16%	33%
Germany	67%	31%		13%	33%
Italy	67%	29%		17%	33%
South Africa	64%	35%		18%	36%
France	59%	37%		20%	41%
Hungary	56%	37%		28%	44%
Poland	56%	37%		18%	45%
Russia	54%	34%		24%	47%

■ Strongly agree　　Somewhat agree　　■ Somewhat disagree　　■ Strongly disagree

Figure 29 Likelihood of taking the vaccine by country

[197] See https://www.ipsos.com/ipsos-mori/en-uk/three-four-adults-globally-say-they-would-get-vaccine-covid-19 or https://cov.cx/a1a94 , which has other interesting data as well. The survey was taken between 24 July and 7 August.

People's attitudes may change when the exact details of a vaccine are known – or maybe not. How many people ask for scientific validation before agreeing to accept a vaccination at present? Probably a very large section of the population will take it as a matter of course – that is perhaps the 50% group. A smaller section will not take it, for personal reasons that probably transcend the medical issues as they are presented. That just leaves the other 25% of undecideds who might assess the risks when a vaccine is finally released.[198]

The Ipsos survey that generated the chart above asked people why they would not take the vaccine. The most commonly cited reason was concern about side-effects, followed by doubting that the vaccine would be effective. One in five mentioned they are against vaccines in general and almost the same number felt they weren't sufficiently at risk to make it worthwhile.[199]

This has interesting implications for herd immunity calculations. If only 60% (for example) are vaccinated, and if the vaccine is only 50% effective, that means we've added a 30% increase to the herd immunity numbers. But with the claimed level of herd immunity generally cited in the order of 60% or more, where do we get the other 30%+ from?[200] This becomes less of a problem if the current leading vaccine candidates do prove to be 95% effective. That would get us to 57% immunity – still not a complete herd immunity, but much closer, and a point where virus growth is greatly curtailed.

There are probably some easy priority choices to make in terms of who gets vaccinated first. Healthcare professionals should get it first. Until a month or two ago, one would automatically say "first responders should come second", but with the moves around the country to defund the police, who knows if that's still a universally accepted view.

---

[198] I'm probably in the undecided category at present (in case you wondered). I'm nothing at all close to being an "anti-vaxxer" in general, but I'm cautious about the rush into totally new approaches to developing vaccines for Covid-19 – things that would be extremely clever if they work, but which might be terrible if they don't. I want to see more studies and to allow more time for testing to prove there are no unexpected side effects.

I also hope that after the headlong rush to get the first vaccine out there, things will continue to proceed with more careful testing of better vaccines that get released some months – maybe even years – later.

[199] Ibid. 60% were worried, 37% didn't think it would work. Note people could give multiple reasons, so the total is greater than 100%. 3% even said they didn't have the time to be vaccinated.

[200] And let's not even start to think about how long immunity lasts and how quickly it fades.....

Beyond that, it starts to get more complicated and confusing. Should there be other categories of "essential infrastructure workers" that get it before "normal people" – and if there should be such people, who would they be? Utility workers? Farmers and meatpackers and other people in the food supply chain? Would that extend to people working in supermarkets? Does "food supply chain" also include truck drivers? And so on.

If you think that is contentious, you haven't seen anything yet. Now we get to decide who among the category of "everyone else" gets it first and last.

For example, should the first people to get it be at-risk elderly people, or young and healthy people? You might say "of course, the at-risk elderly", but there is a rational school of thought that says "If we vaccinate a very elderly person, we might on average add one more year of life for them, but if we vaccinate a younger person, we might add another 20 or 30 years of life for them, so there's more benefit vaccinating the younger person".[201]

Another example would be choosing between wealthy and poor people, or between white and black people. Please keep in mind I'm just relaying the equation here, not advocating or suggesting it. It could be said that wealthy white people should get it first, because they are more likely to contribute more to the economy into the future than poor black people, because the former group is likely to contribute more to the economy and its speedy recovery. Other people are saying poorer black people should get it first because they're more at risk and have less ready access to quality healthcare. So, pretty much for any issue, two opposite perspectives can be considered.

Here's an interesting article that touches on these issues some more.[202]

---

[201] The calculation is a bit more complicated, because you also have to consider the respect chances of getting infected, and the respective chances of dying, but at least to start with, you can see how a "scientific" and dispassionate approach might bring about quite the opposite answer to the expected answer on the basis of traditional values and assumptions.

A real cynic might add to this equation "If a politician gets a vaccine first to a younger person, that younger person will vote for them in more elections into the future than an older person"!

[202] See https://www.scientificamerican.com/article/how-to-decide-who-should-get-a-covid-19-vaccine-first/ or https://cov.cx/a1a95 and also https://www.statnews.com/2020/09/01/u-s-advisory-group-lays-out-detailed-recommendations-on-how-to-prioritize-covid-19-vaccine/ or https://cov.cx/a1a96 which has an interesting table of four priority categories of people.

We also noted what appears to be the priority list for the UK, appearing on the front page of the Daily Telegraph[203] :

1	OLDER ADULTS RESIDENT IN A CARE HOME AND CARE HOME WORKERS
2	ALL THOSE 80 YEARS AND OVER AND HEALTH AND SOCIAL CARE WORKERS
3	ALL THOSE 75 YEARS OF AGE AND OVER
4	ALL THOSE 70 YEARS OF AGE AND OVER
5	ALL THOSE 65 YEARS OF AGE AND OVER
6	HIGH-RISK ADULTS UNDER 65 YEARS OF AGE
7	MODERATE-RISK ADULTS UNDER 65 YEARS OF AGE
8	ALL THOSE 60 YEARS OF AGE AND OVER
9	ALL THOSE 55 YEARS OF AGE AND OVER
10	ALL THOSE 50 YEARS OF AGE AND OVER
11	REST OF THE POPULATION (PRIORITY TO BE DETERMINED)

Figure 30 Possible UK vaccine priority list

This is a fairly unimaginative list with much unexplained – what qualifies as "high-risk" or "moderate-risk"? And note the 11th item on the list, with the note "priority to be determined"!

The National Academies of Sciences, Engineering and Medicine in the US subsequently came up with a suggested framework for setting priorities in the

---

[203] See https://www.bbc.com/news/blogs-the-papers-54882074 or https://cov.cx/a1a97
- note : link still exists, but no longer shows this chart

US. It has only five categories, but is interesting because it shows an estimate for how much of the population falls within each category.[204]

How the COVID-19 vaccine could be rationed

A plan from the National Academy of Medicine places those at highest risk from the virus at the top of the list. Percentages of the U.S. population:

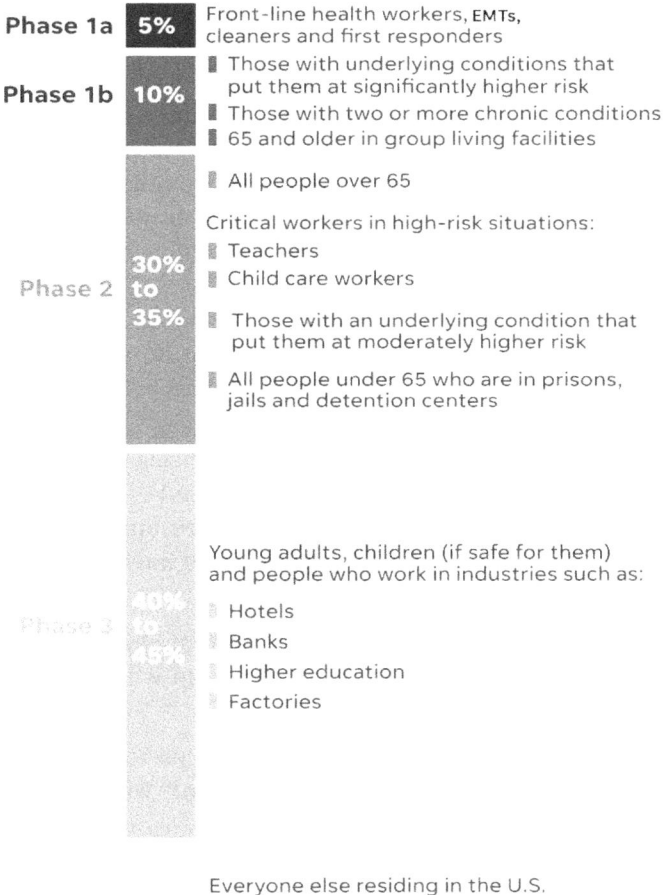

Phase 1a **5%** Front-line health workers, EMTs, cleaners and first responders

Phase 1b **10%**
- Those with underlying conditions that put them at significantly higher risk
- Those with two or more chronic conditions
- 65 and older in group living facilities

Phase 2 **30% to 35%**
- All people over 65

Critical workers in high-risk situations:
- Teachers
- Child care workers
- Those with an underlying condition that put them at moderately higher risk
- All people under 65 who are in prisons, jails and detention centers

Phase 3 **40% to 45%**

Young adults, children (if safe for them) and people who work in industries such as:
- Hotels
- Banks
- Higher education
- Factories

Everyone else residing in the U.S.

SOURCE National Academy of Medicine

Figure 31 Proposed US vaccine priority list

---

[204] See https://www.usatoday.com/story/news/health/2020/11/19/covid-19-vaccines-who-gets-coronavirus-immunization-first/3778098001/ or https://cov.cx/a1a98

This is not yet an official policy, merely a suggested approach. But we did note, wryly, that in the US, between 85% and 95% of the entire population qualify under one of the priority categories, leaving only 5% - 15% of "everyone else".

One more point, just to make a contentious topic even more inflammatory. Should the vaccine be made mandatory? To some people or no-one or everyone?

Before you quickly shriek "No, the vaccine should be optional, any other approach is un-American", I should point out three things.

Firstly, vaccines in effect are close to mandatory, certainly in my state of Washington, if children wish to be allowed to attend public school.

Secondly, and perhaps not so realized, vaccines are also mandatory for teachers, too. Both for their safety and for the safety of the children they are in close contact with. I don't know, but I bet there are other categories of people who also must agree to vaccinations – probably military, maybe healthcare workers, remote workers (ie in far-away-from-hospital type locations), and so on.

If you have children, how would you feel about sending them back to school, with crowded classrooms, lunchrooms, and all the other risk environments? Maybe you don't want your children vaccinated, but are you also happy that every other child and teacher is also unvaccinated?

Thirdly, it is likely that mandatory vaccine policies might come, not from governments, but from private companies. In mid-November, Qantas, the Australian national airline, announced that when it resumes international flying sometime next year, it will require all passengers to have proof of vaccination. Qantas says it expects other airlines will do the same.[205]

An anticipatory article in December observed that employers will be able to legally mandate their employees get vaccinated, and will be able to terminate anyone who refuses to comply.[206]

So even if our federal government can't force us to be vaccinated, other "authorities" in the real world can and almost certainly will.

I'm glad I just get to write about this. I for sure would hate to have to formulate and implement policies on this matter!

---

[205] See https://www.bbc.com/news/world-australia-55048438 or https://cov.cx/a1a99

[206] See https://www.cnbc.com/2020/12/07/covid-vaccine-update-your-boss-can-fire-you-if-you-refuse-the-coronavirus-shot.html or https://cov.cx/a1f86

Cures

The second of the four approaches to reducing the impact of the Covid-19 problem is to develop a cure that makes a case of Covid-19 into no more a problem than a sore throat.

In other words, some sort of medication of the "take a pill twice a day for a week" type - something inexpensive and easily taken, and which changes a virus infection from a severe illness and possibly fatal, making it merely a passing inconvenience, without any need for hospitalization or ICU care.

There are a number of drugs at present that may have some positive impacts on the virus, but none that show any potential to become a "take one twice a day for a week" cure that will work for 99% of all infected people, 99% of the time. Not only do the currently likely treatments not work for everyone, they don't necessarily completely zero out all the symptoms and severity of the virus, maybe just reducing it down to a point where you don't need to go to a hospital, but still feel very unwell at home for a few days.

Some of the treatments being researched are known specialty antiviral drugs. Some need to be administered via IV drip/injection, and some are ideally administered as part of a hospital stay for general supervision. Again, such concepts are far removed from the "just take a tablet for a while" solution we'd all hope for.

Some of the possible treatments are drugs that have already been "out there" and used for other ailments for years or even decades, and which are now showing positive effects when used against Covid-19, too. The good news about these drugs is they are, to some degree, already well known and well accepted, with understood and limited side-effects, and because they were developed many years ago, may even have had their patents expire, reducing their cost. Hopefully, they are commonly available from multiple suppliers and very inexpensive – some can cost less than a dollar or two for a complete course of treatment.

There are also new treatments being researched and developed, but they can be more expensive, and might not be as easy as just taking a course of pills. For example, a six-dose course of remdesivir comes with a drug cost of $3,120, and due to being administered through an IV drip, may require hospitalization to some degree while it is being given. Without considering these associated costs, and even if no hospitalization, the cost of administering six IV shots has to be added to the cost of the drug itself, so the very best-case scenario looks to be $5000 or more. Compare that cost and complex dosing procedure to the existing medicines, costing sometimes less than a bottle of cough mixture or a pack of aspirin, and as easy to take as cough mixture/aspirin, at home.

Other treatments are not revolutionary, but each one of them helps some people in some way, and the disease is becoming more survivable. But "more survivable" isn't quite the same as "inconsequential and unimportant", is it, especially because some of these various developments only benefit people who have become severely infected and have been admitted to hospital and perhaps even the ICU. Sure, if that ends up being you or me, we'll be extremely appreciative to be able to eventually emerge, still alive, but wouldn't you rather have the "magic pill" that prevents the disease from ever becoming that serious?

The "magic pill" is something that can potentially benefit everyone, and be most beneficial to the population as a whole, the healthcare infrastructure, and the economy.

The problem is there are no "big pharma" companies trying to develop $1 treatments using out-of-patent freely available medicines. Big pharma companies need to earn a return on the money they invest into new drugs and new treatments, and whereas it is fairly obvious how remdesivir – a drug which is reputed to cost $9 to make sufficient for a six-dose course, but which is sold for $3120 – may end up being a wonderful money-maker for Gilead[207], the company that developed it, it is hard to see how any company could make a profit on a generic drug which they don't even control the sale of.

There are lots of existing drugs being tested/trialed to see if they might reduce the risk/severity of a Covid infection, and this is an area in which we expect to see continued progress and good news appearing. But we are not confident of any stunning breakthrough that discovers the $1 "magic pill", and we've also no idea for the timing of when less substantial developments will happen.

We were amazed at the speed with which remdesivir was pushed through the testing/trialing process, the lack of any major/massive benefits identified, and the rush to excitedly hail it as a game-changer and obtain FDA approval – an astonishing contrast to the hostile reception (or just total ignoring and pretending they don't exist) and very slow responses which less costly drugs are being given.

So we don't expect a low-cost highly effective cure to appear in the foreseeable future.

---

[207] All the more so because the US Government paid, up-front, $70.5 million of the costs to develop remdesivir, with no requirement for that funding to ever be repaid. How much money will Gilead make from remdesivir? That's imponderable, because we don't know what the future sales of the product will be. Gilead reported $873 million in sales for the drug in the third quarter of 2020, but the carefully curated campaign of optimism about the drug is slowly starting to fade away and to be replaced with the less appealing reality. See https://www.fool.com/investing/2020/11/04/will-gileads-remdesivir-only-be-a-short-lived-succ/ or https://cov.cx/a1ab01

Outbreak Control

The third of the four paths to getting the virus acceptably under control is to be able to quickly identify people with infections, and to win the "race" with the virus – finding and stopping such people from infecting other people, before they become infectious.

Achieving that is certainly very beneficial for everyone else. But the problem with this third "solution" is that it does nothing to reduce the potential severity of the disease, should you be one of the hopefully very few unlikely ones who still acquire it. That's not a reason to ignore outbreak control as a strategy, and outbreak control is enormously beneficial to society as a whole. It has also been a colossally and tragically overlooked part of the US' public health response to the virus.

But outbreak control should never be a primary or sole goal in our fight against the virus.

Outbreak control, in theory, is simple, and it is a huge puzzle and disappointment that we have failed so spectacularly at implementing it. Let me explain how it works because you can and should adopt these measures yourself if you or someone close to you becomes infected. In the simplest form, outbreak control simply means finding and isolating newly infected people before they have a chance to pass the infection on to others.

This would be moderately easy if the way a virus worked was first to very slowly incubate inside a newly infected person, secondly to then start creating obvious symptoms, and only after that, in a subsequent third stage, start to become infectious.

Unfortunately, that's not the way it works in real life.[208] With most respiratory diseases, there may be a short time when you are infectious *before you are symptomatic and realize you are unwell*. This gives the virus a bit of an edge, a bit of a head start in the race.

The Covid-19 disease is no exception, you become infectious before you have any symptoms. Some people never get symptoms and don't even know they have (had) the virus. Some (Many? Most? We're not sure, although the CDC suggests 75%) of these people, while having no symptoms, can still infect other people.

---

[208] And for obvious reasons. Viruses "adapt" to become better at passing themselves on – the scenario I described would see each infected person passing on the virus to very few other people. The most effective transmission involves the virus passing itself on before the infected host person even realized they are unwell. Guess how Covid-19 works.....

So it is necessary to find infected people *before they even know they are infected*.[209] This is a bit of a tall order, isn't it. But it is essential, and for it to work, it requires two things : The first requirement is for people to be randomly and regularly tested, as often as possible, so as to find, to everyone's surprise, the people who are infected without realizing their state. To do this means we need fast, low-cost, and reasonably accurate[210] tests.

The second requirement is that once a person has been identified as being infected, there must be very fast contact tracing to identify who the person has been in close contact with over the last several days. This will hopefully enable us to find who the person caught the infection from (so we can not only have them isolate themselves, but then do another series of contact tracings to find who else they might have infected), and it will also enable us to advise the other people the newly infected person has been with that they are now at risk and need to come in to be tested, too.

It is a race against time, and against the virus, requiring both easy instant testing (and equally instant results) for anyone and everyone, and a contact tracing system that very quickly responds when a newly infected person is found. No part of this process is working well at present, and all parts must work well for effective control of the virus spread.

- *Fast Universal Testing*

We've written about what is happening with tests in several sections below, starting on page 179. The quick summary is that while our record in the US has been appallingly dismal to date, we may have turned the corner, with a growing number of new tests now being made available – tests that promise results within 30 minutes, sometimes within as few as five minutes.[211]

The next issue is to get the cost per test down to a low level. At present, the costs for tests with fast results are sometimes as high as $250 (at Anchorage

---

[209] Do you see the nonsense, now, of the CDC saying that only symptomatic people should be tested for the virus?

[210] Actually, tests don't have to be 100% accurate to be helpful. It is better to have a good test that is fast to administer and give results than to have an excellent test that is more cumbersome to administer and give results, as we explained previously.

[211] Here's a recent article about a "breathalyzer" style testing device.
https://www.studyfinds.org/coronavirus-test-via-breathalyzer/ or https://cov.cx/a1ab02
This is a product still in a pre-production phase, so we've no idea what the cost per test might end up as being, or how quickly the result would be obtained, but presumably the cost will be low and the result quickly provided.

Airport in Alaska) or even $500 (at house parties in the Hamptons[212]). Recently we have seen Costco advertising tests for $130 and $150.

That's a lot to pay for a "just in case" test, and the test is less helpful than one would hope. After you get the test kit from Costco and take your sample, the sample then has to be sent to a laboratory to be analyzed, with results promised to you one – three days after the sample is received at the lab. So, from deciding to be tested to getting a result, you're looking at probably anywhere from three to six days. That's much too much of a "head start" for the virus, if indeed you have an infection.

We need $2.50 and $5.00 tests – we need the cost to drop one-hundredfold (or even more). We need tests that give results in a few minutes, not in many days.

The tests should not only be affordable and fast, but they should also be simple (and as foolproof as possible) too, so that anyone can test themselves, at home, any time they choose to.

As of late October, faster antigen type tests are starting to appear in various places, and we expect they will become more commonplace, potentially to the point where they'll be a pre-requisite to be admitted into office buildings, shopping malls, sports stadiums, airports, and who knows where else.[213]

In addition to better individual testing, at long last – months after the virus became a terrible urgent problem, researchers finally came around to considering and accepting the concept of test pooling, something that I and others had been advocating for a considerable time, and something that has been

---

[212] See https://www.cnn.com/2020/08/22/us/hamptons-parties-coronavirus-tests-trnd/index.html or https://cov.cx/a1ab03

[213] This raises the possibility that a person might end up being tested two or three times in a single day. That is getting to the point of diminishing returns, and probably not necessary or justified. But what type of system can be adopted so that a person can prove they were tested, just a few hours ago, somewhere else, and that their test result was clear/negative rather than positive?

There are plenty of ways that this testing could be coordinated, possibly in conjunction with the mobile phone that almost everyone from pre-teen years and forward carries with them, everywhere, these days. The argument against such things is there is the risk of loss of privacy associated with such data sharing and phone apps.

This is another issue that is more social policy than health science. We all should be able to offer our opinions and suggestions on this matter.

used in other scenarios for many decades.[214] This is discussed further in our section "Test Pooling", below on page 184.

But then in early September, the CDC took an astonishing step, suggesting that access to testing should be limited to people who already have symptoms of the disease.[215] This would make it impossible to find asymptomatic sufferers at all, and impossible to find the people who will have symptoms, but not yet.

It would mean by the time most people came in for testing, they'd have already been infecting people for several days. The race against time to limit the number of people an infectious person infects would be lost before it starts.

The CDC sort of backtracked from that astonishing statement, and in any event, as long as they are not in some way making tests illegal, it is possible to proceed in a sensible direction and just ignore their occasional acts of lunacy.

- *Fast Contact Tracing*

Once we've identified a newly infected person, our focus switches to the second requirement for effective outbreak control – fast contact tracing.

The current "old-fashioned" method of contact tracing involves a contact tracer person contacting a newly infected person and working with them to identify every person they may have come into significant contact with during their time of possible infectiousness, then contacting those possibly at-risk people and encouraging them to voluntarily distance/isolate themselves and be tested.

It is labor-intensive, inaccurate, and unavoidably incomplete. Think about how you'd describe a typical day to a contact tracer. "Well, there was the guy on the bus who I was standing next to, but I don't know his name. There was a woman in the shop who was too close to me while we stood in line to check-out – I don't know who she is, and I don't remember the name of the check-out operator either, I'm sorry. And then there were all the people at work, too, all 150 of them."

---

[214] We don't understand why the authorities have been so slow to accept this excellent and time-hallowed concept.

[215] See https://www.businessinsider.com/cdc-modified-covid-19-testing-guidelines-to-exclude-asymptomatic-people-2020-8 or https://cov.cx/a1b01 . This is an impossible to understand or justify decision, and all the more astonishing now that the country is starting to move to having more tests available, and with lower costs per test. All the people who claim that only the CDC and similar "experts" should be allowed to set and debate public health policy went briefly silent while trying to work out how to justify this unjustifiable statement.

How many of those people will the contact tracer be able to identify and contact? Do you think any employer would like to see their entire staff asked to go into voluntary lock-down any time any employee came down with a case of the virus?

Many people with new infections say they're never contacted by any contact tracing person at all. The system is not working well, if at all, at present.

What is needed is some type of automatic system that somehow knows everyone we've been close to – not only that, but knows how close we've been next to each person, and for how long, so it can create a prioritized list of at-risk people.

You might think, in the previous paragraph, that I'm talking wishfully and hypothetically about something that, alas, doesn't exist and probably is impossible to create. Not so. In this amazing day of universal connectedness, such things are possible already. A simple app added to your smartphone and using the Bluetooth, Wi-Fi, cellular, and GPS capabilities of the phone, would allow the phone to know where you are all the time (this information is already known) and also to know who you are close to – not so much by knowing what other phones were in the same general area, but by knowing which other phones' Bluetooth signals were detected, and how strong their signals were. Because Bluetooth is a low power and limited range service, if a phone can detect a clear Bluetooth signal from another phone, then the two phones are probably close to each other, and therefore, the two phone owners are also probably close to each other, too.

It then becomes the work of a minute or two to download that data from a newly infected person's phone, and after a minute or two of calculation, immediately send text messages to all the possibly now at-risk people's cell phones.

Instead of days of old-fashioned and inaccurate/incomplete contact tracing, you're talking a minute or two, tops.

Several countries are looking at types of tracking/monitoring systems like this, and a group of New Zealanders have also designed a separate standalone device that people could wear around their neck.[216]

It is true these systems would not be 100% perfect, but they don't need to be 100% perfect. All they have to do is help us to ensure that, on average, each newly infected person infects less than one more person, so the virus spread diminishes and dies out, rather than grows. If every fifth person still infected one person, and if every tenth person infected two people, and every 15th person infected

---

[216] See https://www.stuff.co.nz/business/122492568/covidcards-work-but-making-them-mandatory-would-be-an-extreme-last-resort-says-minister or https://cov.cx/a1b02

three people, you still have an R rate massively less than 1.0[217] and each new outbreak quickly dies out.

Some of the concerns about personal privacy would just have to be accepted as a necessary trade-off, and keep in mind that all the shadowy three-letter agencies already have much of this information in their computer databases.[218] Which would you prefer? To die a painful death, drowning from fluid in your lungs, at the hands of the virus? Or to have the state knowing where you were yesterday and the day before?[219]

Regular testing of as many people as possible, and automatic instant contact tracing could stop the spread of the virus, without needing to wait for vaccines that may or may not risk, or develop new wonder-drug cures, or anything much else at all.

• *Current Contact Tracing Apps*

We already have the technology to deploy this type of software. Indeed, there are a confusing plethora of apps already available for more recent Android (version 6 and above) and iOS (version 13.5 and above) phones. The essential element of contact tracing of course is that as many people as possible must participate in the process, and so it is important that everyone is using a compatible app on their phones, and that the app works across both Apple and Android devices.

---

[217] The R rate would be 6/15 or 0.40.

[218] Not only governmental three-letter-agencies. Private companies, too. It is possible to get companies such as Facebook to serve ads to people based on where they are and where they have been. There are multiple databases out there already that store details of where we are (or, more exactly, where our phones are) every minute of every day. I get a report from Google every month telling me where I've been, and how long I've been in various places, maybe you do too.

This is not really a new loss of privacy at all. You can decide which concerns you more – the government or private companies knowing more about you than your employer, partner, parents, and children do.

But, however you feel, we've already lost much of the privacy we think we still have. It is inappropriate to let concern over losing privacy that we've already lost stand in the way of an automatic contact tracing system that could be designed to minimize most of any further privacy loss that it might cause.

[219] Some of the concerns could be ameliorated by keeping data on each person's phone, and only having it downloaded, with their participation and approval, in cases where they've been discovered to have a Covid infection. The phone could also automatically delete data that is more than, say five or six days old.

It seems that after a bit of a "Tower of Babel" to start with, we are now moving to a more integrated process via a process known as "Exposure Notifications Express" in both types of phones.[220] The chances are you've not heard about it, though – I hadn't until researching this section of the book.

Why isn't this better known? Why isn't there a national push to get everyone using this service? Not only is it not well known, but the states themselves are slow to embrace the technology. As of early September, only half the states had some sort of participation in this program.

How many more tens/hundreds of thousands of people need to die while effective and almost free preventative measures are waiting for us to adopt and deploy them?

Lastly on this frustrating point, it is relevant to observe that using phones and their Bluetooth transceivers to evaluate contacts and risks is far from perfect. Some people don't even know how to turn their Bluetooth on. Even if it is on, different phones have different powered transmitters, so it is very hard to match the power of a received signal with the likely distance between the two phones. Signal strength also depends on where your phone is (and where the other phone is). If your phone is in your trouser pocket, it won't send and receive as well as if it is on a countertop.

Plus, just because you're receiving a Bluetooth signal doesn't mean you're close to another person and at risk. You might be in one company's office, and another person might be on the other side of the wall, with your phones close and receiving strong signals, but not only is the person on the other side of the wall, they're in an entirely different company's premises, too.

That's not to say this is bad – it is better than nothing. But is it much better than nothing? Interestingly, Singapore discontinued its phone-based tracking/tracing program and is now replacing it with dedicated devices.[221]

But anything is better than nothing. Give us something – give us anything. Don't leave us with nothing.

- *Diminished Infection Risk*

The effectiveness of a test and trace program can be greatly improved by continuing to maintain some elements of social distancing.

If wearing masks reducing our risk by 30%, if social distancing reduces our risk by 30%, and if contact tracing and testing can catch half of all new infections

[220] See https://9to5mac.com/2020/09/01/how-to-turn-on-off-covid-19-contact-tracing-iphone-ios/ or https://cov.cx/a1b03

[221] See https://www.bbc.com/news/technology-53146360 or https://cov.cx/a1b04

before the newly infected person becomes infectious, and if we start with an R value of, say, 3.0, then we end up with a resulting R value of 0.735. That is less than 1.0, so the virus slows down its spread and stops.

That is also why we say we don't need a 100% effective system. Sure, 100% would be lovely, and seeing the R value drop all the way to zero would be marvelous. But we'll happily accept a value of 0.735 – it is below 1.0.

The big limitation of a test and trace system is that it only works while it is in operation, and it costs money to keep it in operation. If the system is abandoned, then as soon as one new virus infection enters into the country, the virus will quickly return and take over the country again, unless one of the other four measures is also in place, or until the test/trace system is reactivated.

Herd Immunity

The fourth and final path to prevailing over the virus has the benefit and appeal of being an "automatic" thing, and a reward for our suffering. As such, it appeals to both the lazy among us and those of us saddled with the notion of suffering and subsequent redemption.

Herd immunity is a bit like outbreak control through testing and tracing. It depresses the "R" value and means a newly infected person doesn't lead to a massively spiraling upwards new outbreak. But it does not make the virus less dangerous to anyone who still gets it. So it is a secondary and less desirable strategy compared to the first two strategies – vaccination and cures.

We discuss herd immunity in more detail (see "Herd Immunity", below on page 216), in the context of it being a situation that may allow you to avoid infection, and following on from that topic, the topic of how long immunity might last, either after having had the disease or being vaccinated.

So, as subsequently discussed, it seems the length of protection gained from either a past infection or a vaccination could be as short as one month (as was the case for a man in Nevada) or as long as three or four months (the generally discussed time frame and the experience of three other confirmed re-infections in August); and possibly longer – maybe six months, maybe even a year. But it is very unlikely to be lifetime protection, and therein lies the terrible weakness of the herd immunity concept as it might apply to the Covid-19 virus.

The herd immunity concept needs to be modified to reflect that it, in this case, it is "perishable" – it is not the same as everyone who has ever had the disease will never have it again. Rather, some smaller subset of the people who have *recently* had the disease (or been vaccinated) and still have sufficient antibodies to counter a potential second infection will probably not get the disease again, for an unknown number of months, before losing the benefit of their prior exposure and becoming similarly at risk as everyone else again.

At the time of working the following statistics (7 September – the numbers will be different in the future, but the overall concept will be the same) – the US has about 5.8 million people who have had the virus and are now free of it with the expectation of herd immunity. But if we look at a worst-case scenario and assume this expires in as little as three months, that means everyone who had the virus before about 1 June no longer have herd immunity. There were 1.8 million people with the virus back then, so we've possibly got a total of 4 million people with active immunity at present.

The US has 330 million people, so 1.2% of its population has active herd immunity at present. You don't need to do any more sums to guess that 1.2% isn't a game-changer at all, do you. A commonly cited number is that we'd need over 60% herd immunity for the virus spread to stop as a result of herd immunity alone.

There is unlikely to ever be a case where 60% of the population has had the virus within a three- or even six-month period. That would require a steady new case count of 1.1 - 2.2 million cases a day. The worst day ever for the US has been around 125,000 new cases. A 9 – 18 fold increase in daily new cases, and not just on a single day, but every day, all the time, would destroy our healthcare system entirely, and the fatality rate would skyrocket because there'd be no hospital beds for sufferers, and even if there were, there'd be no supplies, no medicines, and insufficient doctors and nurses.

It might be possible to build up to that 60% via vaccination, but if a vaccine only has a three-month effect as well, and keeping in mind that not all vaccinated people will truly get immunity for any amount of time, and that everyone will need two jabs, that suggests we'd need more than 5 million vaccinations to be given every day, forever into the future. That also seems unrealistic.

Now to think about this some more. We said there have been 5.8 million sufferers in the US up until September. All these people, in total, represent about 1.8% of the US population. We know that some parts of the country have had more cases than others, but how to now reconcile the total of 5.8 million recovered people with studies such as this that say one-third of people in the Bronx now show as having virus antibodies?[222]

According to the data, the Bronx borough had about 3600 cases per 100,000 people as of the end of August. That is another way of saying 3.6%.

It is generally thought that 40% of cases are asymptomatic, and for the sake of this calculation, let's assume that all 40% of such cases in the Bronx were never

---

[222] See https://www.msn.com/en-us/news/politics/one-third-of-bronx-test-subjects-have-coronavirus-antibodies/ar-BB189LfZ or https://cov.cx/a1b05

detected or counted in the total case number.[223] So that means we add another 2.4% of people and we now get a total of 6% of people who have had the virus.[224]

How can we reconcile this high estimate of 6% with the claim that 33% of people have virus antibodies? Something is seriously wrong. Is the antibody testing wrong? Can people get antibodies in some other way, beyond having a case of the disease? Is the belief that 40% of cases are asymptomatic wrong, and is it really 90% that are asymptomatic? Or, are the antibody tests not being done on a balanced sample of residents?

The two most likely areas of imprecision are the estimate of how many people don't develop symptoms and the test sampling method.

It is very difficult to accurately guess how many people have the virus without symptoms. One point, in particular, is that some people categorized as asymptomatic were simply pre-symptomatic – that is, at the time of the test, they had the disease but no symptoms, but possibly a day or two later, the symptoms developed. We don't know if any studies check back a day and a week later to see if symptoms later developed. We suspect very few do this, because the data is not so much being obtained by studies as it is by simple evaluation of test results – positive or negative test, and symptoms present or not.

Here is one round-up of studies that shows a huge skew in apparently asymptomatic sufferers (a low of 5% in one study, a high of 80% in another).[225] The CDC updated its estimate in mid-July; previously they had estimated 35% of people have no symptoms, and now they are saying 40%.[226]

If the 40% figure is correct (and of course it isn't all that different to 35% as they previously estimated), we still need some more explanation to reconcile the New York numbers. I guess this is due to sample bias – samples were collected primarily from people who may have had the virus already. There may also be a

---

[223] This is unlikely. New York has had such a high rate of testing that many asymptomatic cases are likely to have been identified and found. But let's allow the assumption because it makes it easier to do something that seems impossible – reconcile the claim of one-third of all people in the Bronx having virus antibodies.

[224] We could now be macabre and reduce this by the number of people who died, but again, let's give the numbers the benefit of the doubt.

[225] See https://www.cebm.net/covid-19/covid-19-what-proportion-are-asymptomatic/ or https://cov.cx/a1b06

[226] See https://baptisthealth.net/baptist-health-news/covid-19-roundup-new-estimate-of-asymptomatic-carriers-use-of-face-coverings-varies-and-update-on-lingering-symptoms/ or https://cov.cx/a1b07

tendency for the antibody test to generate false-positive results – perhaps confusing some other very similar antibody for a Covid antibody?

There are similar puzzling studies elsewhere, too, also reporting apparently much higher numbers of people with antibodies in their blood that suggest they've been "exposed to" Covid-19.[227]   Other studies use more empirical inferences to get numbers that also are in the order of ten times higher than official numbers.[228]

Even the CDC is suggesting the number of exposed people might be ten times higher than the counted number of cases, but if that is so, why – three weeks after the quoted comments from CDC Director Robert Redfield saying so[229] – did the CDC adjust its symptomless prevalence estimate from 35% to only 40%? Why did it ignore its own director's comments and not go up to 90% symptomless? Or in some other official way issue a policy document reconciling officially confirmed cases, symptomless cases, and implied-by-sampling total people exposed to the virus?

These are vitally important questions that demand answers. How many people really have – in some way – "experienced" the virus sufficiently to now have antibodies? Is it 6.5 million (current official case count)? Is it 10.9 million (adjusting for 40% symptomless and assuming none of them were included in the official count)?   Or is it 65 million (based on the "90% undetected" possibility)?

At 65 million, that is almost 20% of the country. That's not enough to get herd immunity, but it is a lot closer than is "only" 6.5 million.

The matter is however not as important as it might seem, because the herd immunity is temporary, rather than permanent. As I type these words on 2 November, whatever the actual number of people with "herd immunity", whether it be in the Bronx or the country in total, will have massively changed from the research that was done in July – indeed, maybe even most of those people have now had their immunity fade away to nothing already.

This brings us back to the assumptions embodied within a consideration of herd immunity.

We are assuming that everyone who has had the virus gets herd immunity for a while, and we might also be assuming that everyone who tests positive for

---

[227] See, for example, https://www.statnews.com/2020/07/21/cdc-study-actual-covid-19-cases/ or https://cov.cx/a1b08

[228] See https://www.nature.com/articles/s41467-020-18272-4 or https://cov.cx/a1b09

[229] See https://www.washingtonpost.com/health/2020/06/25/coronavirus-cases-10-times-larger/ or https://cov.cx/a1b10

antibodies also has immunity. The first of those assumptions is optimistic (because we now know for sure that some people are getting second infections three months or less after their first infection), and is limited by the likely short duration of the immunity received (maybe six months or so on average). The second of those assumptions is even more optimistic still.

Put it all together, and it seems the hope for herd immunity is unrealistic. Because it is only a short-term benefit, we'd need everyone to be getting the virus regularly and repeatedly – a classic good news/bad news scenario : The good news is that after having had the virus, you won't get it again for 3 – 6 months. The bad news is that after those 3 – 6 months, get ready to have the virus again. And then again in another 3 – 6 months. And so on, for the rest of your life – a life that sooner or later may well be shortened by the virus.

Herd immunity is like being with a group of your friends and saying "I hope all of you get the virus very soon because if you do, I am less likely to get the virus too". Isn't it the ultimate act of selfishness, and doesn't it shift our entire focus from wanting our community to beat the virus to instead quietly wishing they'd all catch the virus so that we won't get it too?

We can't sit back, do nothing, and wait for herd immunity to automatically kick in. I don't think it ever will, for the reasons outlined above. We need to pro-actively come up with cures and vaccines, and until then, we need to focus on outbreak control, social distancing, and mask-wearing.

PART TWO : About the Virus

4. How the Number of Infections Increased So Quickly

For most people, the virus suddenly "came from nowhere".[230] One day, all was calm, the next, it was something you read about in China, then it was something happening in an old people's home in the Seattle area (just a few miles from where I live), and then, the next thing you know, President Trump was banning travel from China, much to the outrage of many people, then declaring a state of emergency and we all started talking about "lockdowns" and "social distancing".

The virus burst into our lives suddenly and strongly. Here's just one example of how a single business meeting in Boston in late February resulted in the virus spreading around the country and world in the days and weeks that followed.[231] The virus, in ideal circumstances, can spread far and fast, and the cited example was being silently duplicated, all around the country, back in February and March (and has continued to do so, pretty much without stop, ever since).

People have often exclaimed the virus "caught us unawares". That is both true and untrue.

---

[230] Not to boast, but one of the benefits of being a Travel Insider is that you were getting briefed about and updates on the virus from me way back in January 2020.

[231] See https://www.sfgate.com/news/article/Genetic-data-show-how-a-single-superspreading-15512903.php or https://cov.cx/a1b11

It is untrue because there have been any number of published papers worrying about new respiratory type viruses appearing from nowhere, and the implications such new viruses might have on the world. There are entire departments at a state and national level of people who anticipate, plan for, prepare for, and monitor for such outbreaks. They run "simulation games" that model what would happen if/when such a virus was to appear in our midst.

Most other countries also have people tasked with such duties, and then we have the World Health Organization that is supposed to provide an overall global monitoring and coordination role.[232]

It is, however, also demonstrably true to say the virus outbreak caught us unawares. That is partially because of the way it grows in numbers. It starts slowly but then picks up speed.[233] There's something very counter-intuitive about this. By the time we'd realized the virus was *going to become* a major problem, it *had already become* a major problem.

The rate of growth of an infection depends on several different things. The two key variables are how long it takes from when one person gets infected to when they have in turn infected other people, and how many people each person infects.

Both numbers are of course important.

The longer the length of time between one cycle or generation of infections and the next, the more time we have to respond and react, and that's of course a very good thing. This time measurement is termed the **serial interval**.

But if we had to choose one of these two variables as the more important, it would be the second number – how many people that each infected person in turn infects.

---

[232] We're going to try and avoid dwelling too much on the colossal and catastrophic failures of any element of this infrastructure to respond adequately and quickly to the Covid-19 outbreak. But it is really hard not to sound off on these appalling betrayals of public trust by "experts" who only had one job to do – prepare for and advise on such things.

[233] From the first case in the US to reaching 1 million cases took 96 days. To go from 1 to 2 million cases took 44 days. To go from 2 to 3 million cases took 27 days. To go from 3 to 4 million cases took 15 days. Now it is taking about five days for each new million cases. See https://twitter.com/JHSPH_CHS/status/1334947286762270720 or https://cov.cx/a1f85

The Virus Reproduction Rate

The number of people each person infects is measured by what is known as the reproduction rate or sometimes called the reproduction number. It can be simply thought of as "how many new infections are created by an infected person". It is sometimes termed the Ro or R_o number, although to be exact, R_o refers to the initial rate of reproduction. Another value is Rt or R_t, which refers to the reproduction rate at a specific time.

There are three key things about this "R" measure and the way the virus spreads.

The **first** is that if the value is greater than 1.0, that means the virus is spreading and increasing in number. That should be intuitive – if each person infects more than one extra person, the total numbers grow and grow.

The **second** is that the value can change over time, based on things such as how "easy" it is for each person to pass the infection on – that being something which depends on social distancing, mask-wearing, and how many people have already either been vaccinated or had the virus and become immune to re-infection (assuming that such an immunity is created, something that is currently far from certain).

The **third** and most impactful thing is that this growth is geometric or exponential.[234] The easiest way to think of it is if we use an easy to calculate R number – 2.0.

So, we start with one person infected. At the end of the serial interval (whatever that might be), they have infected two people. Each of those two people goes on to infect two more people (four in total). Each of those four more people infects two more, and so on.

Now for the thing about geometric/exponential growth. It starts slowly but then "catches you by surprise" and risks becoming almost unstoppable.

It is the "catches you by surprise" element that is the most distinctive.

For example, look at this data series (immediately below). It shows the growth of two different objects over five time periods. Let's say you have a system that is capable of managing up to 2,000 events at a time, and you have two different types of events for the system to handle.

Which one do you think is going to be the most significant in the future? Maybe the blue and green lines are the numbers of two different infections in the

---

[234] For our purposes, we can consider the two terms, "geometric (growth)" and "exponential (growth)" as identical and interchangeable. There is a difference, but it isn't relevant to this discussion.

community, but of course, they could be anything and are just made-up for this example.

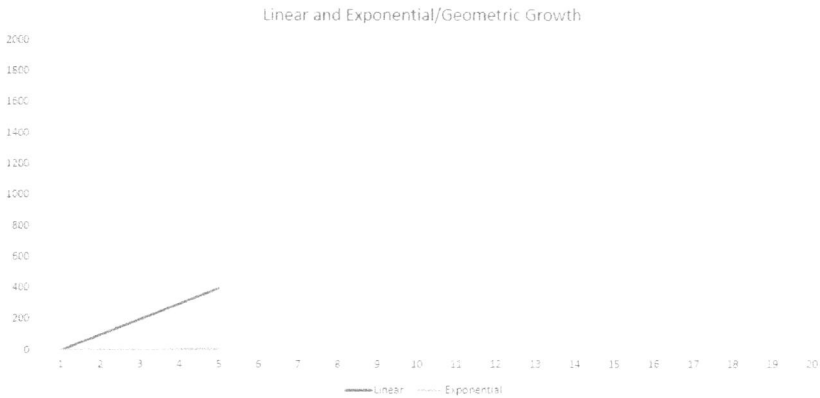

Figure 32 *Linear/Exponential Growth, 5 time periods*

Most people will glance at these two lines and immediately select the blue line as the more significant line, and not worry too much about either at the end of period five. Their perception of the green line is that it is probably also a straight line, but with a much lower rate of increase.

If you were deciding which of these two trends was the more significant and needed more immediate action, the chances are you'd choose the blue one too.

Now, let's extend the data series a bit further. Let's look at ten time periods.

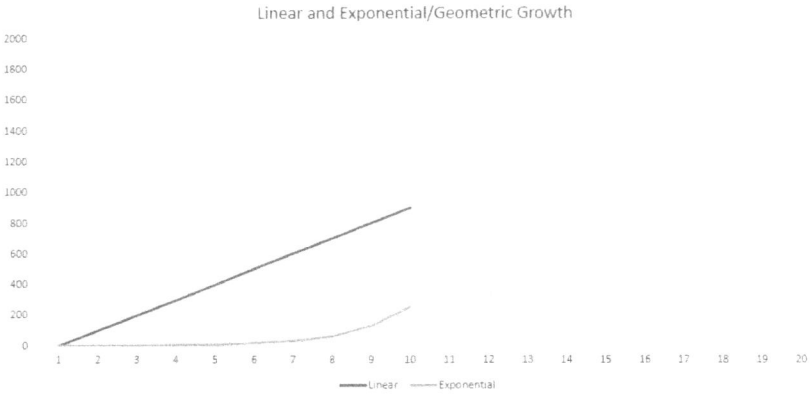

Figure 33 Linear/Exponential Growth, 10 time periods

What do you think now? You can see how the green line is starting to show itself as not flat, but curving upwards, and is steepening, but even at the tenth period it seems to only now be growing the same as the blue line, which has a huge head start over the green line and is reaching close to half of the system's total capacity.

Maybe this is the point where you start to become aware of, interested in, and concerned about the green line, but if you're focusing on "the bigger problem", you'll see that the blue line is showing a number four times greater than the green line.

Let's look at five more periods into this data series.

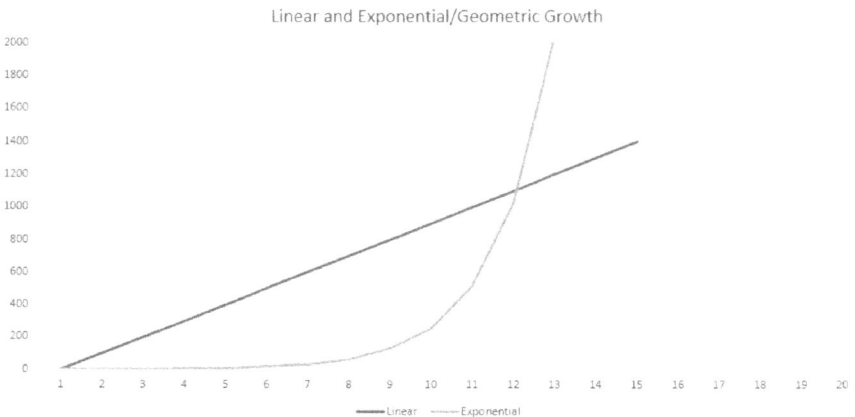

Figure 34 Linear/Exponential Growth, 15 time periods

The green line has now disappeared up and off the scale entirely. At some point in period 13, it went, within that single period, from initially less than the blue line value to "breaking the system" and exceeding its total capacity by the end of the period. It is so far out of the chart and beyond the system's capacity we don't even know where it is by the end of period 15.

Whereas in period 10 the blue line was showing a value four times greater than the green line, part-way through the 13th period, the green line had caught up, and at the end of the 15th period, although you can't see it, the green value is almost six times greater than the blue line – using the same chart scale, that means it stretches up more than another page and a half in this book before reaching its value. That's how far ahead it has gone.

Not only is it six times greater, but in number terms, it is so huge that it has "broken" your measurement scale – or, in real-world public health terms, has become an epidemic/pandemic[235] and is raging out of control.

It has "appeared from nowhere", in other words.

The point is we are usually slow to recognize and respond to geometric growth, and by its nature, it catches us unawares.

It might be helpful to put a real-world value on each of these numbered periods. It seems, for the coronavirus, its serial interval is about 4 days.[236]

That is very short compared to the time it takes to observe, become aware of, and respond to the virus. How long does it take to compile and collate data, and then distribute it to people, have them look at it, consider it, have meetings to discuss it, prepare draft plans, revise them, get approvals, and then act on it? Thinking of the several preceding charts, it is unlikely any "alarm bells" would ring after the fifth period (a mere 20 days from the start of everything). After the tenth period, numbers are still insignificant, and unless you were looking for the outbreak, you'd not see it (particularly because, in real life, China was obscuring what was happening for as long as possible).

Let's say it is the "unlucky" thirteenth period which forces people's attention. In the real world, probably the first thing that happens is that people seek

---

[235] In case you wondered, an epidemic is a disease that affects a large number of people in a region, community, or country. It is localized (although possibly to a large area). A pandemic is declared when a number of different regions, communities, countries, or continents are all suffering epidemics.

[236] See https://wwwnc.cdc.gov/eid/article/26/6/20-0357-f1 or https://cov.cx/a1b12 This is based on Chinese data, which we are reluctant to accept, but there are other studies that also show a similar value, for example https://www.sciencedirect.com/science/article/pii/S1201971220301193 or https://cov.cx/a1b13

verification and validation, during the fourteenth period (which is only half a week). We have a weekend (work stops but not the virus), and hurried discussions during the 15th period, and by the start of the 16th period, policy decisions are starting to be formulated, but then have to be revised due to the continued exponential growth, and now we're already at the 17th period. (And don't forget, after having decided on action, there will be a delay in implementing such actions.) Where are we then?

Just for grins, let's look forward another five data points, and this time, see how we've changed the values on the y (vertical) axis to allow the green line values to stay on the chart.

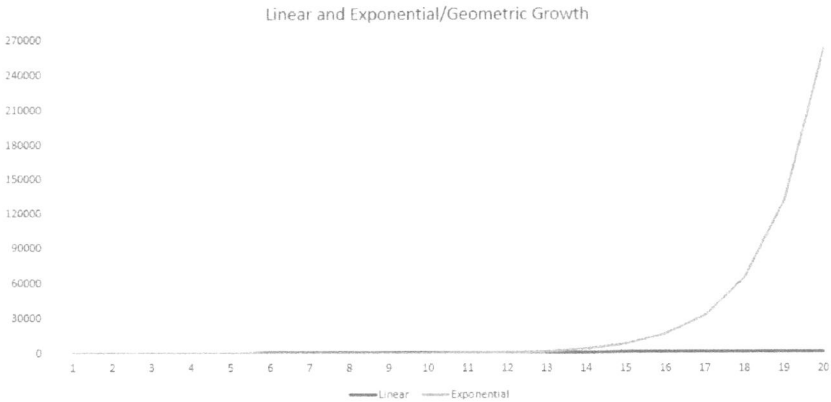

Figure 35 Linear/Exponential Growth, 20 time periods

As you can see, this again shows the "appeared from nowhere" phenomenon. The green line looks to be flat, at almost zero, for thirteen time periods, but then it lifts off and starts soaring up the chart in the next half dozen time periods.

And where now is the blue line? On this scale, the blue line that dominated the first two charts is now lost somewhere in the bottom of the chart, all the way along. The green line value at the end of the 20th period is now 138 times greater than the blue line.

This is so amazing that we'll dwell on it a bit more. The charts above assumed an R value of 2 – a simple doubling every period. What is the actual value of R for the Covid-19 virus? That has changed over time, and these days it is much lower than it was originally because of our social distancing and masks – by making it harder for the virus to spread, its R rate of course decreases.

But in the earlier stages, it was generally thought to be around the 2.5 area, with some studies convincingly showing it was much higher in the earliest times with no social distancing.[237]

Let's look at a table of numbers of infected people with an R value of 2.5 and serial interval of four days, showing the number of weeks it takes to get to each new number of infections.

Of course, as we know, while the virus was growing at that rate to start with, its rate of growth mercifully slowed down.

Weeks	Newly Infected	Total Infected	Note
0	1	1	
0.6	3	4	A single family
1.1	6	10	
1.7	16	25	
2.3	39	64	
2.9	98	162	
3.4	244	406	An entire school
4.0	610	1,017	
4.6	1,526	2,542	
5.1	3,815	6,357	A small town
5.7	9,537	15,894	
6.3	23,842	39,736	
6.9	59,605	99,340	
7.4	149,012	248,352	
8.0	372,529	620,881	
8.6	931,323	1,552,204	A large city
9.1	2,328,306	3,880,510	A small country
9.7	5,820,766	9,701,276	
10.3	14,551,915	24,253,191	
10.8	36,379,788	60,632,979	
11.4	90,949,470	151,582,450	
12.0	227,373,675	378,956,125	The entire US and Canada
12.6	568,434,189	947,390,314	
13.1	1,421,085,472	2,368,475,785	China and India
13.7	3,552,713,679	5,921,189,464	Nearly the entire world
14.3	8,881,784,197	14,802,973,661	
14.8	22,204,460,493	37,007,434,154	
15.4	55,511,151,231	92,518,585,385	Almost everyone who has ever lived

Figure 36 An example of Exponential Growth

[237] This higher value has been vividly confirmed in August in New Zealand, where the country, which had been virus-free for 102 days and had returned to normal life with no need for social distancing at all, discovered that someone one new case of the virus had come into the country undetected. Within a couple of weeks (about four generations), there were over 100 cases discovered, all as a result of that one case, suggesting an R value in the order of 3.

The key point again here is to note that the growth is "below the radar" for most of the time, the same as it was with the blue and green lines above. If unchecked, it would take only three weeks to go from less than a large city to more than the entire US, and less than two more weeks to span the entire world.

This table above clearly illustrates the sneaky way geometric progression evolves. It all happens in the last short period of time. A single week before the US is fully infected, only a fifth of the county is infected, and two weeks before, only about 3% of the country is infected. That is still a lot of people but gives no obvious hint that within two weeks, it will have spread further to the entire country, and then another two weeks on will have taken over the world.

You've heard the proverb "A stitch in time saves nine". Nowhere is it more apt than when it comes to controlling disease outbreaks. It is essential to stop these things before they become unstoppable and before it becomes too late.[238]

The good news, and obviously, we've slowed the rate of disease spread, both in the US and in most other countries. But we've not stopped it.

Now, I know what you're saying. You're saying "David, those are interesting numbers, but it isn't what actually happened. So where is the reality and why?"?

The Actual Serial Interval and Reproduction Rate Values for SARS-CoV-2

Until now, we've been using a simple easy example, with an R value of 2.0 for the charts, and 2.5 for the table.

What are the actual observed serial interval and reproduction rate values for the coronavirus?

---

[238] This is an important concept because it also applies to each person and how they are individually treated. To start with, a person is infected with a low number of virus particles. They replicate and double, then they double again and again and again, and so on. When they are growing by some number of thousand particles per doubling, it is so much easier to fight and eliminate the infection than when they are growing by billions of particles per doubling.

This simple truth explains why it is so important to urgently start treating an infection with anti-viral drugs as utterly soon as possible. But this simple truth is being ignored by our healthcare authorities who tell us just to stay at home and hope for the best if we're infected, and only go to a hospital if our symptoms become severe.

In years to come, when people write books (maybe even me!) analyzing what happened and how we responded to the virus threat; the lack of interest in deploying early-infection treatments will stand out as one of the most colossal of all our many failures.

The serial interval probably has not changed much over time. The serial interval is less variable, and also much less studied – perhaps because it is not as important as the reproduction rate value. A virus will spread (or not) with any serial interval value, it just does it more quickly/slowly. It is primarily the reproduction rate that determines the contagiousness and severity of a disease.

Having said that, some studies show that the serial interval is shorter for infection to close contacts, and longer for infection to strangers. That makes obvious sense – you're living with your family all the time, and probably with no masks or social distancing, so that makes it easy for the virus to move to other family members as soon as it can. Masks and social distancing slow the spread on to other people.

As we looked at before, the value of four days has been cited as a possible serial interval although there's a wide variance around that mean point. Intuitively, this feels a little on the short side, but if we accept it as it is, it surely shows how short the time is between "barely there" and "ranging out of control, everywhere".

Another study suggests a serial interval of 6 – 9 days, but we view that as possibly an outlier at the high end of what should be expected.[239]

The R value in particular has changed over time, which, as we explained before, is to be expected. Not only do social distancing and mask measures reduce the infection rate, but there's another factor as well that starts to kick in later in an infection cycle – the fact that it gets harder and harder for the virus to find new people to infect.

If the virus typically infects three other people, but if one-third of the population has now had the virus, then one of the three possible new infections

---

[239] See https://wwwnc.cdc.gov/eid/article/26/7/20-0282_article or https://cov.cx/a1b14 . Unfortunately, this statement of the serial interval as being 6 – 9 days immediately destroys the credibility of the study. Just like an average is not a range, but a single number, so too is a serial interval a single number, not a range. Giving the serial interval a range means "we really don't know what it actually is so we're guessing". To be kind to the article/study, it too was based on Chinese data, which may be, ahem, "imperfect".

The same study also suggests an R value of 5.7. This is interesting, because calculating either the serial interval or the R value, based on observing the rate of growth of an outbreak of a disease, has the two numbers inter-related. It is sort of like saying "something times something = 60". If the first number is six, then the second number has to be 10, and if the first number is 12, the second number has to be five, and so on. So if they are using a range of numbers for the serial interval, they should be using a range of numbers for the reproduction number, too.

Yes, they do show a confidence interval, but that is a slightly different thing.

no longer happens because the person already is or has been infected, so the R rate drops from 3 to 2, and so on as the number of infections increases (we discuss this further in our section on "Herd Immunity" below – see page 216). For now, however, even with over 10 million cases in the US, we're still so far away from any measurable herd immunity impact that it is best ignored entirely.

You can look at the excellent https://rt.live website and see how the Rt value has changed for each state from March until now. The scales on each chart only go up to 2.0, but the early R values in some states (for example, Illinois) were as high as 3.5 and New Jersey peaked at just over 4.0.

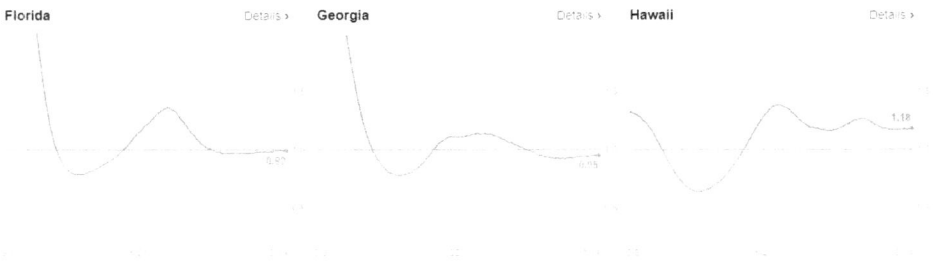

Figure 37 How R values change over time

The above chart, from rt.live, shows how the R value has changed quite dramatically over time in different states. When the value is greater than 1.0, it is shown in red, and this indicates growing rates of new cases every day; when it is below 1.0, it is shown in green to denote shrinking rates of new cases.

In all three states, it could be said that about when social distancing controls were introduced, the R value dropped, and daily new case numbers started dropping. But then, as you know, most states relaxed their social distancing requirements and case numbers started growing again. Some states have now reintroduced social distancing in some form and case numbers have started dropping again.

Whatever the R value is in real life, it seems that without social distancing and masks, it is definitely greater than 1.0 so new case numbers have a propensity to grow in value.

Studies have suggested values ranging between 1.5 and 3.5 as the "normal/natural" rate, but those numbers are so enormously variable as to be without much underlying value.

As a comparison, the seasonal 'flu is often cited as having a reproduction rate of 1.3 (although this can vary a bit from year to year), the common cold is in the range of 2.0 − 3.0, and at the high end of the scale, Mumps, Chickenpox, and Measles all have terrifyingly high rates of about 10 − 12.[240] [241]

Okay, you've probably now got the point, several times over, about geometric growth!

---

[240] See https://en.wikipedia.org/wiki/Basic_reproduction_number or https://cov.cx/a1b15

[241] There are two reasons why these high numbers are so terrifying, one obvious and one more subtle. The obvious reason is because of how quickly the diseases can spread. The subtle reason is that the higher the R number, the harder it is to get herd immunity. We discuss this further in the herd immunity section, further on in the document.

5. How Serious is the Virus?

I t is fair to pause and both ask and attempt to answer the question – is the virus really a problem? Is this book really necessary, and should you even bother reading it? Do we truly need to lock-down our country and spend trillions of dollars fighting it? To wear masks everywhere we go, inside and outside? Or is this all some type of irrational overreaction? A hoax/conspiracy?

Even though that is a huge range of possible interpretations, you'll find plenty of people who sincerely believe every one of those different views.

We can understand how, back in January/February/March, there was a wide divergence of opinion on this matter, because little was known, little had yet happened, and perhaps because people really couldn't comprehend the magnitude of what was threatened. As we said in the previous chapter, it is almost impossible to visualize the future implications of an exponential growth curve, and even harder to accept them.

Back in the early stages of our country's fight with the virus, many people would quote annual deaths from 'flu (typically 40,000 or fewer for a full year in the US[242]) and then compare that to a total number of US deaths from the coronavirus, back in Jan/Feb/March, which by 31 March had only just reached

---

[242] For the last nine years, estimated 'flu deaths have ranged from a low of 12,000 in 2011-12 to a high of 61,000 in 2017-18. See https://www.cdc.gov/flu/about/burden/index.html or https://cov.cx/a1b16

5,000 dead. They would then sneer, laugh, and say "See, this is only one-eighth as serious as the regular 'flu".

That was *never a fair statement to make*. Depending on when you choose to define the start of the US Covid-19 infection, the end of March represented probably less than two months of the outbreak. A better measure, on 31 March, was not the 5,206 deaths accumulated so far, but the 1,101 new deaths reported on that single day.[243] Assuming no further rate of increase (or decrease) that would represent an annual death count of almost 400,000 people. Compare that number to a year's worth of 'flu deaths, and now you get a very different reading of the relative severity of the two diseases. On that basis, Covid is ten times more serious than 'flu, and only cancer and heart disease kill more people a year.

Remarkably, even now, people will say "Only 243,000 people (in the US) have died of the virus; that is unfortunate, but not worth destroying our economy over".

We'll leave the value judgment inherent in equating the respective worth of lives and the economy to others. But the logic and the math of that statement is as flawed and faulty as the earlier statement quoted above.

The thing is, 243,000 people have died as of 7 November, and that is after all the social distancing, closures, mask-wearing, and everything else that has bedeviled our lives for the last eight months. We can only guess at how many more would have died if we'd lived our lives normally with no change, as happens with the seasonal 'flu.

In other words, yes, **Covid-19 truly is a very big thing**. Even after all the measures we've taken, it has still killed 243,000 people so far. The death toll is predicted to possibly reach 326,000 by 1 December,[244] [245] and 410,000 by the

---

[243] There's that exponential thing at work again. The total deaths for two months are 5,206, and of those, 1,101 of them all happened in the previous day.

[244] See https://covid19.healthdata.org/united-states-of-america or https://cov.cx/ihme - this site regularly updates its predictions based on the ongoing data collection and changing current situation. As of its 3 September update, it is showing a projection for 325,907 deaths by 1 December, and 410,451 by the end of the year, with over 2500 more deaths every day to bring us into the new year. Who only knows when and at what number the final total will be.

[245] Good news. A revised projection on 18 September is showing a reduced 378,321 possible deaths by 1 Jan.

And, another update – a projection on 9 October has reduced the forecast further to 321,140. And another update – as of the 29 October projection, the total is now looking to be 326,660.

end of the year (which, while the end of the calendar year, is still less than a full twelve months of the virus outbreak).

Your Risk of Dying

Never mind the "theoretical" numbers above. The thing most of us want to know is will we, ourselves, and our loved ones, live or die?

That's a truly hard question to answer. To be at risk of dying, you first have to catch the virus, and whether you do that or not is anyone's guess and in large part up to you.

There have been observations of the virus "unfairly" impacting some groups of people more than others. This is more likely to be a lifestyle issue than due to genetics. But there is one interesting thing that has been noticed – people with Type O blood seem to be slightly less at risk of catching the virus than people with other blood types.[246] However, there is no indication whether being more at risk of catching the virus transfers to also being more at risk of having a severe infection and of dying. However, another study suggests people with Type A or AB blood are more at risk of complications.[247]

If you follow "best practices" (see "PART THREE : Avoiding the Virus", below) you have a good chance of avoiding an infection completely – even the most gloomy of predictions are not currently suggesting that more than half the population will get the disease.[248] If you do become infected, it seems you've something like a 50/50 chance of getting only a mild infection that you'll barely even notice, and in such cases, with such a mild infection, your chance of dying is very close to zero.

And what about your chances if you do have a noticeable infection? That is an easy question to ask, but a surprisingly difficult one to answer.

Before we go any further, we have to rebut a misapprehension that we've seen in several places. To work out your risk of dying, it is *not* usual to express the **total deaths from the disease as a percentage of the total population**.

---

[246] See https://www.statnews.com/2020/09/14/23andme-study-covid-19-genetic-link/ or https://cov.cx/a1b17

[247] See https://www.hematology.org/newsroom/press-releases/2020/possible-link-between-blood-type-and-covid-19 or https://cov.cx/a1f99

[248] Although one wonders why the projections stop at 50%. Why don't they keep projecting further? A partial answer is they are allowing for herd immunity, but as we increasingly perceive herd immunity to be temporary rather than permanent, there's sadly less reason why one couldn't create a seemingly valid model projecting closer to 100% virus spread.

Certainly, if you do this, it accurately expresses what percentage of the country has died, to date. In early December, that number was 0.09%, which sounds encouragingly low, doesn't it.

But that number doesn't predict the future – the virus is still with us, and the number of deaths and therefore percentage is increasing every day, and so is not a valid measure. It is a helpful measure when a disease has finally run its course, or as a historical measure of a certain period of time, but it doesn't relate to you or your personal and future chances of surviving/dying.

The calculation is mathematically correct but devoid of meaning.

It also shows a very low number, and the problem with that is some people have used the low number as an excuse/justification for engaging in risky behavior. But if you engage in risky behavior, your chance of becoming infected skyrockets up, and so too, therefore, does your chance of dying.

The people who use this faulty logic are in effect saying the same as a person who would reason "my chance of dying in a car crash today is so close to zero as to be impossible to measure, therefore it is safe for me to drive at 100 mph around town after drinking all day"!

What you probably most want to know is "*If I get infected*, what are my chances of surviving or dying". The first part of that question is the implied "Assuming that I get infected" and the question behind that question is "what are the chances of me getting infected"?

Of course, that is an important question too, but whereas we can make some general observations about your chances of surviving an infection, it is very much harder to make observations about your chances of getting infected to start with, because that is very much up to you and your lifestyle and activities. What we do in this book is help you to understand how to minimize the risks and chances of becoming infected - see the part of the book "PART THREE : Avoiding the Virus", below, starting on page 213.

Now, back to your chance/risk of dying, *if you get infected*. A problem with understanding your chances of dying is because about half the people who get the disease don't even know they have it. This means it is hard to know the total number of infected people, which is one of the two numbers we need to get your chance of dying.

The other hard to know number is how many people have actually died of the disease. You might think that is an easy thing to count, but it is surprisingly difficult. For example, what say you were diagnosed with the disease but weren't even in a hospital – it was a mild case. Then one day, you got in a car crash and died in the pileup.[249] Would that be a Covid-19 death? Some states say yes it is,[250] others say no it isn't.

What say you're 102 years old, and in a hospice with terminal cancer. You then catch the virus, and a week later you're dead. What is the cause? The cancer? Old age? Or the virus? Some states blame the virus, others don't.

An extension of that second scenario is to wonder if it is correct to equate the death of someone who has lived a long and full life, and now is frail and with a very short life expectancy,[251] on the one hand, with the death of someone who is in their prime of life, healthy, robust, athletic, and with no reason not to anticipate many more decades of great good health.

It is certainly true that the older you get, the more likely a coronavirus infection is to become fatal. This is not always the case with other viruses – sometimes young people suffer more severe mortality rates, and sometimes, risks are evenly spread.

- *The Imprecision of Death Certificates and Recording Causes of Death*

It is interesting and possibly helpful to understand how deaths are analyzed in the US. Every death requires a death certificate, which records the immediate final cause of death. Beyond that are additional lines to enter conditions that contributed to or caused the ultimate final cause of death, and space for other related conditions that while not a direct cause of death, probably had some bearing on the person dying.

Here are two samples of completed example death certificates that show how this is recorded.[252]

---

[249] A more extreme example – you are mugged and shot/killed by the mugger. In WA state, there are five cases of this happening, and the deaths were recorded as Covid-19 deaths. Most people would not consider that to have anything to do with Covid-19. See https://www.kxly.com/three-percent-of-washingtons-reported-covid-19-deaths-may-be-inaccurate/ or https://cov.cx/a1g02

[250] See https://cbs12.com/news/local/man-who-died-in-motorcycle-crash-counted-as-covid-19-death-in-florida-report or https://cov.cx/a1g01

[251] The expression "One foot in the grave, the other on a banana skin" comes to mind!

[252] See https://www.cdc.gov/nchs/data/dvs/DEATH11-03final-acc.pdf or https://cov.cx/a1b18 for a detailed explanation of how death certificates are filled out and for more complete examples.

CAUSE OF DEATH (See instructions and examples)

32 **PART I.** Enter the chain of events--diseases, injuries, or complications--that directly caused the death. DO NOT enter terminal events such as cardiac arrest, respiratory arrest, or ventricular fibrillation without showing the etiology. DO NOT ABBREVIATE. Enter only one cause on a line. Add additional lines if necessary.

Approximate interval: Onset to death

IMMEDIATE CAUSE (Final disease or condition ---------> resulting in death)	a. Rupture of myocardium Due to (or as a consequence of)	Minutes
Sequentially list conditions, if any, leading to the cause listed on line a. Enter the	b. Acute myocardial infarction Due to (or as a consequence of):	6 days
UNDERLYING CAUSE (disease or injury that initiated the events resulting	c. Coronary artery thrombosis Due to (or as a consequence of):	5 years
in death) **LAST**	d. Atherosclerotic coronary artery disease	7 years

PART II. Enter other significant conditions contributing to death but not resulting in the underlying cause given in PART I

Diabetes, Chronic obstructive pulmonary disease, smoking

33. WAS AN AUTOPSY PERFORMED? ■ Yes No

34. WERE AUTOPSY FINDINGS AVAILABLE TO COMPLETE THE CAUSE OF DEATH? ■ Yes No

35. DID TOBACCO USE CONTRIBUTE TO DEATH? ■ Yes Probably No Unknown

36. IF FEMALE
■ Not pregnant within past year
Pregnant at time of death
Not pregnant, but pregnant within 42 days of death
Not pregnant, but pregnant 43 days to 1 year before death
Unknown if pregnant within the past year

37. MANNER OF DEATH
■ Natural Homicide
Accident Pending investigation
Suicide Could not be determined

Figure 38 Sample Death Certificate 1

CAUSE OF DEATH (See instructions and examples)

32 **PART I.** Enter the chain of events--diseases, injuries, or complications--that directly caused the death. DO NOT enter terminal events such as cardiac arrest, respiratory arrest, or ventricular fibrillation without showing the etiology. DO NOT ABBREVIATE. Enter only one cause on a line. Add additional lines if necessary.

Approximate interval: Onset to death

IMMEDIATE CAUSE (Final disease or condition ---------> resulting in death)	a. Aspiration pneumonia Due to (or as a consequence of)	2 Days
Sequentially list conditions, if any, leading to the cause listed on line a. Enter the	b. Complications of coma Due to (or as a consequence of)	7 weeks
UNDERLYING CAUSE (disease or injury that initiated the events resulting	c. Blunt force injuries Due to (or as a consequence of)	7 weeks
in death) **LAST**	d. Motor vehicle accident	7 weeks

PART II. Enter other significant conditions contributing to death but not resulting in the underlying cause given in PART I

33. WAS AN AUTOPSY PERFORMED? ■ Yes No

34. WERE AUTOPSY FINDINGS AVAILABLE TO COMPLETE THE CAUSE OF DEATH? ■ Yes No

35. DID TOBACCO USE CONTRIBUTE TO DEATH? Yes Probably ■ No Unknown

36. IF FEMALE
Not pregnant within past year
Pregnant at time of death
Not pregnant, but pregnant within 42 days of death
Not pregnant, but pregnant 43 days to 1 year before death
Unknown if pregnant within the past year

37. MANNER OF DEATH
Natural Homicide
■ Accident Pending Investigation
Suicide Could not be determined

38. DATE OF INJURY (Mo/Day/Yr) (Spell Month)	39. TIME OF INJURY	40. PLACE OF INJURY (e.g., Decedent's home; construction site; restaurant; wooded area)	41. INJURY AT WORK?
August 15, 2003	Approx. 2320	road side near state highway	Yes ■ No

Figure 39 Sample Death Certificate 2

So, what does it take on a death certificate for the death to be counted as a Covid-19 death? Is it necessary for the virus to be cited on line 32a?[253] Can it be cited anywhere in the Part I panel? What about the Part II panel? While there's usually no doubt *when* a person dies, accurately categorizing the "why" and "how" of their death becomes more uncertain.

Making the matter even more frustrating is it seems, at least for some of the time, different states have different guidelines for how to report Covid-19, and

253 It would not normally appear here. Physicians advise me the typical cause of death is cited as respiratory failure.

possibly then different federal agencies have different guidelines for how they look for Covid-19 mentions on death certificates.[254]

On the other hand, other reports suggest death numbers are being undercounted. This is usually done by looking at the total number of people dying of all causes and seeing if the total numbers are up or down on last year. If the numbers are up, there is a possibility it is due to virus-related reasons, and if the official count of virus-related deaths doesn't match the overall increase, the logic suggests that therefore the virus-related death count is too low.[255]

So, high or low? I don't think anyone knows, for sure. So even though the numbers mightn't be exactly correct, let's use them with our fingers crossed, and try to get a better handle on your particular chances. [256]

First, if we look at the cases we do know about, late on Thursday 13 August 2020, the US had officially counted 5,397,797 cases and 169,892 deaths. So, a

---

[254] This is not only a problem in the US. In the UK, for example, for the longest time, if you didn't die in a hospital, the public health authorities refused to consider that your cause of death could be Covid-related. This undercounted a lot of elderly/nursing home/hospice type Covid-19 deaths.

[255] See, for example, https://news.yahoo.com/covid-deaths-europe-us-exceed-164917547.html or https://cov.cx/a1b19 and, for the US, https://www.cdc.gov/mmwr/volumes/69/wr/mm6942e2.htm or https://cov.cx/a1b20

Most recently, this 3 December 2020 article suggests the unofficial death toll in the US might be almost 400,000 at a time when the official count is 274,000 – see https://www.mediaite.com/news/staggering-new-cdc-data-suggests-true-coronavirus-death-toll-is-now-near-400000/ or https://cov.cx/a1f59

These types of estimates are very imprecise, however. For example, as a result of less driving, vehicle deaths have dropped during the Covid period. There are probably other dependent increases and decreases too.

[256] This imprecision has inevitably caused some people to believe that there is a deliberate distortion in the official count of Covid-19 deaths. The only problem is, it seems for every person who claims the death count is being deliberately overstated, there's another person who believes the death count is being deliberately understated.

What do I think? I'm not sure there are deliberate policies to under- or overcount the deaths. If there are such policies, it seems the possible cases of over-counting in some jurisdictions are being matched by under-counting in other jurisdictions. Perhaps the two balance each other out? Regrettably, a more likely explanation is simply one of bureaucratic bungling and incompetence.

I guess I'm a simple soul. I'm happy to accept the basic statement "this disease is dangerous and deadly, and a lot of people are dying from it" without demanding to know the exact count.

very simple measure is to say that if you are officially counted as a case, then you have a 96.8% of surviving.

But even that number is far from accurate[257] and doesn't tell the whole story. Look at these two charts, one of daily new cases, the other of daily new deaths.

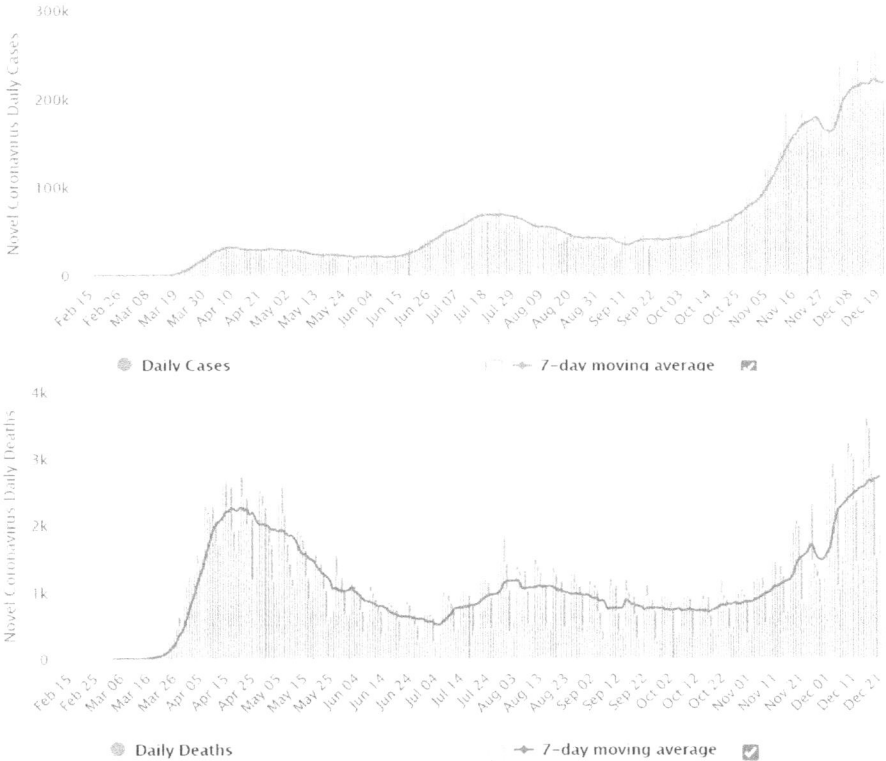

Figure 40 US daily case and daily death rates

What we're showing here is how in April, when new cases were averaging just over 25,000 a day, death rates went as high as 2,000 a day – 8%. In July, new case rates went as high as 65,000 (more than twice the rate in April), but deaths peaked at about 1,000 a day (about half the April rate) resulting in a much lower

---

[257] There are problems with matching all cases with all deaths, especially in the early stages of an infection, but now that we have many months and large numbers, those problems become less significant and for the purposes of this simplified discussion, it is probably acceptable to use this simple approach, because in any event, we are going on to say it is not a good measure!

death rate – a bit under 2.0%. In December, cases are running around 220,000 a day, while deaths are around 2,700, a bit under 1.5%.[258]

Perhaps we have got much better at treating people with the virus, and hopefully this learning curve will continue to improve into the future.[259] So the overall average of 3.2% includes the higher mortality rate when we were still learning how to treat the virus. A better number to look at now is more like 1.75% - or, to see the glass as half full rather than half empty, a survival rate of 98.25%.

There's another "confounding" factor as well. We are testing more people these days, including people who are not yet sure they are infected, so more of the people with "unknown" infections are getting discovered. That means that the average "test-confirmed sufferer" now is not as sick as they were back in April, and is another reason why the survival rate appears to have improved.

---

[258] If you look closely, you'll note that the death curve lags some weeks behind the case curve. That is only to be expected – a person registers as a case usually several weeks before they die. The lag between cases and deaths is made worse by delays in then registering the death as a Covid-19 death. For the purpose of our simplistic analysis here, it is not necessary to drill down into more detail on this point, because there are other much more substantial modifiers that need to be applied to this calculation as well. We discuss these in the following sections.

[259] A key consideration here though is to understand that our improvements in care and the reduction in mortality primarily relate to patients who are most severely afflicted. That's a small percentage of all patients, and a situation we're of course eager to improve. There has been little or no improvement whatsoever in the standard of care and responses offered to patients when they are initially infected and only mildly affected.

Of course we're delighted to see any and all reductions in mortality. But we most want to see a reduction in people who become moderately or severely affected by the virus – a reduction in the number of people who ever need to enter the ICU ward in the first place.

While some researchers are diligently evaluating possible cures and drugs to moderate the severity of an infection, we note the massive unwillingness by most medical practitioners to "think outside the box" and consider, let alone recommend, their patients consider some of the treatments that we detail further in this document. Here we are, 50+ million cases into the disease worldwide, and the standard advice to a newly infected patient is nothing more than to take it easy and drink plenty of fluids. That is appalling.

It is unclear how much of the improvement in survival rates is due to better treatments and how much is due to more testing and the detection of milder cases.[260]

This huge apparent shift in mortality rates – dropping from about 8% down to about 2%[261] (very approximate) causes another problem. Many – most – of the "official studies" were done with March and April data, not with July or October/November data. Clearly, the truth has remarkably changed over the months. If you're doing your own research, you need to keep an eye on what period of time the data you are viewing was obtained.

So with all these disclaimers, let's see if we can't "drill down" a bit and get closer to understanding what your chance of surviving the disease may be.

Never mind the "all men are created equal" concept. When it comes to the virus, there is no equality whatsoever. Some people are ten or even one hundred times more at risk than others.[262]

Age-Related Risk

Probably the biggest influencing factor in terms of disease outcomes is how old you are. The older you are, the worse your chances of surviving it.

---

[260] The charts on the IHME site do a great job of showing estimated daily infections, based on the total number of daily tests and known infections, with the assumption being that the more tests that are done, the more unknown cases are detected, as well as actual daily infections, as do the charts on the rt.live site. See https://covid19.healthdata.org/united-states-of-america?view=infections-testing&tab=trend&test=infections or https://cov.cx/a1b21 and the various state charts from this page https://rt.live/ or https://cov.cx/rtl

[261] Now, in November, you could credibly suggest the case fatality rate is even lower still – perhaps 1.5% these days. It is very hard to say, because of the unknown lag between when cases are reported and when deaths related to the new cases on a given day are reported, and because of the rapidly changing numbers of new daily cases.

[262] Or, if you prefer, some people are 100 or more times *less* at risk than others.

Interestingly,[263] the CDC hesitates to correlate age and death, but they are willing to match age with the likelihood of being hospitalized.[264]

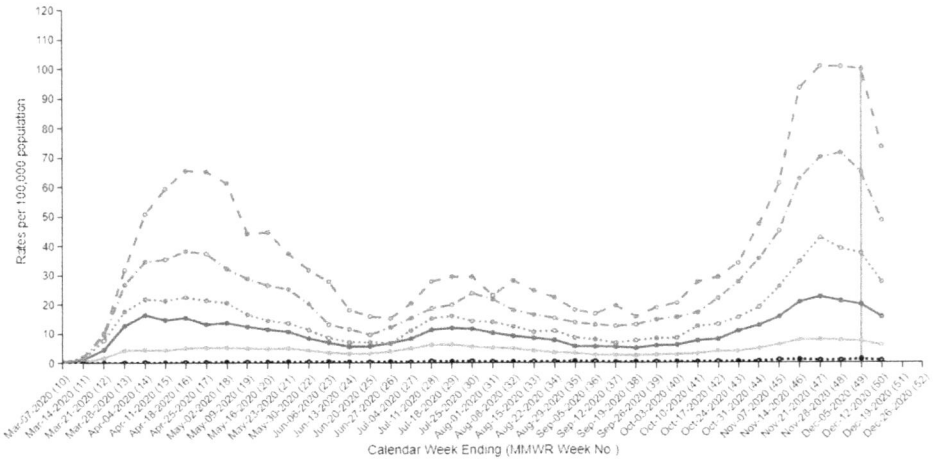

Figure 41 Hospitalization rates by age

To explain, the lines from top to bottom are for 85+ yr olds, 75-84, 65-74, 50-64, 18-49, and under 18.

These are not entirely meaningful numbers, unfortunately, because we don't know what percentage these numbers are of all people getting the disease in each age group.

Any hospitalization first requires you to get the disease and then to become sufficiently seriously unwell and require being admitted to a hospital. To tell us the overall number of people being hospitalized is a great example of a statistic

---

[263] And frustratingly. While it is interesting to know what our chances are of being hospitalized, surely the ultimate issue we all most want to know is what are our chances of living or dying. Our western aversion to anything to do with death, while understandable, needs to be kept out of a discussion that is necessarily all about death (and its happier twin, survival)!

[264] See https://gis.cdc.gov/grasp/COVIDNet/COVID19_3.html or https://cov.cx/a1b22

that may be perfectly correct, but which is also unhelpful to the point of being meaningless![265] [266]

This second chart is also a bit puzzling, but it gives a very vivid depiction of the bottom-line impact of age on death rates.[267]

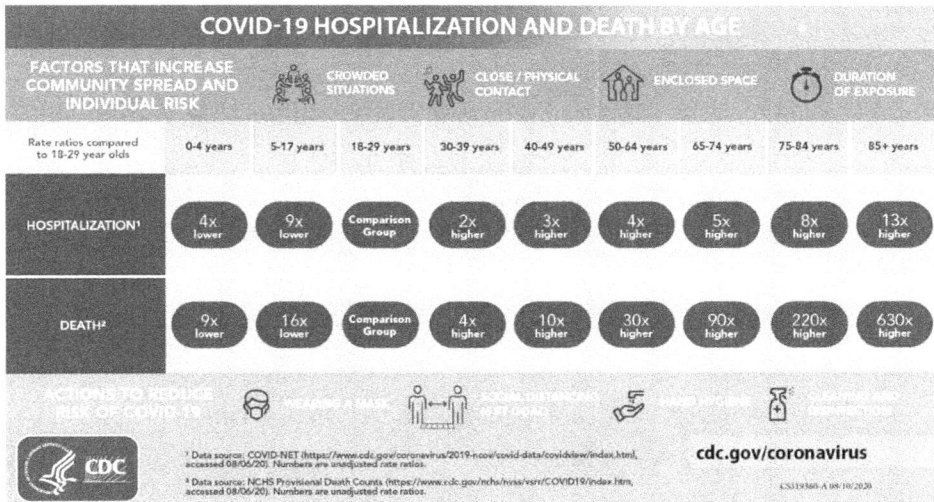

Figure 42 Hospitalization and death rates by age

---

[265] That's a bit like a table of bungee jumping deaths by age group. That's not something most of us never need to worry about, because we're unlikely to voluntarily go bungee jumping!

If you don't jump, you have no risk at all. The relevant measure is what percentage of people who jump will die, rather than what percentage of everyone will die from a bungee jump (whether they ever actually jump or not).

Oh, in case you're wondering, bungee jumping, while appearing to be risky and terrifying, is actually quite safe. It has a very low fatality rate – about one in every half-million jumps. And, yes, I have jumped. Once, but for sure, never a second time!

[266] If that phrase and concept "a statistic that may be perfectly correct, but which is also unhelpful to the point of being meaningless" sounds familiar, it is because we used it just a few pages before when talking about total deaths per million people. This is a subtle trap in data analysis – citing numbers that sound exact and important, but which are actually meaningless.

[267] See https://www.cdc.gov/coronavirus/2019-ncov/covid-data/investigations-discovery/hospitalization-death-by-age.html or https://cov.cx/a1b23

Compared to people aged 18 – 29, if you are 65 – 74, you've a five times greater rate of being hospitalized and a 90 times higher risk of dying. And if you're over 85, the number is astonishingly greater again.

It can also be derived from this chart that the risk of dying, after being hospitalized, goes up with age as well. You see that 30 – 39 year-olds have twice the chance of being hospitalized, but four times the risk of dying, while 50 – 64 year-olds have four times the chance of being hospitalized, but not four times the risk of dying, but a massive 30 times more.

These numbers are helpful, but there's still a vital pair of data points missing. What is the risk of hospitalization or dying for the benchmark 18 – 29 yr old? We can't conveniently determine that from this chart. So yet again, while we know the risk is much higher or lower depending on your age, it is difficult to put an exact number on it, and of course, that's what most of us instinctively would wish to have.

We need to point out something that is little appreciated. While it is true that very few children seem to contract severe or fatal cases of Covid, that does not mean they are not at risk. There are a couple of important considerations.

First, an infected child can still pass their infection on to other people.[268]

Second, there is increasing awareness of recovered children now showing signs of various lasting harm and damage to their arteries and veins.[269]

Another source[270] studied the chance of patients dying in a number of countries. The word "patient" isn't defined, but we assume it means "someone who has been admitted to hospital" rather than referring to everyone known to have been infected.

There are surprising differences in death rates in different countries (huge differences – in some countries you have a ten times greater chance of dying than in other countries) so we hesitate to consider the numbers in the study as anything other than indicative and confirming the general concept that older people are much more at risk.

---

[268] See, for example, https://www.mana.md/can-children-spread-covid-19/ or https://cov.cx/a1f93

[269] See https://www.studyfinds.org/children-with-covid-blood-vessel-damage/ or https://cov.cx/a1f92

[270] See https://www.sciencedirect.com/science/article/pii/S1525861020304412 or https://cov.cx/a1b24 Note also this study was based on data collected on 7 May. There have been major changes in treatment plans and survival rates since that time, and so the data now might be very different from how it was back then.

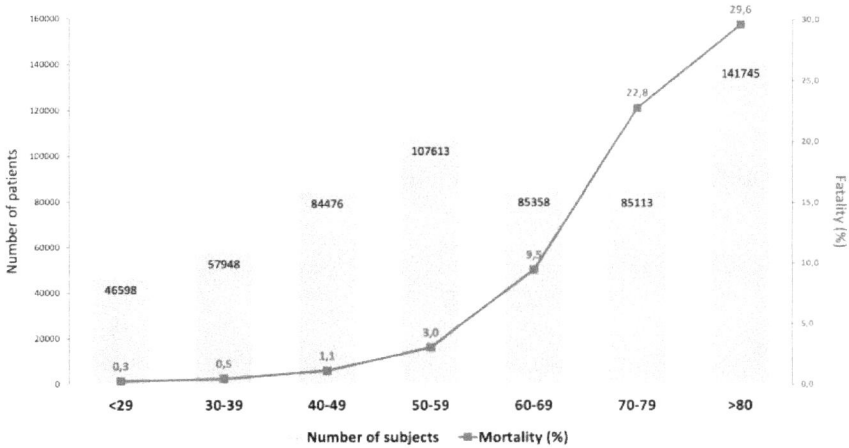

Figure 43 Mortality rates by age

As you can see, there is a similar massive increase in mortality with age. The actual values are unfortunately quite different from the previous set of data (why?), but the concept of major increases in risk/mortality with advancing age is consistent.

There's one more thing to keep in mind. We don't know for sure (not yet, anyway!), but we'll guess that when you're over 80, your chances of dying if hospitalized for any illness are very much greater than if you're half that age. So are the higher numbers we're seeing here "just because that is how it goes for everyone and every disease" or are they truly/significantly higher because the coronavirus is more dangerous? That's something that would be helpful to know, but not something any of the studies we've seen have chosen to consider.

Okay, enough about age. There is more to your risk of dying than just age alone, which brings us to the next point.

Comorbidities

If you already have some types of illnesses and conditions, you are more at risk than if you are fit and healthy in all respects. That's probably not an altogether surprising situation. These other conditions and illnesses are termed comorbidities.

This CDC chart shows the most impactful comorbidities as they apply to Covid :[271]

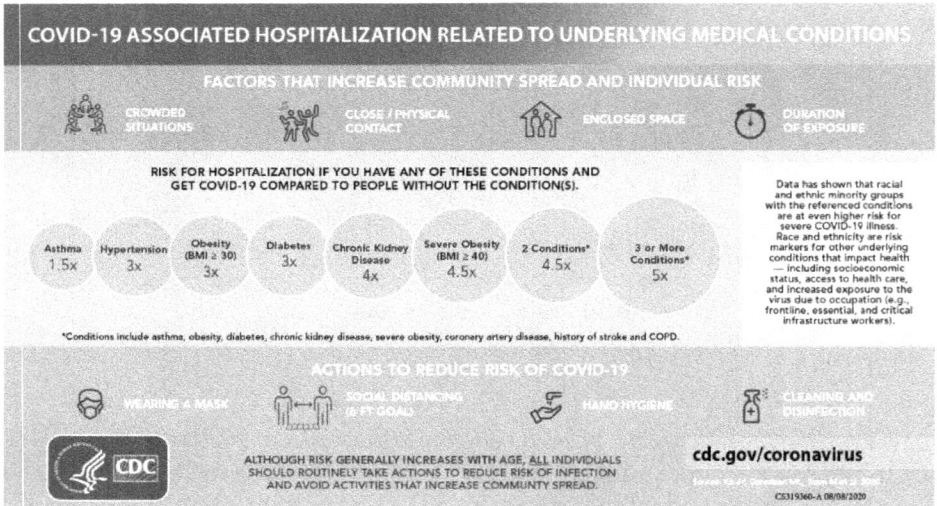

COVID-19 ASSOCIATED HOSPITALIZATION RELATED TO UNDERLYING MEDICAL CONDITIONS

FACTORS THAT INCREASE COMMUNITY SPREAD AND INDIVIDUAL RISK

CROWDED SITUATIONS   CLOSE / PHYSICAL CONTACT   ENCLOSED SPACE   DURATION OF EXPOSURE

RISK FOR HOSPITALIZATION IF YOU HAVE ANY OF THESE CONDITIONS AND GET COVID-19 COMPARED TO PEOPLE WITHOUT THE CONDITION(S).

| Asthma 1.5x | Hypertension 3x | Obesity (BMI ≥ 30) 3x | Diabetes 3x | Chronic Kidney Disease 4x | Severe Obesity (BMI ≥ 40) 4.5x | 2 Conditions* 4.5x | 3 or More Conditions* 5x |

Data has shown that racial and ethnic minority groups with the referenced conditions are at even higher risk for severe COVID-19 illness. Race and ethnicity are risk markers for other underlying conditions that impact health — including socioeconomic status, access to health care, and increased exposure to the virus due to occupation (e.g., frontline, essential, and critical infrastructure workers).

*Conditions include asthma, obesity, diabetes, chronic kidney disease, severe obesity, coronary artery disease, history of stroke and COPD.

ACTIONS TO REDUCE RISK OF COVID-19

WEARING A MASK   SOCIAL DISTANCING (6 FT GOAL)   HAND HYGIENE   CLEANING AND DISINFECTION

CDC

ALTHOUGH RISK GENERALLY INCREASES WITH AGE, ALL INDIVIDUALS SHOULD ROUTINELY TAKE ACTIONS TO REDUCE RISK OF INFECTION AND AVOID ACTIVITIES THAT INCREASE COMMUNTY SPREAD.

cdc.gov/coronavirus

CS319360-A 08/08/2020

Figure 44 Comorbidities and their impact on hospitalization rates

Alas, like all the CDC charts, it only goes part-way to answering the question which, truly, everyone most wants to know : "What is my chance of dying?".

The above chart shows how your chance of being admitted to hospital increases,[272] but being admitted to hospital is not the same as dying, and we do know there is a range of outcomes once hospitalized – your chance of surviving/dying is not constant.

A more complete list of factors that might make your Covid-19 experience more serious can be found on another CDC page. Currently, in order from the most-clear evidence supporting the comorbidity as a factor leading to higher hospitalization and presumably, therefore, death rates to least (note that the

---

[271] See https://www.cdc.gov/coronavirus/2019-ncov/covid-data/investigations-discovery/hospitalization-underlying-medical-conditions.html or https://cov.cx/a1b25

[272] There is a subtle aspect to these statistics though. A person is more likely to be admitted to a hospital just because they have a comorbidity, so these statistics are not accurately reflecting only the severity of the Covid infection.

items within each category are in alphabetical order rather than in further sequenced progression of risk), the list comprises[273]

Strongest Evidence (ie most serious)

- Serious heart conditions
- Cancer
- Chronic kidney disease
- COPD
- Obesity (BMI > 40)
- Sickle cell disease
- Solid-organ transplantation
- Type 2 diabetes mellitus

Mixed Evidence

- Asthma
- Cerebrovascular disease
- Hypertension
- Pregnancy
- Smoking
- Use of corticosteroids or other immunosuppressive medications

Limited Evidence

- Bone marrow transplantation
- HIV
- Immune deficiencies
- Inherited metabolic disorders
- Liver disease
- Neurologic conditions
- Other chronic lung diseases
- Pediatrics
- Thalassemia
- Type 1 diabetes mellitus

You'll also note on the chart a mention of racial/ethnic factors. That's a subject that one has to handle with extreme delicacy these days, and it seems the point being very carefully hinted at on the chart is that it is hard to know whether the greater hospitalization rates experienced by some demographic groups are directly due to race/ethnicity, or due to other factors that correlate to

---

[273] See https://www.cdc.gov/coronavirus/2019-ncov/need-extra-precautions/people-with-medical-conditions.html or https://cov.cx/a1b26

race/ethnicity.[274]   There is however an interesting study that shows there are some genetic links (without mentioning race/ethnicity) to risk factors.[275]

There is one more "sickness" that seems to greatly impact on your survival chances. Your gender. Men are more likely to die than women.[276]

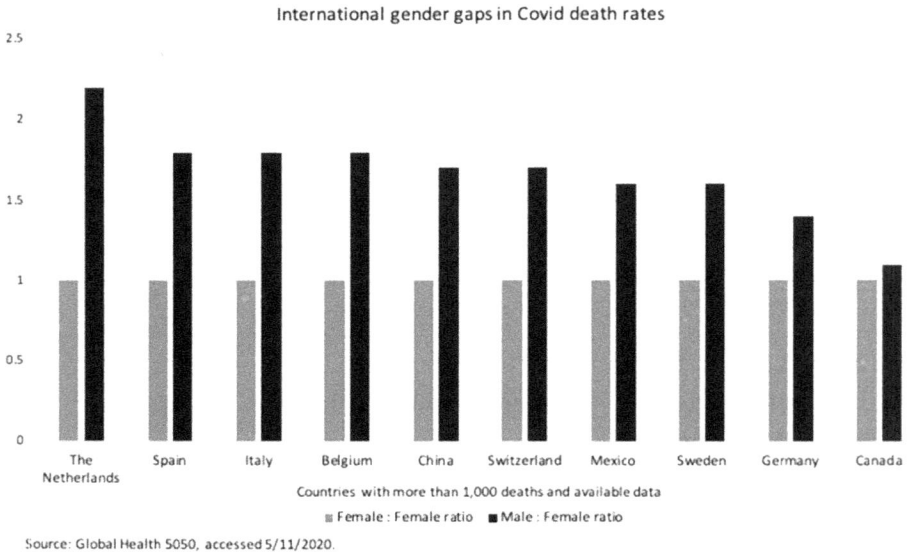

Figure 45 Gender influence on death rate

---

[274] These "other factors" might be the things you'd expect such as quality of healthcare, or tendency to various lifestyle-related illnesses and comorbidities, or they might be surprising "confounders" such as different diets or other unstated reactions/responses to becoming unwell.

It is not just being politically correct to be careful when observing a difference in different demographic groups, because there can be all sorts of related/linked factors over and above the obvious visible "color of their skin" type issue.

[275] See https://science.sciencemag.org/content/370/6515/eabd4585 or https://cov.cx/a1g03

[276] See, for example, https://www.brookings.edu/blog/up-front/2020/05/15/covid-19-much-more-fatal-for-men-especially-taking-age-into-account/ or https://cov.cx/a1b27 and https://www.studyfinds.org/men-more-likely-to-die-from-covid/ or https://cov.cx/a1b28 and newly presented research in December, https://www.cnn.com/2020/12/09/health/men-covid-19-icu-admission-wellness/index.html or https://cov.cx/a1f91

Our commiserations to Dutch men, and we envy the men in Canada. It is very puzzling and would be very helpful to understand why Dutch men have twice the risk of Dutch women of dying, but Canadian men have pretty much the same chance. If we knew the answer to that question, it might help us in treatments for everyone.[277]

Another study[278] listed eleven possible comorbidities and found a significant increase in risk for (from greatest risk increase to least)

* Chronic kidney disease
* Congestive heart failure
* Hypertension
* Diabetes

Also mentioned was cerebrovascular disease, but the higher risk rating wasn't statistically significant.

Interestingly, some potential comorbidities were deemed by that study not to add appreciably to risk – chronic liver disease, COPD, asthma, and HIV/AIDS.

So, if you have, for example, COPD, do you get to pick either the study rating it in the most serious category of comorbidity or the study that says it makes no difference?

How can we trust either study if they show such different findings?

Which Strain of Covid-19 Do You Have?

I came across a fascinating article that classified the disease into six different categories, marked by different symptoms and different degrees of severity.[279]

I treat this study with caution because nowhere does it say they have isolated the virus and determined there are six different strains of virus associated with these six different clusterings of symptoms and severity. This is something that

---

[277] Keep in mind also that we don't know at all, from the data shown in the table, whether the varying factor is in male deaths or female deaths. We are assuming, from the way the data is shown, that female rates are less varying while make rates change widely. But maybe, actually, it is the opposite way around. That would really be interesting to know.

Yes, you guessed it. Here's some more data that, while interesting, is also incomplete and, as shown here, almost meaningless.

[278] See https://journals.plos.org/plosone/article?id=10.1371/journal.pone.0238215 or https://cov.cx/a1b29

[279] See https://covid.joinzoe.com/us-post/covid-clusters or https://cov.cx/a1b30

in theory could be done, but not so much in their "after the fact" analysis of course, and it is something that really should be done to advance this type of analysis further.

I also noticed some other correlations – people in the more severe clusterings "coincidentally" also had other comorbidities.

But, since there seems to be some correlation between groups of symptoms and likely hospitalization/survival rates, perhaps we all just accept it at face value without digging deeply into the causality of the clustering.[280]

I talk about these six clusters more in our section, below, on "Symptoms". See page 173.

How Severe Are Your Symptoms?

Your experience with the virus will be whatever it is, but you might find it helpful to understand where on the continuum from mild to wild your symptoms are.

The National Institutes of Health have issued guidelines for categorizing Covid-19 cases into five categories.[281]

* **Asymptomatic or Pre-symptomatic Infection** : Individuals who test positive for SARS-CoV-2 by virologic testing using a molecular diagnostic (eg, a polymerase chain reaction "PCR") or antigen test, but have no symptoms.
* **Mild Illness** : Individuals who have any of the various signs and symptoms of COVID 19 (e.g., fever, cough, sore throat, malaise,

---

[280] Cluster analysis is something to always be very cautious with because the clustering is an artificial construct that someone has created to try and get sense from the raw data; and there's always a massive danger that the logic of the clustering is actually being determined by a desire to get clear results, rather than coming up with independent justifiable clustering logic and then seeing if results follow the clustering.

Clustering can be helpful but is a dangerous technique, and while it is usually adopted to try and make data patterns more obvious, it may also end up creating patterns where none really exist. It can also obscure true patterns – for example, by collecting an assortment of different symptoms and placing them in clusters, it obscures the relative importance of each of the collected symptoms. Are seemingly different symptoms linked to each other and a different virus strain? The clustering might seem to assume that, but it is an assumption that needs to be tested and validated, rather than accepted at face value.

[281] See https://www.covid19treatmentguidelines.nih.gov/overview/management-of-covid-19/ or https://cov.cx/a1b31

headache, muscle pain) without shortness of breath, dyspnea, or abnormal chest imaging.

  ◆ **Moderate Illness** : Individuals who have evidence of lower respiratory disease by clinical assessment or imaging and a saturation of oxygen (SpO2 – ie using a pulse oximeter) ≥94% on room air at sea level.

  ◆ **Severe Illness** : Individuals who have respiratory frequency >30 breaths per minute, SpO2 <94% on room air at sea level, ratio of arterial partial pressure of oxygen to fraction of inspired oxygen (PaO2/FiO2) <300 mmHg, or lung infiltrates >50%.

  ◆ **Critical Illness** : Individuals who have respiratory failure, septic shock, and/or multiple organ dysfunction.

The NIH has no treatment recommendations for the first two categories of illness, but if you move to the third category of moderate illness, you definitely need to involve your doctor in your treatment.

We'd go further than that and urge you to **involve your doctor right from the very first level**, and talk through the treatment options we detail below. If it is good enough for President Trump to immediately get a large variety of treatments – many of them being low cost and not even requiring a prescription – then surely it is good enough for you, too.

Summary

So, what are your chances of dying from Covid-19? As you have seen, your chance of dying – always recognizing the first assumption, ie, that you catch the disease in the first place – varies enormously depending on your age, your health, even your gender, possibly your race/ethnicity, and also (not shown above but a factor[282]) where in the world you live.

If we start from the assumption you've got the disease, and if you're in the US, you start with probably slightly less than a 2% possibility of dying (perhaps kinder to say, a better than 98% chance of living!).

You're more likely to be severely afflicted if you are older, if you have comorbidities, and if you're male.

Getting to the point where you need hospitalization means that your disease experience and risk is moving up the scale. This happens to about 9% of all

---

[282] See for example the data on this site https://www.worldometers.info/coronavirus/ or https://cov.cx/w-c and the huge skew in death rates, both as a percentage of the population as a whole, and more helpfully, as a percentage of case rates

people infected.[283] But that's not a reason to avoid going to a hospital! You'll get better care in a hospital than at home, so if you are at the point of feeling the need for more care, act on that and quickly. When you reach that level of impact, your chances have already deteriorated, and going to a hospital will help you rather than hinder your recovery.

Once you're in hospital, if they then decide to move you to the ICU, that is again a double-edged sword. It means your infection has escalated further up the severity scale, but it does you no good to try and manage in a regular ward and hospital room. If you need the greater degree of personal care that an ICU offers, then hurry to move there and appreciate the opportunity to do so.

The next big step is if you need to be intubated – ie, coupled up to a ventilator. That means you're now scoring very high on the disease impact scale.

It seems that, back in the March time frame, hospitals hastened to put people on ventilators, because they observed low oxygen levels and breathing distress, and it seemed like an obvious thing to do and was a familiar technique that had been used with some success in other types of treatments of other types of diseases (ARDS in particular).

There's also another terrible truth that is rarely spoken of. The alternatives to ventilators were deemed riskier – but not in the sense you might think. They were deemed to be riskier for the healthcare workers – there was feared to be a greater likelihood of aerosolized virus particles being released into the air with other types of supplemental oxygen assistance, and so for the benefit of the doctors and nurses, rather than for the benefit of the patients, people were being placed on ventilators, perhaps unnecessarily.

Now there's a growing realization that ventilators are a stressful experience (both physically and mentally), and while attempting to address a symptom aren't helping with the underlying problem, nor even helping much with the symptom either! You should encourage your doctors to delay that step as long as possible, using other forms/sources/delivery methods for extra oxygenation instead.[284]

---

[283] Most of the way down this article is interesting data about the percentage of people who, after becoming infected, are hospitalized. It says that about 9.5% of cases needed hospitalization in August and September, reducing in October, but this reduction, the article suggests, is due to lack of hospital resources rather than cases being milder. See https://www.theatlantic.com/health/archive/2020/12/the-worst-case-scenario-is-happening-hospitals-are-overwhelmed/617301/ or https://cov.cx/a1f89

[284] See https://www.aarp.org/health/conditions-treatments/info-2020/ventilator-use-older-coronavirus-patients.html or https://cov.cx/a1b32 and also

(continued on next page)

However, if they have tried other types of oxygenation and your oxygen levels are still very low and you're struggling to breathe and distressed by shortness of breath, you probably have to accept what the ICU team recommends and agree to intubation.

Even at that high level of severity, it seems these days your odds of beating the virus remain better than 50/50 most of the time.

You can also take encouragement from the steady drip, drip, drip, of new discoveries and new treatments. None of them are profoundly impactful by themselves, but overall, in total, they are improving recovery rates all the time.

---

https://www.inquirer.com/health/coronavirus/coronavirus-covid-19-ventilator-patients-survival-rates-increase-20200703.html or https://cov.cx/a1b33

6. How to Know if You Have the Virus

So you wake up one morning, with the start of a sore throat, and feeling a bit unwell. In happier times, you'd either grumble a bit then get up and on with your life, or choose to treat yourself to a day in bed and hope to be back to normal the next day.

Nowadays, and pretty much whatever it is that causes you to feel less than 100% well, it is hard not to start wondering if you're coming down with Covid-19. And instead of perceiving the worst that can happen is needing to endure the hassle of a visit to a doctor, making the copayment, and then filling a prescription for a course of antibiotics to clear up your sore throat, you've got the specter of the virus hanging over you, possibly implying an extended period of hospitalization, ventilation, and maybe even death. The stakes have become much higher.

Which of course means you're understandably keen to know, as quickly as possible, is this the start of something to worry about, or is it nothing worse than it ever has been in the past.

In theory, the simplest and best thing to do is go and see a doctor if you feel unwell. We're absolutely not arguing against the good sense of that. In addition, if you have difficulty breathing, or any other symptom that may be life-threatening or alarming,[285] consider calling 911 for advice and probably immediate help.

But what if you're just the very slightest bit off-color, and you'd not normally go see a doctor in such minor cases but are now worried it might be the start of a virus attack? What if your doctor says they can't see you for several days or is closed for the weekend? Do you go to an Urgent Care Clinic or an Emergency Room (with its much higher copay requirement), or wait to see your doctor?

When Should You Go to Hospital?

Let's "triage" this question by considering the most important element first. What symptoms signal "get to hospital soonest"?

The official list of virus symptoms that should see you going to a hospital has five entries[286] :

- Trouble breathing
- Persistent pain or pressure in the chest
- New confusion (mental fuzziness)
- Inability to wake or stay awake
- Bluish lips or face (and/or low oxygen levels)

The CDC unhelpfully says this is not a complete list and other symptoms may also require immediate hospitalization.[287] That's definitely so, of course, and any time you're concerned about a development in your illness, you should first try to discuss it over the phone with your doctor, and then follow their guidance.

Depending on your doctor's style, and how well they know you, they may tell you to head either to their office or hospital, or just tell you to suck it in and stop worrying about it!

Note – if you do feel the need to go to visit either your doctor or a hospital or any other sort of medical facility, it is a good idea to call them first and ask how they want to receive you. Some facilities have special entrances they prefer infected patients to use, or might meet you in the car park and escort you in, or

---

[285] You know yourself, your general health, and your general attitude to ailments. If you truly feel alarmed – "I've never felt like this before" or "Last time I felt this way, I ended up really sick for many days" – or any other similar sort of feeling, don't ignore your feelings.

[286] See https://www.cdc.gov/coronavirus/2019-ncov/faq.html#Symptoms-&-Emergency-Warning-Signs or https://cov.cx/a1b34

[287] A classic example of official "CYA" actions at work!

test you in the car park. That's not "for your convenience" but rather for their safety!

Give a call and find out what to expect and do.

How Quickly Can You Get Very Sick?

So maybe you do have the virus, but your doctor tells you not to worry and just to take it easy and drink plenty of fluids at home, and to keep away from other people.[288]

Do you have to hover anxiously, in your car, close to a hospital, in case things take a turn for the worse? How quickly can the virus go from just a thing in the background of your life to a life-threatening challenge that needs urgent medical intervention?

The good news is that it is exceedingly rare for the virus infection to suddenly escalate from a tolerable malaise to a life-threatening illness. You don't go from having a sore throat and some pain when breathing to suddenly being "unable to breathe" in a couple of minutes.

Although there are articles talking about patients quickly moving from mild to severe illness,[289] we've never seen a definition of what "quickly" actually means.

We suggest you keep a diary to track your progress through the illness. Several times a day, take your temperature, check your blood oxygen level, and describe the severity of other symptoms and your general state of wellness/sickness.

The checking of your blood oxygen level with a pulse oximeter is particularly important because you'll not consciously notice changes in your blood oxygen level until it drops down to an unusually low level. If you see a trend of "at first I was at 99%, then 98%, then 97%, then 96%", you know that when it next reads 95% this is a meaningful indicator that things are getting steadily worse and

---

[288] As you read further into this book, you'll discover that the "do nothing" advice may not be the best advice and you'll have the information and data you need to have a more focused discussion on that point.

[289] For example, https://www.healthline.com/health-news/mild-covid-19-symptoms-can-quickly-turn-serious or https://cov.cx/a1b35

you're approaching the point of needing to head off to the hospital for oxygen supplementation.[290]

Even though a diary record is a mix of objective (ie, your temperature, blood oxygen level) and subjective (I feel sick, my chest hurts, etc) data, it will help you better remember how you were, and see how you are progressing. It makes it easier to spot trends.

There are also many anecdotal stories shared by doctors of how patients misremember the timing and sequencing of their symptoms. Having it all written down eliminates any such errors.

Seeing a Doctor Probably Won't Help Your Survival Chances

There's one other thing to keep in mind, and which might temper your eagerness to get a doctor to help you as soon as possible. Although almost all health-care sources advocate seeing a doctor if you're at all concerned with your health, they then go silent when it comes to explaining why you should do that and what the doctor will do for you.

Based on the first-hand accounts of Covid-19 sufferers as well as the oblique "what to expect" commentaries on health sites, if you do go to see some type of health-care professional, and if you are diagnosed with a *mild* case of the virus (ie, not something that needs hospitalization), the chances are *the doctor will do nothing* and not give you any type of prescription medicine to treat the infection.

This should not come as a surprise. Remember, Covid-19 is a virus, not a bacteria. Viruses are notoriously difficult to treat. They don't respond to antibiotics (although they may in time create secondary infections that do need antibiotics).

Currently, there are no universally accepted treatments or cures for a person who has the virus in a mild form. Even the much boasted about remdesivir is only used as a treatment for hospitalized patients (it is taken intravenously for five days) and acts to speed a recovery rather than prevent an infection from becoming serious in the first place.[291]

---

[290] Blood-oxygen levels are a bit misleading. You might think "anything over 50% is a pass", but actually, optimum levels are in the high nineties percent. At about 94% or so, it has already become a cause for serious concern and possibly hospitalization.

[291] Remdesivir is too expensive, not available in sufficient quantities, and too resource-intensive to administer to everyone who tests positively, and may not be helpful in the early stages of an infection in any case. The overall value of this much talked about drug is no longer as clear in any event, with WHO now arguing against its use.

The doctor will likely just tell you to let him know if your symptoms worsen, give you a printed sheet about how to keep away from other people, and possibly suggest you get some cough mixture if you're coughing, and maybe a fever reliever if you have a fever (both being drugs you can buy without a prescription). In other words, he will treat the symptoms rather than the actual virus itself. And of course, he'll offer you some general platitudes about taking it easy, getting plenty of rest, and drinking plenty of fluids.[292] He'll close with some generic reassurances, and that's all you'll leave with.

But while antibiotics are useless against viruses, there is another category of drugs – antiviral drugs – that are most helpful in fighting a virus in its early days. There are a growing number of possible treatments and newly identified medicines showing antiviral properties that are receiving growing bodies of evidence to support their use in early treatment stages.

Sadly, few physicians seem either up to date with the latest development or willing to "stick their neck out" and prescribe you medications that haven't been officially endorsed as appropriate for Covid-19 cases, or which have the whiff of controversy or uncertainty about them. We discuss some of the specific treatments that may bring benefits in our chapter "15. Non-official Treatments to Consider".

Indeed, you'll not even leave the doctor's office with the sure and certain knowledge that you do have the virus. The most that is likely to happen is the doctor will say you could have the virus and tell you where to go to get a test for the virus, a procedure that has sometimes seen you waiting a week or even two to get the results back.

Note these comments refer to the early and moderate stages of a virus infection. If you start to be severely afflicted, then hospitalized treatments can help counter the worst side-effects of the virus infection and can help balance your body's attempts to fight its virus invader. As soon as your health deteriorates to a point where you're seriously unwell (particularly having trouble breathing[293]) you need to get yourself checked in to a hospital.

But, before that terrible point, which hopefully you'll avoid entirely (most people do), let's have a look at what types of symptoms are associated with having

---

[292] These are indeed typical platitudes but are also valid, appropriate, and important things to do. But maybe there are some other things that actually can be done to help, as well.

[293] Covid can cause blood-oxygen levels to drop even without the patient being aware or experiencing difficulty in breathing. You should have a pulse oximeter available so you can monitor your blood oxygen level – see our chapter on "17. Medical Equipment & Supplies You Should Have" which discusses these and other devices, below.

the virus. The good news is there are one or two unusual symptoms that might help you to identify your situation.

Symptoms

If there is one thing that can't be stated too many times, it is that this virus and the illness it causes is peculiar and different from just about any other virus out there.

It manifests itself with a wide range of different symptoms, some but not all of which appear in most patients. And, don't forget, it is thought that almost half of all infected people experience no symptoms at all.[294]

The illness might finish after a short time or inexorably continue for months. In some people it is mild, in others it is deadly. Some people recover completely, others end up with lasting damage to their brain and other organs (including heart and lungs).

The chameleon-like nature of the virus makes it hard to state a short and definitive list of symptoms. Amazingly, new symptoms are being discovered, even now, after over 38 million cases have already been registered, worldwide, and with more than seven months of focus on the disease by medical experts everywhere.

Every symptom of the virus is never present in all cases. But some are more common than others, and are more unusual and so are less likely to be a symptom of some other disease instead.

The timing of when symptoms appear is another thing that varies. The disease itself can become impactful after as little as maybe two or three days after you acquire an infection, or it can take two weeks to incubate and become apparent.

Each symptom might only appear briefly for a day or two before disappearing again, rather than being present all the way through your illness.

---

[294] Some people suggest the "almost half who experience no symptoms" actually don't have the virus at all, and it is just a false positive result from the virus test process. We're not sure about this, because some studies seem to suggest that a good percentage of the symptomless people are actually infectious and can pass the virus on to others, meaning they obviously are infected, themselves. We talk more about testing further on in this chapter.

There are also some studies suggesting that some people may even have longer than two-week incubations.[295] This throws the concept of two-week quarantines into question – depending on your tolerance for risk, should we consider a longer period?[296] The two-week duration was probably chosen as being a convenient round number to understand, not as any sort of "magic" number, and – like all public health measures, as a necessary compromise between being 100% safe (a month or longer in quarantine) and 0% safe (no quarantine at all).

In other words, a 13-day quarantine would only be slightly riskier than a 14-day quarantine, a 14-day quarantine does not guarantee that all infections have time to appear and be detected, and a 15-day quarantine would be only slightly safer than a 14 day one. Similar statements apply to 12 and 16 days, and so on.

To start with, the early onset of the virus might feel like you are getting a severe cold or a case of the 'flu. We discuss how to tell the difference between a cold, the 'flu, and the Covid virus in the next section, below.

Common symptoms of the virus include :

- (Dry) Cough (reported in 68%[297] of cases)
- Fever – generally considered to be a temperature of over 100.4°F or 38.0°C (88% of cases) or chills[298]

---

[295] See, for example,
https://www.medrxiv.org/content/10.1101/2020.10.20.20216143v1 or
https://cov.cx/a1b36 - this article examined the literature and found reports of cases appearing after as long as 34 days in quarantine. Maybe one or two cases could be overlooked and be explained as bad data or accidental late infection from some unknown source, but there are multiple reports of infections appearing more than 14 days after an event that may have transferred the virus to a person who then quarantines.

[296] The answer to that question is complicated and depends a bit on the situation. For example, if you are New Zealand, and fighting to keep your entire country totally free of the virus, it is essential not to allow it back into the community, and so you could justify a longer period of quarantine because the stakes are higher. If however, you're in a community with multiple active clusters of infection, the downside is not so severe and perhaps you can be more tolerant of shorter quarantines.

[297] Percentages are taken from this document
https://www.vox.com/2020/7/29/21327317/symptoms-of-covid-19-coronavirus-fever-cough-toes-rash-loss-of-taste-smell or https://cov.cx/a1b37

[298] This article correlates how high your fever goes with how serious an infection you have : https://ccforum.biomedcentral.com/articles/10.1186/s13054-020-03045-8 or
(continued on next page)

- Fatigue (38%)
- Congestion or runny nose (33%)
- Shortness of breath (19%) or difficulty breathing[299]
- Muscle or body aches
- Sore throat (14%)
- New loss of taste or smell
- Diarrhea
- Headache (14%)
- Nausea or vomiting
- Skin rash, especially on your fingers and toes. This is a new symptom, only officially noted in August, which is surprising because it is present in "up to" 10% of cases[300] or even higher (see previous footnote)

You might have some of these symptoms, maybe even all of them (unusual) or possibly none (in which case you're unlikely to even think you might have the virus, of course!).

New research published in mid-August[301] offered an interesting new insight. It found significance in the order in which symptoms appeared, saying the most important sequence was to first have a fever, then a cough, then muscle pains. Next might be nausea and possibly vomiting, and next again, diarrhea. If you

---

https://cov.cx/a1b38 Does that mean that you should take an antipyretic drug to lower your fever? The answer to that is a resounding "don't know". It seems to us that the fever is probably showing the degree with which your body is desperately battling the virus, and controlling the fever is merely attacking a symptom/result rather than the cause, it might even be harmful. As the article concludes, (much) more research is needed.

[299] Shortness of breath can be described variously as

- A tightness in your chest
- Inability to catch your breath
- Can't breathe deeply
- Not getting enough air into your lungs
- A feeling of suffocating or smothering or drowning,
- Needing to consciously make an effort to breathe in or out
- Needing to breathe in again before you've finished breathing out

[300] See https://covid.joinzoe.com/us-post/skin-rash-covid or https://cov.cx/a1b39

[301] See https://www.studyfinds.org/coronavirus-symptoms-order/ or https://cov.cx/a1b40

have the 'flu rather than Covid-19, your first symptom is more likely to be a cough.

There are other possible symptoms, too. This article[302] cites five new symptoms (as of early August) that have some possible association with the virus – hiccups, itching, hair loss, hearing loss, and numbness. Of course, all of these (and just about all other) symptoms can mean many different underlying causes, so don't stress if you find yourself with one of these symptoms. But when you're getting three or four, then the chances of it being the Covid-19 disease start to become more significant.

We mentioned in the section on "Which Strain of Covid-19 Do You Have?" (above on page 163) about an analysis that categorized symptoms into six clusters or groupings.[303] These six clusters also had significantly different levels of hospitalization and ventilation.

The six clusters, their primary symptoms, and the outcomes are as follows:

* **Cluster 1 ('flu-like' with no fever)** : Headache, loss of smell, muscle pains, cough, sore throat, chest pain, no fever. *16% hospitalized, 1.5% required breathing support.*

* **Cluster 2 ('flu-like' with fever)** : Headache, loss of smell, cough, sore throat, hoarseness, fever, loss of appetite. *4.4% required breathing support.*

* **Cluster 3 (gastrointestinal)** : Headache, loss of smell, loss of appetite, diarrhea, sore throat, chest pain, no cough. *3.3% required breathing support.*

* **Cluster 4 (severe level one, fatigue)** : Headache, loss of smell, cough, fever, hoarseness, chest pain, fatigue. *8.6% required breathing support.*

* **Cluster 5 (severe level two, confusion)** : Headache, loss of smell, loss of appetite, cough, fever, hoarseness, sore throat, chest pain, fatigue, confusion, muscle pain. *9.9% required breathing support.*

* **Cluster 6 (severe level three, abdominal and respiratory)** : Headache, loss of smell, loss of appetite, cough, fever, hoarseness, sore throat, chest pain, fatigue, confusion, muscle pain, shortness of breath,

---

[302] See https://bestlifeonline.com/strange-new-covid-symptoms/ or https://cov.cx/a1b41

[303] See https://covid.joinzoe.com/us-post/covid-clusters or https://cov.cx/a1b42

diarrhea, abdominal pain.   *Almost 50% hospitalized, and 19.8% required breathing support.*

This is an interesting set of groupings, but we should also point out that these six clusters do not cover every different possible collection of symptoms. For example, all six of these clusters include the symptom "loss of smell". But this is not a universal symptom. In this study,[304] 65% of people who tested positive for the virus reported loss of smell – but so too did 23% of people who tested negative for the virus!

We make two inferences from this – one-third of people who have the virus don't experience loss of smell, and also that a loss of smell, while strongly indicative of having a Covid-19 infection, has about one-quarter of cases where the loss of smell did not mean the person had the virus.

As we said in the introduction, things are seldom black and white!

The Key Differences Between 'Flu, a Cold, and Covid-19

We've always struggled to tell the difference between a cold and the 'flu, so this is a helpful checklist for us.

We're not sure that it makes the diagnosis obvious and certain though, especially when many symptoms are shared across all three ailments, and we've tried to focus on the symptoms most likely to be experienced and/or most likely to help you understand which of these three ailments you might be coming down with.[305] [306]

Symptom	Cold	'Flu	Covid-19
Fever	Very rare	Almost always, can last 3 – 4 days, usually in	Very common

---

[304] See https://www.nature.com/articles/s41591-020-0916-2 or https://cov.cx/a1b43

[305] We also observe, wryly, how the vast majority of people persist in describing their colds as "the 'flu". 99% of the time, they are wrong. They don't have the 'flu. They have a common ordinary cold. But they feel more self-important by describing it as 'flu, and perhaps more justified in staying in bed.

[306] Taken from various sources, including https://www.cdc.gov/flu/symptoms/flu-vs-covid19.htm or https://cov.cx/a1b44 - the list above is not complete

		the range of 100 − 102°F	
Cough	Common	Common	Very common, a dry cough
Sneezing	Common	Rarely	Rarely
Headache	Rarely	Common, and usually quite strong	Rarely
General aches and pains	Uncommon, mild	Common, sometimes severe	Sometimes
Fatigue, weakness	Rare, mild	Can be severe, can last up to two weeks	About half the time
Shortness of breath	Very rare	Very rare	About one in five people have this
Symptom Onset	Gradual	Abrupt	Varies
Loss of Taste or Smell	Very rare	Very rare	Sometimes

Figure 46 Comparison of symptoms

In creating a "What Do I Have" decision tree, we'd focus on :

Fever : If you have a fever, it is unlikely to be a cold, but could be either the 'flu or Covid-19. If no fever is present, you almost certainly do not have the 'flu but might have either a cold or Covid-19.

Loss of Taste or Smell : If this happens, it is almost certainly Covid-19 rather than a cold or 'flu (other than for the secondary diminution of these senses from a blocked nose). But remember that 25% of people reporting a loss of smell don't actually have Covid-19. If this symptom doesn't occur, it could be any of the three things.

Sneezing : If you're sneezing, you probably have a cold (or an allergy), rather than the 'flu or Covid-19.

The most certain way to know if you have Covid-19, however, is always to be tested for it, although – as we explain in the section just ahead on testing, even that is not always reliable and certain.

Distinguishing Allergies from Covid-19

It is also possible to confuse an allergic reaction with a cold or 'flu or Covid-19. You can try and analyze your symptoms to determine which it is, but for us (we are an occasional allergy sufferer), we've a quick and easy way of finding out : If the problem goes away after taking a Claritin tablet, then it is an allergy. If it doesn't, then it could be one of the other three.

If you suffer from allergies, you surely know what they do to you, and hopefully you also have a great allergy treatment to stop the reaction. So if you are experiencing something that might be an allergy, or might be something else, cross your fingers, hope it is an allergy, and reach for your regular anti-histamine and see if it works the same as always.

Testing

Being tested is of course an important part of determining if you have the virus or not. It is also much more than that. Extensive testing allows for the early detection of newly infected people, allowing for the disease to be better controlled.

You're familiar with the concept of testing for diseases already. You've probably at some time or another needed to give a throat swab to test for a throat infection, maybe a urine sample, maybe a blood test, or some other type of test.

In all these cases, the sample is taken, and, a short while later, someone phones you with "The Results". Usually, the results are an easily explained trivial sort of thing – "Yes, you have Strep Throat" or "No, you don't have a bladder infection" or whatever.

You'd expect that testing for the coronavirus would be similar, wouldn't you. Provide a sample, wait for a result, and be told that you either do or do not have the virus. End of story. Get on with your life.

Alas, that is completely not the case. Every part of testing for the virus has been badly managed, and test results have been unreliable, to an almost unbelievable degree.[307] We repeat – testing for the virus should be, and in truth is, a simple process. In theory, yes; but alas, it is not a simple process in practice, especially in the US.

That is why we say testing is an important part. But it is not the only part. You might get a positive test, but not have the virus. Or you might get a negative test, but have the virus.[308] Testing is helpful, but unfortunately is not 100% authoritative (getting a second test to confirm the first test, especially if the first test result is not what you expected it would be, is always desirable).

There is also an important distinction – there are tests for two different things. There are tests to see if you **currently have** an infection or not, and there are tests (antibody tests) to see if you had an infection **in the past** and now developed some possible resistance to a future re-infection.[309]

Understanding if you had an infection in the past is interesting in some contexts,[310] but for our purposes, the key test is probably the one to see if you currently have an infection.

---

[307] This 14 Aug article quotes a Harvard Professor of Epidemiology as saying "The incompetence [of the CDC in particular] has really exceeded what anyone would expect". The article goes on to point out that we are now testing fewer people each week, but with more problems in administering the tests. How is it possible that we are getting worse rather than better? See https://www.theatlantic.com/health/archive/2020/08/how-to-test-every-american-for-covid-19-every-day/615217/ or https://cov.cx/a1b45

[308] This is a great article that discusses testing through the lens of a woman who repeatedly tested negative for the virus, while having a severe infection, even needing hospitalization and oxygen. https://www.gq.com/story/julia-ioffe-false-negative-covid-testing or https://cov.cx/a1b46

[309] That's a very important distinction, and obviously so. But, unbelievably, for a while, both the CDC and some states (PA, TX, GA, VT, possibly others) in the US were reporting tests for current infection numbers and including the other type of tests – tests for past infection numbers – in those results. That of course skewed the national understanding of virus activity numbers until it was discovered. See https://www.theatlantic.com/health/archive/2020/05/cdc-and-states-are-misreporting-covid-19-test-data-pennsylvania-georgia-texas/611935/ or https://cov.cx/a1b47 and https://www.wlrn.org/news/2020-05-20/cdcs-national-dashboard-includes-covid-19-data-that-expert-says-mixes-apples-to-oranges#stream/0 or https://cov.cx/a1b48

[310] The main two points are to try and understand the difference between "known patients" and "total patients", and also to identify what level of potentially growing herd immunity might be present in a community. We discuss herd immunity later on in this document.

Several different types of tests can be used to determine if you currently have the virus or not. From our point of view as patients, you would expect the only difference is in what type of sample is required, and how long it takes to get a result.

Samples are most commonly taken by sticking a long stick with cotton wool a very long way up and into your nose – further than you'd think it can or should go! Some other methods will swab inside your mouth, or even have you spit into a container. Happily, these alternate types of sample-taking are becoming more common.

The most common test (a "PCR" or polymerase chain reaction test) almost always requires your sample to then be sent to an officially approved laboratory for analysis. Running the test takes a few hours of laboratory time.

So, in theory, you could be tested in the morning, and if you are close to a lab, could have the result by the end of the day. But, in practice, it is more likely your test sample and many others will be gathered together and couriered all at once to the lab at the end of the day, and received by the lab in time for the start of the next day.

So far so good – your test gets to a lab the next morning. Now for the bad news. All the labs seem to be struggling to meet the demand for test results, and so rather than working on your sample immediately, and sending the result back to whoever tested you later in the day, it might take several days for your turn in the testing queue. The best-case scenario seems to be a two-day wait, and some people have reported two-week waits for their results to come back again.[311]

This is totally useless. Fast results are essential if you're trying to control outbreaks, and if you need or wish tested people to modify their behavior (ie self-quarantine) based on the outcome. If you think you might have the virus, or if you think you are now clear of your infection, you want and need results asap, so you know how to modify your behavior – to self-quarantine if infected, or to return to normal if the result shows your infection has cleared.[312]

---

[311] Test turnaround times have varied from month to month. Sometimes, they have been fast, other times they have been appallingly slow. So our description, while a sadly true depiction of some of the time, is not accurate for every day between March and now. But it is not true to say "after problems, things improved and now are much better. In mid-November, new reports of problems with testing started surfacing. See https://apnews.com/article/us-covid-19-testing-strained-holidays-db20ebbcc1fa8a411be8f9ebc241af3b or https://cov.cx/a1b49

[312] Knowing you are clear and can return back to normal aspect is almost as important as knowing you are infected. If you've had to self-quarantine, and if you can't work, you'll be very keen to be able to end your quarantine and get back to your normal life.

Very fast test results are also essential when it comes to trying to track and trace other people who might also have become infected. In the two weeks between sending in a test and getting the answer, you can have an infected person infect a group of other people, then those people five days later turn around and infect more groups of people, then another five days later, the second groups infect more groups of people, and by the time contact tracers start to go through the first person's tree of contacts, the third group of people will have in turn infected a fourth group. Furthermore, who can accurately and completely remember where they were and who they met, two weeks ago?[313] The contact tracing concept breaks down entirely, well before two weeks.

If we say one person infects two, they infect four, they infect eight, and they infect sixteen, that means one person caused thirty new infections. That is a terrible rate of virus growth, all because our healthcare system can not get its testing done efficiently.

This brings about an interesting thing. **A fast test result is better than an accurate test result**. A fast inaccurate test result could be repeated a second and if necessary, a third time, perhaps all in no more than an hour's total elapsed time, whereas the more accurate result is still pending.

This is a classic case of "the excellent is the enemy of the good". In our obsession to get highly accurate test results, we've lost focus of the ultimate objective, which is controlling the virus spread. That ultimate objective is better achieved by multiple inaccurate but fast tests (although of course, there is a limit to how inaccurate a test can be before no amount of repeated fast testing is helpful!).[314]

---

[313] I remember one time there was a high-profile arson event in New Zealand, and the police ended up asking anyone and everyone remotely connected with the business and its location where they were on the night of the fire. They asked me because, like probably hundreds of other people, I'd worked in the building some years before, and at first, a flash of panic came over me. I had no idea, and couldn't remember. I had no alibi, and of course, in the tv detective shows, having no alibi unerringly makes you the guilty person.
With what I'm sure what a look of pure guilt on my face, I told the two policemen that I didn't know and couldn't remember. They looked at each other, shrugged, and one of them handed me his card. "Give us a call if you remember," he said. They left. I never called, and they never came back. My guess was most of the people they were contacting, some weeks later, were telling them the same thing. Perhaps only guilty people have alibis?

[314] This article quotes experts as saying test results need to be received in 2 – 3 days to be of any value. Maybe, indeed, after three days they are useless, as the expert

(continued on next page)

There have been, in the past, other types of tests that promised results in a couple of hours or less – sometimes even as little as 15 minutes or so, and which could be processed at the site you were tested at. So, a nearly instant result, while you wait. The promise of these tests is only now (in October) starting to translate to reality because it seems that most of the non-PCR fast type tests were originally not as accurate as PCR testing, which is about to become the next point we look at.

There are also new tests promising very fast results, just now being released and hopefully with better accuracy levels.[315]

Here's an example of a new test that was approved by the FDA in mid-August. It still requires lab processing, rather than "do it yourself" on the spot, but is beneficial because it is less unpleasant to administer, and much cheaper – a $5 cost and possibly $10 fee.[316] This single new test won't transform our testing process and delays, but it is still a welcome element of progress.

Even more exciting, later in August another new test was released, this one selling for $5 and taking 15 minutes.[317] While another positive step forward, there are three quibbles that one could express.   It still requires the uncomfortable nasal swab, it will probably only be sold to healthcare professionals, not to ordinary people, and has a 98.5% correct negative rate (and a 97% correct positive rate), which will mean there will probably be more false positives than true positives. We'll explain that in the next section, below. Abbott Laboratories says it plans to ship "tens of millions" of the tests in September, and 50 million in October. That is good news, but we need, most of all, tests available everywhere, not just in doctors' offices.

---

described, but the two-day delay needs to be understood as being massively less desirable than one or zero days of delay, too. See https://www.cnbc.com/2020/08/15/forty-percent-of-us-covid-19-tests-come-back-too-late-to-be-clinically-meaningful-data-show.html or https://cov.cx/a1b50

[315] Most exciting of all is a new test that promises results in 30 seconds. See https://www.jpost.com/israel-news/india-israel/india-israel-30-second-coronavirus-test-in-very-last-stage-649372 or https://cov.cx/a1b51

[316] See https://www.statnews.com/2020/08/15/fda-clears-saliva-test-for-covid-19-opening-door-to-wider-testing/ or https://cov.cx/a1b52 and https://www.fda.gov/news-events/press-announcements/coronavirus-covid-19-update-fda-issues-emergency-use-authorization-yale-school-public-health#:~:text=Today%2C%20the%20U.S.%20Food%20and,testing%20for%20COVID%2D19%20infection. or https://cov.cx/a1b53

[317] See https://www.msn.com/en-us/health/medical/fda-authorizes-abbott-s-fast-5-covid-19-test/ar-BB18pgyi or https://cov.cx/a1b54

Our dysfunctional approach to testing is harming our ability to control the spread of the virus. The government has spent $8 billion on vaccine development, but only $248 million on testing.[318] Whereas virus development will probably bring some benefit in an uncertain future time frame, spending to improve testing protocols and speeding up testing results brings instant and positive results in terms of controlling the disease spread. We feel the government has incorrectly set its spending priorities.

- *Test Pooling*

Here's one more approach to "mass producing" tests – a very clever concept that is also, surprisingly, not a very new concept. It has been around since World War 2. We can't start to guess why it hasn't been adopted already for Covid-19 testing.[319]

The newer approach in the second article link works a bit like a RAID disk array if that helps explain the concept to you. Or error-correcting memory. The linked article explains it further.

Test Accuracy

Now for a very interesting point to appreciate. Let's say you've been tested for the virus, and the result comes back as positive. The test itself claims to be accurate 98% of the time, and the rate of virus infections in the community is running at about one in every 2,000 people (these are numbers reasonably similar to what you'd expect from a PCR test and the US rate of infected people).[320]

---

[318] See https://www.theatlantic.com/health/archive/2020/08/how-to-test-every-american-for-covid-19-every-day/615217/ or https://cov.cx/a1b55

[319] See https://www.theatlantic.com/health/archive/2020/08/how-to-test-every-american-for-covid-19-every-day/615217/ or https://cov.cx/a1b56 . Since that article, there has been a great further development that now means that pooled testing doesn't need to have multiple tests run on people when one of the pooled test samples is positive, making the process even faster and more beneficial. https://www.pressreader.com/usa/chicago-tribune/20200824/281715501993620 or https://cov.cx/a1b57

[320] You might note that while I'm pointing to a community infection rate of about one in 2,000, if we look at the test results, we see that about one in every 13 is testing positive – see https://www.worldometers.info/coronavirus/country/us/ or https://cov.cx/w-us - I'm using the results on 30 August. Why the huge difference?

(continued on next page)

What are the chances, therefore, that you truly have an infection?

You might think that with 98% accuracy, your chances are therefore 98% that you have the virus. You'd be wrong. You've about a 2.5% chance of actually having the virus.

Wow! Isn't that astonishing. How did 98% accuracy get down to 2.5% accuracy? The short answer is because of Bayesian probability. If that doesn't immediately ring a bell, let's look at it carefully.

Consider, for example, if we test a group of 10,000 people. We know that five of those people (based on the one in 2,000 average we are using) have the virus.

We also know that with 98% accuracy, the test is almost certain to detect all five of those people.

But, wait. That's not the end of the story, although many people think it is. There's another very important consideration : What about the other 9,995 people who are also tested, but who don't have the virus?

The 98% accuracy means that two out of every hundred of those people will get a false positive result. Over the 10,000 people, that means 200 false positives.

So in total, from our 10,000 person group, we get the five correct positives, and another 200 false positives. You have five chances in 205 – about a 2.5% chance – that your positive result is a true positive rather than a false positive. That's a worse than useless situation.[321]

The difference is because at present, in most cases, you have to think you have the virus before you can be tested for it. So of course, most people who think they have the virus, and usually have been prescreened by a physician, will test positive. But as the country gets more testing facilities, and with more people being truly randomly tested (for example, prior to being allowed onto a plane or into an event), testing will shift from "mainly testing sick people" to "testing everyone, sick or not", and the percentage of positive tests will start to more closely reflect the prevalence of the virus in the population as a whole.

[321] This is a footnote you can skip unless you're keen on the underlying details, or if you think you've spotted an error in my reasoning. At present (early September), based on actual reported numbers, there have been 87.4 million tests done in the US, and there are a total of 6.5 million Covid cases. So, it might seem that rather than one in 200 people having the virus, more like one in 13 people do. That would massively reduce the number of false positives, of course.

This is simultaneously right and wrong. How can something be both right and wrong at the same time, you ask? Welcome to the wonderful world of statistics and sampling! At present, the thing is that most people being tested are almost certainly infected – it is very difficult for ordinary healthy people to be tested. But if truly random people were being tested, rather than already sick people, the one in 200 number becomes closer to reality and so too does the overwhelming number of false positives. In other words, if

(continued on next page)

Maybe your test is 99% accurate. That's starting to get close to the practical limit of any/all tests.[322] But your false positive count is still 100, which means there is now only a 5% chance of your positive result being correct.

Go up to an unthinkable 99.9% accuracy, and now you have the five true positives and ten false positives. You still only have a 33% chance of the test result being correct.

How do you solve for the problem of false positives? Rather than trying to impossibly perfect the test, it is better to simply test people twice (or three times).

Using our example above, and the 98% accuracy, we test the 205 people with a first positive result a second time. This time, we almost certainly still get the five true positives, and we get four false positives – now there's almost exactly a 50/50 chance that your positive test is correct.

An interesting observation to make here is that this result is better than a single test with an incredibly 99.9% accurate testing procedure. So why not do two fast $5 tests, rather than one expensive slow test that takes several days for results to come back? As we said above, a blinkered focus on highly accurate testing (which in any event might be much less than highly accurate) has blinded healthcare experts to how less accurate (but more frequent) testing can end up with a better outcome.

If you're absolutely demanding 100.000% accuracy, you'd need to do a third test that is likely to eliminate the four remaining false positives.

Now think about that in the context of an unpleasant test procedure, and a week or longer delay between being tested and getting the result. Everyone who tests positive the first time needs to be tested a second time because there are 40 times more false positives than true positives. The first test does a great job of eliminating 9,795 of the 10,000 people, but it is totally unhelpful in terms of exactly identifying the truly infected.

And when you ask the 205 "possibly positive" people to come back, you're unlikely to have all of them show up. After a hassle the first time – travel, waiting, slightly unpleasant experience, then waiting a week, the motivation to come back a second time will be much weaker. And even those people who do come back might not come back immediately, they might delay their second visit a day or two, adding still further to the mess of it all.

---

you think you have the virus, and a test shows you do, the test is probably correct. But if you don't think you have the virus, and are surprised to see a test result saying you do, the test result is probably wrong.

[322] Human factors and other random errors always intrude on perfection. So while you'll see some tests claiming higher degrees of accuracy, it is important to acknowledge that in the "real world" things are never as good as the theory hopefully suggests.

A Better Measure of Test Accuracy

So far we've deliberately simplified how accuracy is measured by just talking about a single number, the percent accuracy. But there are actually two different measures – often they are similar in terms of their percentage values, but sometimes they are not.

In these types of test scenarios it is important to consider all possible outcomes from the test :

- Outcome 1 : An infected person is correctly identified
- Outcome 2 : An infected person is incorrectly declared uninfected (false negative)
- Outcome 3 : An uninfected person is correctly identified
- Outcome 4 : An uninfected person is incorrectly declared infected (false positive)

A test's accuracy is typically described in two ways, not just one.

The first measure is the percentage of correct positive test results compared to false negative (missed positive) test results among people who truly do have the condition you are testing for. This is called the test's **sensitivity** – ie outcomes 1 and 2.

The second measure is the percentage of correct negative test results compared to false positive (missed negative) test results among people who don't have the condition you are testing for. This is called the test's **specificity** – ie outcomes 3 and 4.

Ideally we want virus testing that is not only fast and easy but also simultaneously very sensitive and very specific. Sadly, that type of testing does not seem to exist.

Inaccurate Tests Are Still Helpful

As mentioned above, while we'd ideally like a test that is 100% sensitive and 100% specific, we don't need one. We can accept some imprecision and imperfection, especially if the trade-off is faster testing.

For example, it seems the fastest tests that can be done immediately, at the testing location, are less accurate than the formal PCR testing that is taking so long to get results back from. But which is better from a public health and disease control point of view? A test that is 98% or even 99% perfect, but which takes a week or even two to get the results from, or a test that is 80% perfect, and with results in 15 minutes?

There are situations where a fast but imperfect answer is better than a slow and better answer.

Now for the interesting thing about inaccurate testing and how it is almost as helpful as accurate testing. One of the key things about the virus is that we – surprisingly – don't need to identify and intercept every last infected person. All we need to do is catch enough people, soon enough, that we can reduce the ability of the virus to keep infecting more and more people (ie, we want to bring the R rate down below 1.0). In part this is brought about by herd immunity and (in the future) vaccination, in part it is brought about by masks and social distancing, and in part it is brought about by identifying people who might be infectious and ensuring they don't pass their infection on.

We discuss these issues in detail in the chapter about disease transmission and growth (see "4. How the Number of Infections Increased So Quickly" and "Herd Immunity", starting on page 50). If we can catch half the people with infections, and if we continue our social distancing and mask-wearing, we'll have done all we need to see the disease steadily dwindle and eventually die out (except for new introductions of the virus of course from external locations, ie, people coming into the country from other parts of the world, and bringing fresh new virus infections with them).

We've tried to get exact data on how accurate different tests are, but it has proven very hard to obtain. Some sources say, without attribution, that the "best" PCR tests can be 100% accurate, other sources say, also without attribution, that "of course" no tests are ever 100% accurate.

Beyond that point, we're not talking about small seeming differences between tests in the mid-nineties percent range and tests in the 99%+ range. Some tests have proved to be as little as 30% accurate. We also think (but don't know for sure) that tests have improved in accuracy over time,[323] so accuracy levels reported some months ago may no longer be correct, now.[324]

It seems that PCR type tests are usually more accurate (but slower than) antigen type tests. But there have been credible concerns expressed that the PCR testing has been set to a "too sensitive" level and it may be creating more false

---

[323] Probably due to three factors – better test design, better test administration, and better lab work.

[324] This is most vividly exemplified in the unattributed comment that early PCR accuracy may have been in the range of 66% - 88% in the real world in this article : https://nymag.com/intelligencer/2020/06/how-accurate-are-covid-19-tests.html or https://cov.cx/a1b58

positive results than we realize – perhaps some/many of the people who are currently being described as asymptomatic are in reality not infected at all.[325]

Here are some articles reporting on test inaccuracy. We cite them more to show we're not being lazy, and also to show the confusion that exists, rather than to give you truly helpful data!

https://www.healthline.com/health-news/how-accurate-are-covid-19-diagnostic-and-antibody-tests#Two-tests-that-diagnose-an-infection or https://cov.cx/a1f80

https://www.wbur.org/commonhealth/2020/07/30/shira-doron-covid-19-testing-types-accuracy or https://cov.cx/a1f81

https://www.npr.org/sections/health-shots/2020/05/01/847368012/how-reliable-are-covid-19-tests-depends-which-one-you-mean or https://cov.cx/a1f82

https://nymag.com/intelligencer/2020/06/how-accurate-are-covid-19-tests.html or https://cov.cx/a1f83

There's another element at issue when it comes to testing, too. Please keep reading.

Test Timing

By "test timing" we mean the relative time between when you acquired an infection and when you are tested for it.

The way the virus works is that you first get some virus particles into your system (in this case, usually by breathing them in), and there is then an initial struggle between your body and the virus to see if the virus can survive and grow. If the virus wins that initial struggle (the outcome is based not only on you but also on how many virus particles you have acquired –you need to have more than a certain minimum number for the virus to become viable) it then starts steadily growing and becoming more numerous, and at some point, you probably become infectious, and at some subsequent point, you probably start to suffer from symptoms of the virus being present (initially in your nasal and oral cavities, subsequently in your lungs and more generally in your body).[326]

---

[325] These concerns have been expressed even by the man who invented PCR tests, many years ago. We discuss this issue in the introductory comments to our "daily diary" article on 19 November, see https://thecovidsurvivalguide.com/2020/11/297-2.htm or https://cov.cx/a1b59

[326] One of the unusual things about this virus is that it seems to be at its most infectious *before* the infected person even realizes they have been infected.

The time from when the first viral particles get into your body, until when you start to become infectious to others, can be anywhere from a day or two through to a couple of weeks. The time from when you start being infectious to when you start to experience symptoms can also vary widely (but normally this happens about 2 – 3 days *after* you've become infectious). It is common for most people to start to experience symptoms 4 – 5 days after being infected, but there is a wide range of timings, some shorter and some a lot longer than that.[327]

The point of this is now to ask the question "From when I get an infection, to when I become infectious to others, and from then on to when I start to suffer symptoms myself – at what point will a test for the virus in my system reliably register its presence?".

This is a key question. If you test too early, there might not be enough virus in your system for a test to detect it. This article suggests it takes at least 3 – 5 days after being exposed to the virus before a test can be expected to detect your infection.[328]

But notice the phrase "at least". That makes the numbers that follow only weakly reliable, rather than definitive. "At least" includes all numbers larger, without any limit.[329]

Proving that point is this article which says that even eight days after you have become infected, testing might still fail to detect 20% of infections.[330] It adds that after four days, only 33% of people were correctly detected as being infected.

Here's another article citing two "experts" – one of whom says to wait at least two days and to be tested in the 2 – 14 day period after possibly being infected, and the other says to get tested 3 – 7 days after possible infection.[331]

This is a vivid example of how experts can be simultaneously correct but also utterly unhelpful. Saying "2 – 14 days" or "3 – 7 days" is totally unhelpful. Hours

---

[327] See, for example, https://www.foxnews.com/health/coronavirus-covid-19-highly-contagious-days-symptoms or https://cov.cx/a1b60 and https://www.webmd.com/lung/coronavirus-incubation-period or https://cov.cx/a1b61

[328] See https://www.msn.com/en-us/health/medical/here-s-how-long-it-takes-to-test-positive-for-coronavirus-after-exposure/ar-BB14SvmO or https://cov.cx/a1b62

[329] That's a bit like advertisements with the weasel words "up to", isn't it. "Enjoy up to 50% better fuel economy" can also mean "enjoy only 0.1% better fuel economy"!

[330] See https://gulfnews.com/lifestyle/health-fitness/covid-19-testing-too-soon-gives-false-negative-result-says-study-1.1591799861871 or https://cov.cx/a1b63

[331] See https://www.self.com/story/coronavirus-testing-protests or https://cov.cx/a1b64

count in the critical rush to identify infected people before they can pass their infection on.

We need to know when is the soonest that a test can be expected to have a meaningful result? Sure, after 14 days it would be pretty much guaranteed to pick up your infection (unless of course you had been cured by then), but as the Asst Professor of Epidemiology who made that suggestion should understand and appreciate, the value of the test then is close to worthless, because by then most people have done all the infecting of other people they're going to do and their infectious level has greatly subsided.

Testing, to be helpful, not only has to be accurate but also has to be done as early as possible (and give you the results urgently quickly too).

Here's an interesting illustration showing one opinion on when an infection can be detected.[332]

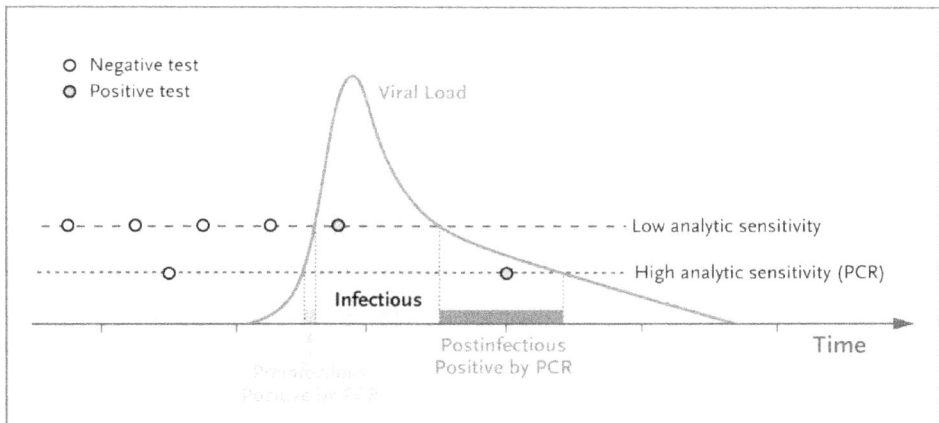

Figure 47 When can an infection be detected by a test?

It suggests a very short time between when a PCR type test may detect an infection and when the person becomes infectious. The main concept of the article is that regular testing with less sensitive tests (the top horizontal line) is more likely to more quickly detect an infection than less regular testing using the PCR process (the lower horizontal line). The PCR process is likely to always be slow and expensive, whereas the less sensitive antigen tests are becoming very quick, simple, and affordable.

---

[332] See https://www.nejm.org/doi/full/10.1056/NEJMp2025631 or https://cov.cx/a1b65

The best answer would be to get tested after two days, then again the next day (3rd day) and the next day (4th) and the next day (5th).[333] And maybe a few more tests, too! At $5 a test, that's prudent and affordable.

The nation doesn't (yet) have the capacity to provide that quantity of testing kits, and so there are compromises every which way, which in turn rely on our comment above about inaccurate tests still being helpful, and also provide one reason why our continued uncontained level of virus infection throughout the country is worse than most other countries.

There is another dimension to test timing as well. Testing is important, initially, to tell people when they have the virus. But it can also be important to tell people when they are free of the virus.[334]

Unfortunately, the main test – the "gold standard" PCR type of test – struggles to identify when a person is free of an active viral infection, cured, and no longer infectious. The problem is simple – a person likely continues to have some dead or inactive virus particles in their system for a considerable time after they have been cured.   The PCR test can not distinguish between an active/live/dangerous virus particle and a dead/inactive/"safe" virus particle, and so is giving "false positive" readings for people who have been cured and are completely safe.[335] This is shown in the illustration, above – a PCR test is as likely to detect the virus after a person has ceased to be infectious as it is to detect the antibodies during a person's infectious period.

That false positive can be guessed at to start with. But the false positives might continue for up to three months after an infection (possibly longer). If you

---

[333] But do you spot the weakness in this "best answer"? It assumes we know when we might have been infected. Sometimes that can be the case – if we spent several hours in close quarters, indoors, with a person who was then shown, the next day, to be infected, we'd have reason to worry. But most people at present are becoming infected not as a result of a known risky experience, but as a result of just general life and living. In other words, for most of us, in most cases, we don't know when to start getting tested.

[334] Unfortunately, a "you don't have the virus" test result is also plagued with imprecisions, in particular, the fact that it takes a number of days between when you are infected and when a test will register the virus' presence. So a negative (ie "you're not infected") test result is never going to be up to date or conclusive. It can never be more than indicative (unless you've been in isolation with no possibility of recent infection).

[335] There's a great explainer in this article https://www.theatlantic.com/health/archive/2020/08/how-to-test-every-american-for-covid-19-every-day/615217/ or https://cov.cx/a1b66

have been cured of the virus, then for some reason get tested again three months later and are shown to be positive, who is to say if it is a false positive as a result of your earlier infection, or a new fresh infection?

Testing Bottom-Line

If you think you have the virus, you should try to get tested. Ask what the test's sensitivity and specificity rates are – I can help you interpret them.

But, in general, and assuming high accuracy rates on both sensitivity and specificity, you can say, as a rule of thumb, that if your test is positive, you might be infected, especially if you also are experiencing typical symptoms, but if you have no symptoms, you probably are not infected, even with a positive test result, and so you should ask for a second test to confirm (actually, in a perfect world, the testing center should recommend a second test to you). If the second test is negative, you probably truly don't have the virus.

But beyond that, I hope this "glimpse under the hood" has shown you how the testing process is beset with imprecisions and inaccuracies and is nowhere near the nice simple and conclusive tool that most people think it is.

Now that we've looked at testing in some detail and also carefully looked at logical fallacies under several different headings in the opening chapter on "1. An Unfortunate and Unnecessary Controversy", it might be interesting to close this section with an analysis of the claim, repeatedly made, that "The US is leading the world in testing and is testing more people than any other country".

First, if we simply look at the numbers of tests by country, using Worldometers[336] as a source, the US today (17 August) is reporting a total of 71.5 million tests. But China, if it is to be believed, claims to have done 90.4 million tests, so right from the start, the claim the US is leading the world is uncertain rather than accurate.

However, wouldn't you agree that a more accurate measure than "total tests" is "tests per unit of population"? Of course countries with more people will probably have more tests more than countries with fewer people. Isn't it more important to know how widespread within the population testing has become?

Using that measure, we see the US has had testing equivalent to 21.6% of the population.[337] China, on the other hand, has only tested 6.3% of its population.

---

[336] See https://www.worldometers.info/coronavirus/ or https://cov.cx/w-c

[337] This is not the same as testing 21.6% of the population. Some people get many tests, so the actual percentage of the population tested is considerably lower.

But before we now call victory for the US, Worldometers reports that, by the measure of tests as a percent of population, the US drops to 18th place.[338] Sure, some of the countries with better testing rates are very small, but there are also large countries like the UK and Russia, and medium-sized countries such as Israel, Singapore, Denmark, and UAE all scoring significantly better than the US.

Wait! There's still more. Not all tests are equal. Surely what matters is how many tests give their test subjects the results back in a meaningful time period. There's no international ranking of countries by the timeliness of their test results, but our sense is the US would not be well placed if there was.

For example, over the weekend, we were sent an email from a guy in Canberra, Australia. He decided, on Saturday, to get a test. So he drove to a testing center that morning, waited 45 minutes to provide a sample, then went home again. Before the end of the day, he had received his test result via a text message on his phone. That is standard for Australia but almost unheard of in the US.

And there's still more. How about the accuracy of the test results? What is the value in doing lots of tests if they're not accurately reporting on if the test subjects are infected or not?

This is a factor that we can't guess about at all, but it is an important issue and in seeking to evaluate a country's overall testing program, is something that should also be considered.

---

[338] Update, in mid-October, the US had slipped further down to 20th place. However, by mid-December, it was back at 18th place again.

7. How Long Does an Infection Last

I t is helpful to understand how long a typical infection takes; to know what to expect and to understand if you are doing better, the same, or not as well as most other people.

Unfortunately, the first thing to appreciate is that this is a very unusual illness, and there are a very wide range of different experiences.

For example, look at this table of symptom duration[339] – there isn't a tight grouping and "peak" where most people's experiences lie.

---

[339] Taken from https://covid.joinzoe.com/post/covid-long-term or https://cov.cx/a1b67

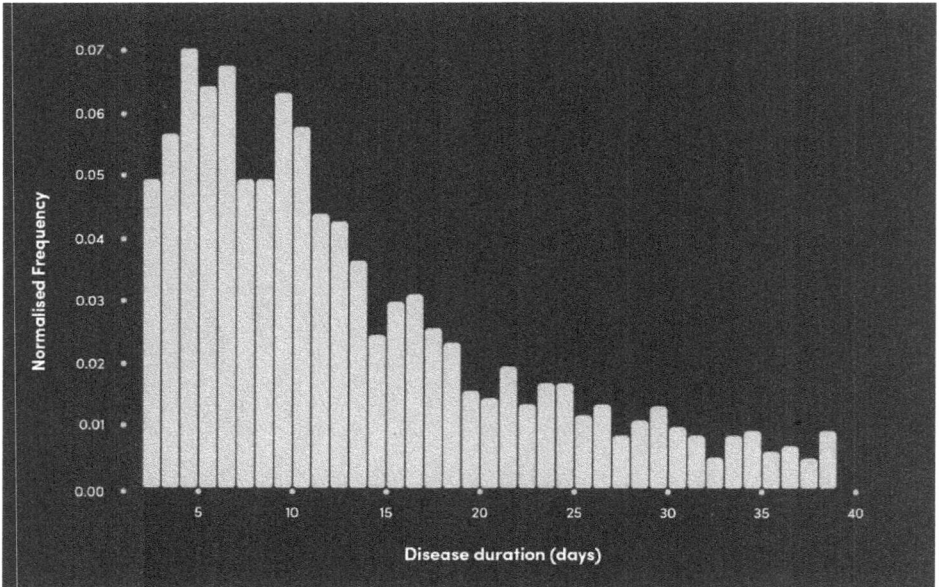

Figure 48 Incidence of disease duration

Not only does the length of illness vary by a very wide margin, but some people have the disease without any symptoms or illness at all. How many people have the disease without any symptoms? We don't know – guesses range from maybe slightly less than half of everyone who has the disease does so with no symptoms, to other estimates saying maybe three in every four people or even nine in ten people have no symptoms.[340]

It is hard to know for sure, of course, because of the lack of symptoms! (And also because testing is so difficult to arrange.)

In General

In general, it seems most people can expect to have their symptoms resolve and go away after about two weeks, and extended illnesses are usually over within

---

[340] We're very uncomfortable with these concepts. If you have no symptoms, do you really have the disease at all? We'll accept that for some people, the disease is so mild that the symptoms are barely noticeable at all. But in some cases, the definition of "has/had the disease" is based purely on not-always-accurate testing for the current or past presence of the virus, making these numbers far from exact.

about six weeks.[341] If you're fortunate, it could even be as short as one week.[342] Another study says that if you have a fever, it may last for about 8 – 11 days.[343]

Beyond that, we can't really say. Have another look above at the chart showing the very wide spread of time it takes for symptoms to go away. You might be anywhere on that chart; we hope it will be on the left side, of course!

This is frustrating. Yes, there are many web sites offering day by day guides as to how a coronavirus infection typically progresses. We hesitate to create such a guide, although we understand the potential and theoretical usefulness of such things. Our hesitation is based on the wide range of "typical" times (look again at the chart above).

An example of the uselessness of some of these tables can be seen in one such table, full of vague and contradictory information within it.[344]

It says that Day Three of an infection is typically when patients in Wenzhou were admitted to a hospital, but Day Seven is typically when patients in Wuhan were admitted to a hospital. Why the huge difference? And, assuming you're not in Wenzhou or Wuhan, what should you expect, here in the US?

It says that by Day Eight patients with severe cases will most likely have developed Acute Respiratory Distress Syndrome (ARDS), requiring intubation, but also says one study found that it takes 12 days in Wuhan until patients get admitted to the ICU.

It says that on average people in Wuhan either recovered or died between 17-21 days after symptom onset. But an average is never a range of numbers. An average is the mid-point of a range, not the range itself, so we've no idea what the article is trying to tell us. It also says the average hospital stay for Wenzhou patients is 27 days – but it says that on Day 27, although patients were typically admitted on Day Three. So do they mean Day 30? Or 24 days in hospital from Day 3 until Day 27?

Okay, we've probably made our point. Be very wary of these types of tables. They're as likely to be wrong than right.

---

[341] See https://www.webmd.com/lung/covid-recovery-overview#2-4 or https://cov.cx/a1b68

[342] See https://www.msn.com/en-us/health/medical/how-long-does-it-take-to-recover-from-the-coronavirus/ar-BB15hPBf or https://cov.cx/a1b69

[343] See https://www.popsugar.com/fitness/how-long-does-fever-last-with-coronavirus-47392121 or https://cov.cx/a1b70

[344] See https://www.businessinsider.com/coronavirus-covid19-day-by-day-symptoms-patients-2020-2 or https://cov.cx/a1b71

A Common Timeline for a Covid-19 Illness

However, we know you want a timeline, so after all the excuses and criticisms, here's a very approximate one.[345] Please keep in mind that your experience will almost certainly not fit exactly within these times, and it is neither good nor bad if things are happening faster or slower. It just is what it is - our sense is the key issue is more the severity of symptoms, not the speed with which they come and go.

Day 1

This is defined as the first day you notice you have some virus symptoms. They may be very mild to start with.[346]

Days 2 – 3

There may be slow growth in symptoms during the next two days. Maybe some new symptoms appear, or existing ones become more prominent and impactful.

Days 4 – 6

If you're lucky, nothing new happens at this point. You are probably now sufficiently developed with your symptoms to be likely to get an accurate positive test if you take a virus test (you might be able to get a positive test sooner, but it is only now that the chances of the test accurately detecting your illness rise close to 100%).

If you're not lucky, you'll start to feel worse around now. Your fever will be steady, you might have assorted aches, a cough, and an inability to get comfortable.

Possibly (especially for younger people) you might develop some type of skin rash or swelling/blistering.

Days 7 & 8

This is about the soonest you can expect your symptoms to start to subside, but don't be alarmed if they persist longer.

Other people might stay the same or even get worse, and a few will briefly feel better, only then to have a relapse and become worse than before.

Days 8 – 12 (other sources suggest days 5 – 10)

---

[345] Largely copied from this article
https://www.nytimes.com/2020/04/30/well/live/coronavirus-days-5-through-10.html or https://cov.cx/a1b72

[346] Remember our recommendation to keep a diary of your symptoms. Be sure to start it right away.

This is the point where your infection *might* get really bad. It is sometimes referred to as the "second-week crash".[347] Keep an eye on your blood oxygen levels (see our chapter on "17. Medical Equipment & Supplies You Should Have", starting on page 398).

If things are not improving, and particularly if they are getting worse, this is the period where most people tend to get admitted to a hospital. If you get past this period and still haven't been admitted to a hospital, your chances of subsequently needing hospitalization are now starting to decline.

Days 13 & 14

If you had only a mild illness, you have probably recovered by now.

If you had worse symptoms but managed to keep your oxygen levels up, you should be feeling better, even if not completely recovered.

But if you had severe problems and possibly lower oxygen levels, you may still be going through the process.

Day 15 and beyond

Your mileage may – will – vary. See again the chart at the top of this chapter (on page 196).

Long-Haul Illness

Talking about the concept of day 15 and beyond, some unfortunate people have long-lasting effects and problems, sometimes exceeding three months in duration.[348]

This article suggests 12% of Covid-sufferers still have some symptoms 30 days after symptoms first appeared, and – in the UK – 2% of Covid-sufferers still have symptoms after 90 days.[349] An Irish study suggests a much higher number – it

---

[347] See https://www.stuff.co.nz/national/health/coronavirus/300001328/coronavirus-secondweek-crash-is-time-of-peril-for-some-covid19-patients?rm=a or https://cov.cx/a1b73

[348] See https://www.vox.com/2020/7/14/21324201/covid-19-long-term-effects-symptoms-treatment or https://cov.cx/a1b74 and https://www.stuff.co.nz/national/health/coronavirus/122431932/coronavirus-i-think-i-have-long-covid-but-im-struggling-to-be-diagnosed or https://cov.cx/a1b75 and https://www.theguardian.com/commentisfree/2020/jun/28/coronavirus-long-haulers-infectious-disease-testing or https://cov.cx/a1b76

[349] See https://www.trialsitenews.com/so-called-long-covid-a-bigger-problem-than-many-know/ or https://cov.cx/a1b77

isn't clear to us exactly how random their sample selection process was, so we simply observe that the study showed a high prevalence of ongoing fatigue, which is the most prevalent lingering condition.[350]

It is unclear why some people have chronic ongoing symptoms, and the medical community is only slowly starting to accept the existence of this phenomenon as a specific thing. In October an interesting article speculated that the reason for the illness is not so much the virus, but "misbehaving" antibodies that are now attacking your otherwise healthy body, even though the virus has long since been overcome. In comparing this to the lupus disease, the article omits the mention that a common treatment for lupus is hydroxychloroquine, a treatment that many have advocated for the early stages of Covid-19, too.[351]

Another possible explanation is due to damage to the lungs in particular.[352] Probably there are several different underlying causes – sometimes it might be one issue, other times another, and perhaps on occasion a combination.

Of course, with the virus still very new, it is hard to know if people who have suffered ongoing symptoms for three or four months will continue to suffer them indefinitely, or if it is just a long slow but definite fade away of the symptoms ending in a return to normalcy.

Here's a somewhat click-baity article that claims to list the 98 (!!!) different symptoms that might persist for an extended time.[353] It shows the percentage of people reporting each symptom. This is based on a self-reported group of 1,567 sufferers who described their symptoms in their own words, hence the similarity in some of these entries.

The article starts with the least common long-lasting symptom, and requires you to click countless times to get to the more common ones. To save you some of the bother, here are the top 25 entries.

[350] See https://www.medrxiv.org/content/10.1101/2020.07.29.20164293v1 or https://cov.cx/a1b78

[351] See https://www.nytimes.com/2020/10/27/health/covid-antibodies-autoimmunity.html or https://cov.cx/a1b79

[352] See https://www.reuters.com/article/health-coronavirus-lungs-int-idUSKBN27K00X or https://cov.cx/a1c19

[353] See https://www.msn.com/en-us/health/medical/the-98-longest-lasting-covid-symptoms-you-need-to-know-about/ss-BB17W417 or https://cov.cx/a1b80

Symptom	Prevalence
Fatigue	100%
Muscle or body aches	67%
Shortness of breath/difficulty breathing	65%
Difficulty concentrating or focusing	59%
Inability to exercise or be active	59%
Headache	58%
Difficulty sleeping	50%
Anxiety	48%
Memory problems	46%
Dizziness	42%
Persistent chest pain or pressure	39%
Cough	37%
Joint pain	36%
Heart palpitations	32%
Diarrhea	32%
Sore throat	32%
Night sweats	30%
Partial or complete loss of smell	30%
Tachycardia	29%
Fever or chills	28%
Hair loss	27%

Blurry vision	27%
Congested or runny nose	26%
Sadness	26%
Neuropathy in hands or feet	26%

Figure 49 Long-lived symptoms

More scholarly details of the study and analysis are also available online.

If you are suffering long-term extended issues, we recommend you join the group that is coordinating the experiences of all such people.[354]   Our sense is this remains a somewhat overlooked aspect of the disease and needs further pressure to encourage more attention.

Post-Covid Syndrome

There's a related nastiness, too, that seems similar and may or may not be another form of a long-haul illness, which has the unofficial name of post-Covid syndrome. Some people are reporting, after having gone through an infection, then feeling better and getting an "all clear" negative test, that a few weeks after that, they start to feel unwell *again*.

They start to be easily fatigued, maybe suffer shortness of breath, get a cough again, and perhaps lose their sense of smell.

According to data from patients of the Caduceus Medical Group in Southern California,[355] about 15% of their recently recovered Covid patients are experiencing this. They report the most common symptom is very bad fatigue, and they surmise that it seems to be more a factor in people who didn't take it easy and rest a great deal while fighting the disease initially.

They assist their patients by treating symptoms, but the underlying mechanism that causes this is not well understood.

---

[354] See https://www.survivorcorps.com/ or https://cov.cx/a1b81 for more information

[355] I've been very impressed with the material they are sending to their clients on how they are responding to the challenges of Covid-19. If you're in their service area and you need Covid help, they'd be a great resource. See https://www.caduceusmedicalgroup.com/ or https://cov.cx/a1b82

There are also reports elsewhere of new auto-immune diseases appearing in people seemingly recovered from Covid (Caduceus mention Hashimoto's, Lupus, and Sjogren's) but these remain relatively uncommon, so far.

How Long Does a Person Remain Infectious

If you know you have the virus, how long are you infectious and capable of passing the virus on to other people?

Most people are at their most infectious in the early stages of the disease – and most alarmingly, are at their maximum degree of infectiousness before their symptoms have started to appear.

While the infection risk starts to diminish after that maximum, it doesn't vanish for some time.

The CDC says that most research suggests that *most* people remain infectious for no more than ten days after their symptoms appear and that all people stop being infectious after 20 days.[356]

The CDC also says that the infectious stage does not go away until at least 24 hours after the patient's fever subsides without the use of fever-reducing medicines. It adds that your other symptoms should also be improving before you can be considered no longer an infectious risk.[357]

One point of clarification, in case needed. There is a difference between no longer being infectious and no longer having the disease. As implied immediately above, you can still have all manner of Covid-19 symptoms, but no longer be infectious.

---

[356] See https://www.cdc.gov/media/releases/2020/s0814-updated-isolation-guidance.html or https://cov.cx/a1b83

[357] See https://www.cdc.gov/coronavirus/2019-ncov/if-you-are-sick/end-home-isolation.html or https://cov.cx/a1b84

8. How to Know if You are Cured

This is perhaps the happiest question in the entire book! But, like everything else, it is surprisingly hard to answer succinctly and exactly.

It takes a lot more than just the simple passing of time to be cured. As we mentioned above in the chapter "7. How Long Does an Infection Last", starting on page 195, it can take days, or weeks, or even months for a person to finally work their way clear of their infection.

Hopefully, at some point, you'll start to feel better. When can you say that you are now cured, and – very importantly – no longer infectious and a risk to others?

You'll not be surprised to learn that, like everything to do with the virus, the answer to this is somewhat vague.

It also is important to distinguish between being no longer infectious and being cured. You can be no longer infectious well before you are cured.

But in general, if you feel better, that's the first point and perhaps even the most important point. Consider that reaching first base.

The second point is you no longer have a fever (and are not taking anti-fever meds) and have been without a fever for at least one or three days.[358] When that describes you, please advance to second base.

---

[358] The CDC had been using three days with no fever as part of its "you are no longer infectious" tests, but then shortened it to one day. Maybe split the difference and call it two?

You reach third base if it is at least ten days since you first started suffering from virus symptoms.

This "wait ten days" part is somewhat arbitrary. So we suggest one more thing.

To complete your home run, you should speak to your doctor and possibly get tested to see if you still have the coronavirus in your system. The best practice is to get two tests, at least a day apart, with both of the tests showing you to be clear.[359]

In some cases – if you have an impaired immune system – your doctor might advocate continuing to take it easy.

And in all cases, it is important not to over-stress yourself during your recovery. If you do this, there is a clear danger that you'll relapse.[360]

So, the answer to the question seems to be that it will take at least ten days before you're free of the virus, and possibly considerably longer.

But note this process assumes you had symptoms. It seems almost half of people officially deemed to have the virus never show symptoms. If you're fortunate enough to have had a symptomless case of Covid-19, then you immediately pass first and second base on our three-base/home run analogy.

The two key points remaining for people who never had any symptoms might be "at least ten days from your positive test results" and your doctor's opinion and tests showing you to now be clear of the virus.

---

[359] We tell you this because it is official advice. But for much of the last eight months, this suggestion has little connection to reality. Hopefully, the growing number of fast and inexpensive tests will start to make this a practical suggestion at long last.

We'd also not obsess too much if you are getting PCR type tests and they show the virus is still present. This may be a "false positive" result by the test, caused by the test being unable to distinguish between the active live virus particles and the dead remnants of the virus that is now "safe" and no longer active.

[360] See https://www.cdc.gov/coronavirus/2019-ncov/hcp/disposition-in-home-patients.html or https://cov.cx/a1b85 and https://www.cdc.gov/coronavirus/2019-ncov/hcp/disposition-hospitalized-patients.html or https://cov.cx/a1b86

9. Self Quarantining

If you do have a case of the virus, you must do all you can to prevent passing it on to others. Hopefully that goes without saying.

Unfortunately, there's a strong possibility that you may have already passed it on, during the early stages of your infection, when you didn't yet have symptoms and so were unknowingly passing the virus on to other people around you. But what's done is done, you still need to fairly focus on ensuring you don't pass it on to any more people, please.[361]

---

[361] There can be very selfish as well as altruistic reasons to do this. If you are careless, maybe you infect someone else you know, then they in turn infect other people that you both know, including possibly others of your immediate family and closest friends. The disease heartlessly travels through groups of people, and just because you have been careful not to infect your closest family members doesn't mean you haven't infected someone else, who in turn infected someone else again, and that person now meets your close family members and brings the virus right back home again.

Remember the concept of "everyone is no more than six connections away from anyone else in the world". It is the same with the virus, and usually, rather than six connections, the number is much smaller.

So if the thought of saving the lives of strangers isn't strong motivation, keep in mind that your careful quarantining may be both directly and indirectly also saving the lives of those people closest to you.

Your Recent Contacts

You should *urgently* contact anyone you might have had "risky contact" with for the previous few days before your symptoms first appeared and recommend they also self-isolate and get tested to see if they now have the virus, too.

How many days back should you go? Many official contact tracing programs go back two days. We'd suggest three or even four, but probably no further - the chances of you being infectious fall off drastically when you go further back than this.[362]

Be also aware that as well as maybe you giving your new infection to these other people, perhaps one of them was the person you picked up the infection from – another reason for all your recent contacts to check themselves out.

A "risky contact" would be someone you had close contact with. If you both were not wearing masks, the risk factor goes up, if the contact was indoors, the risk factor goes up, and the longer you were together, yet again the risk factor goes up.

As you contact these people you should also suggest they might want to start giving "heads up" warnings to the people they are in the most regular and close contact with. It is only by reaching aggressively back that we have a chance of trying to reduce the virus spread.

Some people have said they feel awkward and embarrassed at doing this. There is no reason why you should feel that way. In large part, the virus is a "no-fault" phenomenon; there is no need to feel guilty or embarrassed at telling people you have the virus. It is a short-term temporary situation for you, and hopefully soon enough you'll emerge fully recovered and back to normal once more. There shouldn't be any stigma before, during, or after being infected, and all people with any degree of sense will appreciate your calling to tell them of their possible risk and thank you for doing so.

But if your feeling of social discomfort might prevent you from contacting everyone you can, maybe you can ask for a friend or family member to do it for you.

Some public health services offer some degree of "contact tracing" whereby they'll do all this for you. But we've heard some dismaying stories about how ineffective those services are – the phrase "too little, too late" sadly springs to mind much of the time. Yes, certainly cooperate with any such service that might

---

[362] It seems that in general 42% of all infections are passed on by people before they have any symptoms, and 35% of infections are passed on the day symptoms are first noticed or the following day. See https://www.stuff.co.nz/national/health/coronavirus/300105935/covid19-most-coronavirus-transmission-isnt-being-caught-in-time or https://cov.cx/a1b87

be offered, but don't rely on it entirely and at least call the people you've had the highest risk contacts with, directly, yourself.

The Quarantine Period

In most cases, how you quarantine will be a compromise between the ideal and the practical. But that is not a reason to not bother at all, it is a reason to try your very best to make your quarantine as effective as possible.

If you are sharing a residence with other people, there is of course a very good chance that you have already shared the virus with them. But be positive, and hope they don't yet have it,[363] and so do everything you can to keep it from them now.

Ideally, you will be able to shut yourself off from other people in your residence. Live in your own private bedroom, and if possible, have your own private bathroom too. If you have to share a bathroom, please make sure you always lower the lid on the toilet before flushing. An extraordinary amount of aerosol particles and droplets erupt up in a plume from the toilet bowl when flushed, and because virus particles have been detected in feces, this could be creating a cloud of infectious particles. Lowering the lid helps reduce the volume of that cloud.[364] Of course, if the bathroom has a window, open that, assuming the airflow will then cause the contaminated bathroom air to flow out, rather than for air to come in the window and therefore speed the contaminated air to flow into the rest of the house. Otherwise, use the expeller fan if it exists - run that for a while. But, if it is possible, try and find where the fan exhausts to. Some of them just blow the air into the voids in the walls and between floors. That's not nearly as beneficial as one which has an exhaust duct that goes to the outside.

Many houses have multiple exhaust fans – for laundry, kitchen, bathrooms, and maybe elsewhere too, so there might be many exhaust openings around the side of your house. Walk around with the fan running and see if you can work out if any of the openings relate to that fan – maybe a louver will be slightly open when the fan is running, so compare the state of them when the fan is running and not. Sometimes you can hear the fan through one of the openings but not others, too. But if there's no airflow and no sounds, perhaps the bathroom fan

---

[363] Of course they should act with caution and get tested to see if they have the virus so they know what they should be doing themselves. But don't all quarantine together if you are a mix of infected people and people who don't yet know their status.

[364] This is a fascinating article with amazing pictures of the clouds that come up from a toilet flush. https://www.studyfinds.org/what-happens-when-you-flush-with-toilet-lid-up/ or https://cov.cx/a1b88

just blows the air into the building spaces. Even that is better than nothing, but not as good as an open window or a true exhaust fan.

This would be a great time to ask the others who live with you to cook for you,[365] and to leave meals outside your closed door, on paper plates with plastic knives and forks. Put all refuse into trash bags and every few days (the longer the gap between times, the less risky contact your roommates need to engage in) put your trash outside your room for them to take out.

Give thought to the airflow in your room. Air flows are one of the main paths for the virus to pass from one person to others. Many homes have a central forced-air heating/cooling system. Heated or cooled air is ducted around the house from the central furnace/cooler and blows into your room through a register in the floor or walls or ceiling. It travels around your room to heat or cool it, and then usually goes out the door (under the door if it is shut – that is why there is an appreciable space at the bottom of most internal doors) and flows to a central return register somewhere, at which point the air is taken back to the furnace/cooling coil, reheated or recooled, and recirculated again.

That means the virus particles you are breathing out and into the air are swished along with the airflow, through the central unit, and then distributed all through the house. These aerosol particles are thought to be the main way the infection spreads, and you've just made it much easier for them to find the other people living with you.

Yes, there'll be a filter in the main return line just before the furnace/cooling coil, but that filter is not designed to filter out tiny virus particles. It is more to prevent larger particles – things you can see with the naked eye – from getting into the furnace/coil.

You can get higher quality filters, but even then we'd not trust them entirely. Sure, a better filter won't hurt and might help, although you then have to be certain to replace it on the recommended schedule or else it becomes less effective.

Air filters typically have a MERV (Minimum Efficiency Reporting Value) rating. The lowest rating is 1, and the highest is 20. ASHRAE (the American Society of Heating, Refrigerating and Airconditioning Engineers) recommends using filters with a rating of 13 or 14 to have an impact on reducing aerosolized virus particles and stopping them recirculating around your home. Filters with ratings lower than (or equal to) 10 do not claim to trap any particles smaller than 1.0 microns. Filters rated 17 or higher are HEPA type quality.

---

[365] And, absolutely – and truly for medical reasons – to do all the washing up, too! Who said there aren't upsides to having the virus…..

Here's a fairly honest set of claims for what to expect from MERV filters.[366] Some tables show "less than 20%" for lower-rated MERV filter capabilities, and while, strictly speaking that is true, in reality the less than 20% usually means 0%.

MERV VALUE	The filter will trap Average Particle Size Efficiency 0.3 - 1.0 Micron	The filter will trap Average Particle Size Efficiency 1.0 - 3.0 Micron	The filter will trap Average Particle Size Efficiency 3.0 - 10.0 Micron	Types of things these filters will trap
MERV 1	-	-	Less than 20%	
MERV 2	-	-	Less than 20%	Pollen, dust mites, standing dust, spray paint dust, carpet fibers
MERV 3	-	-	Less than 20%	
MERV 4	-	-	Less than 20%	
MERV 5	-	-	20% - 34%	
MERV 6	-	-	35% - 49%	Mold spores, hair spray, fabric protector, cement dust
MERV 7	-	-	50% - 69%	
MERV 8	-	-	70% - 85%	
MERV 9	-	Less than 50%	85% or better	
MERV 10	-	50% - 64%	85% or better	Humidifier dust, lead dust, auto emissions, milled flour
MERV 11	-	65% - 79%	85% or better	
MERV 12	-	80% - 89%	90% or better	
MERV 13	Less than 75%	90% or better	90% or better	
MERV 14	75% - 84%	90% or better	90% or better	Bacteria, most tobacco smoke, proplet Nuceli (sneeze)
MERV 15	85% - 94%	90% or better	90% or better	
MERV 16	95% or better	90% or better	90% or better	

Figure 50 MERV filter ratings

There are two immediate problems with high-rated filters. The first is that most MERV ratings are self-calculated by the filter manufacturer, and so you are relying on them to be accurate in their rating.

The second is that most commercial systems are designed to work with lower-rated MERV 6 – 8 filters. The higher-rated filters impede the airflow more than the lower-rated filters, and this may stress your system and reduce its efficiency and effectiveness.[367]

---

[366] Taken from this site https://www.minnicks.com/learning-center/indoor-air-quality/what-does-merv-rating-mean-on-a-furnace-filter-why-should-i-care/ or https://cov.cx/a1b89

[367] This is a potentially big deal. A reduced airflow means that the heat exchanger in your system isn't transferring as much heat between itself and the air blowing over/through it. If you are in cooling mode, this could mean your coils freeze over, and then transfer less cooling to the air, which makes the system work harder, and ultimately you could have liquid rather than evaporated coolant going back to the outside compressor, which would be very bad. If you are in heating mode, the heater unit

(continued on next page)

For these reasons, it is probably better that you shut off any central air system registers in your room. Use an in-room radiant heater for heating, if you need cooling in the summer, your ideal solution is an "in the window" unit. That way you keep your air separate from the air in the rest of the house.

Also consider adding a HEPA filter equipped air purifier in your room, not so much for your benefit, but more as a courtesy for other people (check our chapter, below, "17. Medical Equipment & Supplies You Should Have" for specifics on how to choose all the things you should have and might need).

Any time you need to venture out of your room, please wear a proper mask – a surgical mask rather than a fashion mask. If anyone comes close to you, they should wear a mask too.

If you are sharing utensils with other people, they should be first disinfected and then washed. Any surfaces that you might touch should also be disinfected, and you should regularly wash your hands.

When can you end your quarantine? We discuss that in the section "8. How to Know if You are Cured", above on page 204.

Pets

There are a very few cases where it seems cats[368] and dogs (also mink[369] and possibly ferrets) may have become infected with the virus, too. Cats seem to be more susceptible than dogs, and generally, if a dog does get infected, it seems unlikely to be life-threatening.

There is very little evidence to suggest that animals can pass the virus on to other animals (it seems this is most likely with cats for some reason), and similarly, there are only very weak suggestions that animals can in turn infect humans.[370]

The terrible thing (and I've a lovely German Shepherd – she and I are inseparable, 24/7) is that, if you have the virus, it behooves you to consider

---

might get too hot and crack, and possibly then allow carbon monoxide (assuming you have a gas furnace) into the airflow. Possibly your unit has a way of varying the fan speed to adjust for the thicker density of higher-grade filters. See https://www.energyvanguard.com/blog/unintended-consequences-high-merv-filters or https://cov.cx/a1b90

[368] Both in the sense of domestic pets, and also larger cats such as lions and tigers, too

[369] See https://www.studyfinds.org/mink-study-first-covid-transmission-animals-humans/ or https://cov.cx/a1b91

[370] See, for example, https://www.cdc.gov/coronavirus/2019-ncov/daily-life-coping/animals.html or https://cov.cx/a1b92

keeping away from your pets, at a time when you likely will most benefit from their comfort and companionship, and at a time when they'll be anxious about what is happening to you.

If you can't or won't keep away from them, you should at least minimize your contact with them. Try not to, ahem, exchange any bodily fluids with them – I don't mean this in the intimate sense, but don't let them lick you and of course, don't give them a "kiss" either. Don't give them the scraps off your plate.

Wash your hands regularly and consider even wearing a mask around your pet.

That is all heartbreaking, of course, but not as bad as watching your pet become infected and die as a result of your wrong choices.

On the other hand, there are only a very few known cases of this happening, and with over 8.2 million virus cases so far (15 October) in the US, and 67% of US households having some type of pet, we'd think there'd be many more cases and publicity about pet infections if it was a definite strong risk.

New research has ranked different types of animals in terms of their theoretical risk of becoming infected by the virus. Cats, sheep, and cattle ranked as medium risk, dogs, pigs, and horses were low risk, and mice were very low risk.[371]

---

[371] See https://medicalxpress.com/news/2020-08-genomic-analysis-reveals-animal-species.html or https://cov.cx/a1b93

PART THREE : Avoiding the Virus

10. How to Avoid Infection – In General

Note – this is the first of four chapters on how to avoid or minimize your risk of catching the virus. We've tried to split the topic into four helpful pieces, but we urge you to read all four chapters as an entirety, because elements of each chapter and the recommendations within it apply to the other three chapters, too.

We'll start this chapter off with some medical theory. Skip it or skim through it if you prefer, we start to get into the real "meat" of the chapter when you get to the section "The Three Main Infection Routes" starting on page 231.

Perhaps we should commence with a question (and answer) – should you even bother trying to avoid the virus? Some people have clearly decided there is no point in trying to avoid an infection. Some are young and foolish (and, as we know or remember, the young have little appreciation of risk and their own mortality), but others are of more mature years and are more likely to have an awareness of such things.

There are also cases where groups of people get together to have a virus party, and hope they'll become infected, to "get it over and done with". Is that a good idea?

We've seen in our section "5. How Serious is the Virus?", above, starting on page 146, some data on what the risks of dying from it might be. Young healthy people have little to worry about, and the older and more generally frail you become, the more serious a threat Covid-19 becomes.

But there is a huge additional factor that perhaps we've not stated clearly enough so far. Simply surviving the virus is not the only thing to worry about and hope for. Some people will suffer continued symptoms and problems for an extended period – we don't know yet how long because the virus is still so new. We discuss this in the section "Long-Haul Illness", see page 199, above.

Other people will *never* make a complete recovery and will suffer lasting damage to their lungs, or heart, or brain, or other organs/aspects of their health. We don't yet have a sufficient statistical base to know about the prevalence of such things, for example, this report[372] simultaneously talks about 77% of Chinese patients with lasting lung damage of varying severity, 19.7% with heart damage, and another study suggesting 12% with cardio-vascular damage of various types.

This article[373] provides another perspective on these concerns, and adds an extra point – even asymptomatic people are likely to experience long-lasting or permanent lung damage.

The good news about lung damage? For many sufferers, it might eventually heal. The bad news? According to this article, it could take 15 years for recovery to be completed.[374]

This article reports that kidney problems have also been experienced.[375] Another article reports on long-term and possibly permanent loss of smell and taste.[376]

We could continue throwing articles at you, but hopefully you get the point. <u>You really want to avoid the virus if at all possible.</u>

Plus, you also want other people to avoid the virus. Because, if other people become infected, that increases the chance/risk that you'll interact with them

---

[372] See https://www.advisory.com/daily-briefing/2020/06/02/covid-health-effects or https://cov.cx/a1b94

[373] See https://www.vox.com/2020/5/8/21251899/coronavirus-long-term-effects-symptoms or https://cov.cx/a1b95

[374] See https://www.independent.co.uk/news/health/coronavirus-long-term-health-disease-covid-19-lungs-heart-brain-a9546671.html or https://cov.cx/a1b96

[375] See https://web.archive.org/web/20201031053240/https://www.today.com/health/coronavirus-long-term-health-covid-19-impact-lungs-heart-kidneys-t178770 or https://cov.cx/a1b97

[376] See https://www.usnews.com/news/health-news/articles/2020-06-04/loss-of-smell-taste-might-be-long-term-for-some-covid-19-survivors or https://cov.cx/a1b98

and catch the infection, too. The way the virus spreads is such that when a person decides to allow themselves to get infected, they are likely in turn infecting some number of extra people too – people who might not be as young or healthy, and who might not be as eager/willing to be infected.

On the other hand, those people with their foolish behaviors and "virus parties" might actually be helping sensible people like you and me. If they should now develop immunity after their virus illness, that might possibly benefit us through a phenomenon known as "herd immunity".

We'll talk about herd immunity – something we've teased you with the mention of several times already – in just a minute. It is important because, at least at present, it presents as the only hope most of us have to finally get clear of the threat of this disease (we wrote further about vaccines in the chapter "3. When Will the Virus Finally Go Away?", starting on page 104).

But first, there's one other question that we should at least acknowledge, even if not completely answer.

Herd Immunity

The phrase "herd immunity" is being used a lot currently, and usually in a sense that is more wishful than real. It refers to the situation whereby the virus stops growing in numbers once a certain number of people have either been vaccinated or caught the virus and survived, and, in both cases, acquired immunity as a result.

The concept is quite simple. Let's assume that the average infected person meets 50 people while they are infected, and has a 4% chance of infecting each person they meet.

That means, to start with, each infected person will pass the infection on to (50 x 4% =) 2 more people. You might recognize this as being the "R number" that we discussed way back on page 136.

Now for the herd immunity concept. What happens in our example if 20% of the population have already had the virus and so are not vulnerable to re-infection?"

The infected person still meets 50 people, but 10 of them (ie 20%) have now had the virus, and so only 40 are liable to be infected. That means that the infected person now passes the virus on to (40 x 4% =) 1.6 people. The virus is still growing but at a slower rate.

Let's continue this thought exercise and say the virus has been present for a while longer, and now 50% of the population have already been infected.

Now when an infected person meets their 50 people, only half of them – 25 – are still vulnerable to infection, and the infected person infects (25 x 4% =) one new person. The virus is now at a steady-state, neither growing nor shrinking in terms of new case numbers. Each infected person infects one more person.

In a while, the total infected percentage will grow to say 60%. That means that only 20 of an infected person's contacts are at risk of infection, and the number of new infections is now (20 x 4% =) 0.8 new infections.

The virus is now starting to die out. Each infected person infects less than one more person – in this example, every five people infect four more people, and so on. Herd immunity has been achieved.

The more infectious a virus is, the higher the level of already infected people that are needed to achieve herd immunity. The coronavirus is sometimes suggested to have an "R" rate of about 2.5, and that calculates out to requiring about 60% or so of the population to have gained herd immunity for the virus to then start dying out rather than staying at a steady level or, as in the early days, growing in numbers.

There is a formula for calculating the necessary level of herd immunity (h) to stop a virus from growing. It is happily simple :

$$h = 1 - \frac{1}{R}$$

So, if we say R = 2.5, then this formula calculates as

$$h = 1 - \frac{1}{2.5} = 0.6 \; ie \; 60\%$$

In other words, we need six out of every ten people, or 60% of the population, to have immunity for the virus to stop growing if its R value is 2.5. If the R value goes up, so too does the level of herd immunity needed to stop the growth of the infection (for example, if R = 3, then we need 67% of the population to have acquired herd immunity, if R = 1.5, we only need 33%).

Herd immunity can also be gained through vaccination. It is the same thing, either way – as long as you reduce the number of potential new infection opportunities, you are moving to a herd immunity point.

So, yes, that also means that wearing masks and social distancing also provides a type of herd immunity, because it reduces the number of potential new infection opportunities.

The weakness of this form of herd immunity, and why it isn't considered in simple calculations, is it only lasts as long as people continue to wear masks and socially distance. It is an active and temporary measure, rather than a passive and possibly permanent measure.

Talking about weaknesses, there is one very important thing to keep in mind about herd immunity. As you now know, it acts to slow down the spread of the virus and to make it harder and eventually impossible for the infection chain to continue to grow. That is the good news.

The bad news? Herd immunity does not give you any personal medical super-powers. If you've not yet had the virus, *you are still as much at risk of becoming infected if you encounter someone with the virus as you ever have been.* Herd immunity reduces the rate of spread, and when the rate of spread and therefore the count of active infections starts to go down, the chances that each person you'll interact with might currently be infectious goes down, too. But if you strike it unlikely, you'll still get the virus yourself, exactly the same as before.

This brings us to the second weakness of herd immunity. *If you do become infected, your experience will be as severe and life-threatening as it always has been.* That should be obvious, but we think not everyone understands this because we just don't understand why people are embracing herd immunity so enthusiastically – especially in the unstated hope that herd immunity means that other people will do what needs to be done, rather than needing to do something oneself.

In Russian roulette, it is like playing the game but the revolver now has more than six chambers in its cylinder. Maybe it now has nine, or twelve, or whatever. You pull the trigger, and your chances of hearing a click have improved, but if there's a bang instead, the impact on you is the same as always.

There are some other aspects to herd immunity too. This brings us to the next point.

Not All People Are Equally At Risk

There is an obvious difference in terms of risk between different people, based on lifestyle alone. Think, for example, of a person who stays at home and lives alone, and only goes out once every two weeks for a careful bit of hurried grocery shopping. Now compare that to a young person who commutes to work on a crowded bus every day, works alongside many colleagues, interacts with the public during the day, and goes out many nights a week eating, drinking, and dancing with friends (and strangers). To make the difference starker, the stay at home person always wears a mask and uses hand sanitizer galore, the other person never wears a mask or washes their hands.

Some high-risk people are termed "super-spreaders" because they, unsurprisingly, infect very many more people than other infected people do. (The term also applies to people who for puzzling reasons seem to be more infectious than other people.)

The interesting thing about this is that the second person is more of a risk factor both in terms of their likelihood of getting the disease and in terms of their likelihood to spread the disease. That seems obvious, doesn't it. This is significant.

The weakness of the original concept of herd immunity is that it assumes everyone is the same, with the same risk of contracting and spreading an infection. But as we've just shown, that is not true.

People with high-risk lifestyles are more likely to be among the first people to contract the disease, because of their high-risk lifestyles. Remember our example, above, where we talked about a person who interacts with 50 people a day? If 50/day is normal (it doesn't matter if it is or not for this example) then the high-risk people might interact with 200 (pick a number, any number) of people, unsafely, every day.

On the other hand, the low-risk person we cited above might only interact with five people every day.

The high-risk person is four times more likely than average, and 40 times more likely than the low-risk person, to get the virus, and also is likely to in turn spread it on to 4 or 40 times more people.

Once the high-risk people have had their infections, the people who remain are lower risk, and because they are lower risk, the R number reduces as does also, therefore, the calculated need for herd immunity.

Allowing for this, some studies suggest that if there is an inequality and imbalance as to who acquires immunity, instead of needing, for example, 60% of the entire population to become immune, once the "super-spreaders" have acquired immunity, and it is thought that by definition, they'll be among the first people to be infected, then that will be enough for the entire population. The percentage of super-spreaders is somewhat conjectural, as is the difference in spreading rates, but studies suggest herd immunity could be reached if only 10% of the population in Portugal or 20% of the population in the UK – the super-spreaders in each case – get the disease.[377]

This is an interesting example of how the abstract theory and consideration only of averages can be and perhaps should be massively adjusted to reflect the real-world issues and implications.

So there has been a refining of the concept of herd immunity to allow for a spread of different risks, with the result that whatever it actually is – a matter for some debate, perhaps – it is likely that real-world herd immunity might be lower than theoretical "everyone the same" herd immunity.

---

[377] See https://www.medrxiv.org/content/10.1101/2020.07.23.20160762v1.full.pdf or https://cov.cx/a1b99

There is another huge assumption built into herd immunity. It is such a huge assumption that it is paradoxically easy to miss it. This assumption is that people actually do get immunity after an infection. But is that true? Alas, immunity is neither guaranteed nor necessarily long-lasting.

Can You Get the Virus a Second Time?

Most people have hoped that getting a Covid infection means they would develop immunity and not have it a second time. That is an essential ingredient of herd immunity.

But there has never been any promise this would happen. The WHO website says "There is currently no evidence that people who have recovered from COVID-19 and have antibodies are protected from a second infection."[378]

It had seemed, based on analysis of antibodies in recovered people's bloodstreams, that some degree of immunity was being created, although knowing how strong that immunity was or for how long it would last required a theoretical estimate, because no researchers would deliberately try to re-infect recovered people, and because we still don't have enough time to start to get a sense for how the antibody levels hold up and/or the rate at which they decline.

Perhaps surprisingly, it seems that people who have mild experiences are more likely to have acquired immunity than people who had the most severe and dire experiences.[379]

This 16 August NY Times article[380] gave a good round-up and links to more scientific articles[381] in support of their summary finding, which is that some

---

[378] See https://www.who.int/news-room/commentaries/detail/immunity-passports-in-the-context-of-covid-19 or https://cov.cx/a1c01 . This was a dubious statement when first made – "no evidence" is a very absolute statement to make, isn't it. And to still be saying this in mid-August is becoming another example of where WHO is either asleep at the switch or allowing political considerations (its egalitarian dislike of "immunity passports") to interfere with medical reality.

[379] Actually, this is not as counter-intuitive as it may seem. People with mild cases clearly have very effective immune systems. People with severe cases clearly have very ineffective immune systems and their struggle against the virus has needed to be aided by lavish applications of every possible modern medical technique and medicine.

[380] See https://www.nytimes.com/2020/08/16/health/coronavirus-immunity-antibodies.html or https://cov.cx/a1c02

[381] As examples, and in case the NYT article is no longer online, this paper https://www.cell.com/action/showPdf?pii=S0092-8674%2820%2931008-4 or
(continued on next page)

degree of immunity is acquired, and for some as-yet-unknown time. Yes, that is very vague, isn't it.

At present, the best thinking, as per the NY Times round-up and as may have also been stated by the CDC in mid-August,[382] seems to be that people can expect at least three months of immunity after recovering from Covid-19. The CDC seemed so certain that they were saying any test for infection that showed positive within three months was almost certainly just detecting traces of the earlier infection.[383]

We also wonder what the phrase "at least", means. In the linked article, this is explained as meaning "probably six months, possibly a year". Of course, no-one yet knows, because the virus is so new. It is only now starting to be possible to test for six months of immunity because there are so few people who have been recovered for six months and available to participate in a study.[384] This will change over time. Three months ago, the number of recovered people was over a million, so it becomes much easier to start new studies drawing from the much larger pool of people who have had the virus more recently.

Even if immunity does result from an infection, it is common for acquired immunity – either as a result of a past infection or a vaccination – to fade over time. Not only does the specific immunity for the specific viral infection fade, but the viruses evolve/mutate. As they change, in their new altered forms they may end up being viewed as a different infection that your existing immune processes (and vaccines) no longer recognize and effectively combat.

---

https://cov.cx/a1c03 and this paper https://www.medrxiv.org/content/10.1101/2020.08.11.20171843v2 or https://cov.cx/a1c04

[382] I've not been able to find their official statement, but consider its paraphrase here as being reliable https://www.cbsnews.com/news/transcript-scott-gottlieb-discusses-coronavirus-on-face-the-nation-august-16-2020/ or https://cov.cx/a1c05 . Update – the CDC is either clarifying or walking back its earlier statement (which is perhaps why I can't now find it). This is their apparently current official opinion : https://www.cdc.gov/coronavirus/2019-ncov/if-you-are-sick/quarantine.html or https://cov.cx/a1c06

[383] A new article is now quoting a study of nearly 20,000 patients in New York, finding that there were stable levels of protective antibodies for three months. See https://apnews.com/article/virus-outbreak-archive-310caebd08336e2df27c468dfc79f9b8 or https://cov.cx/a1c07

[384] Six months ago, in early February, there were barely a dozen cases in the entire US.

Until mid/late August, there were also occasional examples cited in the press about patients who have been cured and then come down with a second Covid-19 infection some time – weeks or months – after they'd been cured the first time.

Until recently, the best thinking about such examples offered several explanations. A thought to be most likely explanation is they were never cured, and have the "Long-Haul" version of the illness (see page 199). Alternatively, perhaps their initial ailment was not the Covid-19 virus – it might have been regular 'flu instead. Less likely is that their "second" experience is not Covid-19, because it seems reasonable to infer that due to the unusual nature of their situation, they'd be very carefully tested.

Talking about careful testing provides another likely explanation. Even if they tested positive the first time for Covid-19, the dismayingly inaccurate tests that have sometimes been out there and in use make a single test far from conclusive, and even two or three tests can still have a significant number of false positives remaining.[385]

There's still another possibility. Maybe the person had two different strains of the virus, with any immunity against one strain not applying against the other strain.

An interesting case that was identified in Hong Kong in August, of a man who has **definitely been re-infected**. The reason for the certainty is because his second infection involves a different strain to the first infection.[386] [387]

The article rightly cautions against making too many certain conclusions from this single case. But the one case is more significant than it might seem. The article seems to reason "because there is only one case, it is obviously very unusual and the exception rather than the rule".

---

[385] See the section on Test Accuracy, above. We showed how a 98% accurate test could still come up with 40 false positives for every true positive. With some tests having only a 50% accuracy, those numbers become even more extremely biased in favor of false positives.

[386] See https://www.theguardian.com/world/2020/aug/24/case-of-man-with-coronavirus-for-second-time-stokes-reinfection-fears-hong-kong or https://cov.cx/a1c08

[387] However, it is important to stress that the reason for his reinfection can not be said to be because of the different strain of the virus that infected him a second time. There is no clear evidence (at least, not yet!) that the two different strains are treated differently by the body's immune system. The only relevant point is that this man had been exactly confirmed to have a specific strain of the virus the first time, and we therefore exactly knew, when he was found to be with the virus again, and it was a different strain, that it wasn't a "long haul" illness simply flaring up again, but a fresh new illness.

I disagreed at the time this happened.[388] While the article doesn't supply exact details, it tells us that on 15 August, the man was diagnosed with a second infection, more than four months after his first. So that means he had his first infection on/before 15 April, and at that time, no more than 1,000 people in Hong Kong had been infected. Hong Kong has a population of 7.5 million. It also seems likely that the new strain the man has is the G614 strain and his first infection has the H614 strain (see below, Figure 51 Change in virus strains over time, on page 226). Most infections now are G614, and so there are not many people with the H614 infection out there, and even now, Hong Kong still does not have many people with the virus – 4,692 in total.

So, in round figures, what are the chances that one of the first maybe 1500 people in Hong Kong, with the H614 strain, would now catch the G614 strain? Let's say after these people were cured, there have been another 2,500 new infections. So there is a (2,500 x 1,500) chance in 7.5 million of one of those people being re-infected, ie one chance in two, possibly a bit less because I overstated the likely total number of infections.

From that, we then have to wonder what the chances are of the second infection being able to be exactly confirmed and being reported, which might make the odds slightly longer in terms of the case ending up on an English newspaper, but even without that adjustment, having only one person with two infections – in Hong Kong – is close to exactly what you'd expect at present. It is not unusual and an exception, it is exactly what would be expected, and it confirms re-infection likeliness rather than presenting an awkward exception case to be explained away.

The broader question might be "Sure, one person being re-infected in Hong Kong might be what you'd expect, but why are there not more people elsewhere in the world reporting second infections?"

Well, the short answer (keep reading for a longer new answer) to that is *there are other people*, as mentioned above already, but we've been tending to dismiss those cases as being due to an error or anomaly, rather than being genuine re-infections.

Maybe they are all genuine re-infections?

One final explanation is to accept that effective immunity is never a 100% guarantee, and as mentioned above, some people's immune systems are unusually weak in the first place.

Until the Hong Kong man's case confirmed a real true 100% re-infection, it had seemed fair to consider the other rare cases as being meaningless anomalies

---

[388] And went on the record with my disagreement. I'm not now trying to be wise after the fact.

rather than valid indicators of everyone being at equal risk of re-infection as they were of infection before being infected by the Covid-19 virus.

Now we have one clear and certain example of a person being infected twice, albeit with slightly different strains of the virus. This seems to be bad news, no matter how you choose to view it.

The Hong Kong case was disclosed on 24 August. The very next day, news broke of two more people confirmed to have been re-infected – one in Belgium and one in the Netherlands.[389] We don't know much about these two new cases – we don't know if they have the same strain or a different strain, and how long since their first infection. But it seems to now be increasingly confirmed that a first case of the virus can, in some cases, give only short immunity.

We know the Belgian case is a woman who had the virus in March and again in June, so there are about three months between her infections.[390]

Professional reassurers switched gear again. First, they'd been telling us to ignore early reports of people getting a second infection. Then they told us that one case in Hong Kong was insignificant.

When two more cases inconveniently put the lie to that second line of reassurance, they then focused on how these three cases appeared to be milder than the first case and also pointed to the patients as being older and perhaps more susceptible to re-infection due to their age. They also happily pointed to the three or more months between the first and second infections, telling us that at least an infection was providing some period of immunity.

And then, oops. A young 25-year-old man in Nevada had a second case, within a month of the first case. And, wait, it gets worse. His first case was mild, his second case saw him needing to be hospitalized and given supplemental oxygen.[391]

So, let's think about what we were told and what reality now shows :

---

[389] This was mentioned on The Guardian's live blog. Hopefully this link will take you to it : https://www.theguardian.com/world/live/2020/aug/25/coronavirus-live-news-gaza-in-lockdown-following-first-local-cases-hong-kong-man-re-infected?CMP=share_btn_tw&page=with:block-5f44e7c38f08767dd7f0e657#block-5f44e7c38f08767dd7f0e657 or https://cov.cx/a1c09

[390] See https://www.stuff.co.nz/national/health/coronavirus/300091506/coronavirus-two-cases-of-covid19-reinfection-in-europe-with-more-likely or https://cov.cx/a1c10

[391] See https://www.msn.com/en-us/health/medical/nevada-man-had-covid-19-twice/ar-BB18tZF0 or https://cov.cx/a1c11

We were told	The truth now is
❖ More than three months immunity	❖ Less than one month
❖ Milder second case	❖ More severe second case
❖ Primarily older people	❖ Young people too

Of course, this is all based on one man in Nevada. There might be any number of other "confounding" considerations that caused him to be re-infected so soon and so seriously.

Now (early October) there have been a growing number of other confirmed "double infection" cases, and sadly, the Nevada man's experience of a second infection being worse than the first infection has been repeated several times.[392]

Most dramatically of all, a person who survived a first infection had a second infection and died of it.[393]

The SARS-CoV-2 virus does mutate and has mutated, although it is not clear if second infections are because of a mutation invalidating any immunity first gained. There may be other reasons why a person gets a second infection.

Below is a fascinating chart showing the shift in prevalence between two different strains of the virus.[394]

---

[392] See https://www.theguardian.com/world/2020/oct/06/flurry-of-coronavirus-reinfections-leaves-scientists-puzzled or https://cov.cx/a1c12 and https://www.dailymail.co.uk/news/article-8889269/Russian-professor-69-infected-Covid-19-twice-says-herd-immunity-impossible.html or https://cov.cx/a1c13

[393] See https://www.webmd.com/lung/news/20201014/dutch-woman-first-to-die-after-covid-19-infection or https://cov.cx/a1c14

[394] Taken from https://medium.com/microbial-instincts/what-the-d614g-mutation-means-for-covid-19-spread-fatality-treatment-and-vaccine-7dda1c066f0d or https://cov.cx/a1c15

Global Transition

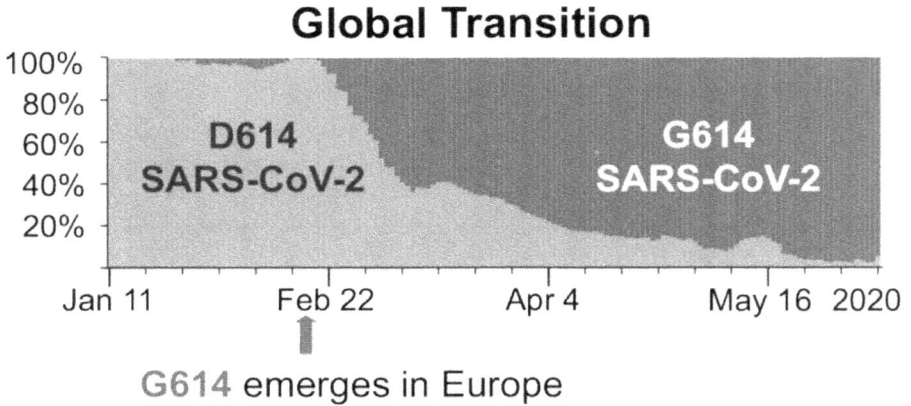

Figure 51 Change in virus strains over time

As an aside, some people assert that the virus will naturally go away because it will mutate and evolve to become less harmful. The mutation shown below was from a less harmful to a more harmful type, and as you can see, the more harmful type quickly displaced the less harmful type, all around the world.[395]

In other words, while sometimes it is true that viruses have mutated to less harmful strains which have then displaced the more harmful strain, this is not a guarantee and not something we should be waiting for or expecting as our eventual (and only?) solution.[396]

---

[395] Maybe the mutation was from less to more harmful. Or maybe not. This recent article says it was a mutation from less to more infectious, but possibly at the same time, from more lethal to less lethal. You'd think this might be obvious, or at least carefully studied to understand, but instead it is yet another example of the confusion that surrounds so much of the virus and its properties.
https://news.trust.org/item/20200818024342-3xads or https://cov.cx/a1c16

[396] The main reason why harmful viruses evolve to become less harmful is in cases where the virus is "too harmful" and quickly kills off its host person before the person has had a chance to go around spreading the virus to other people.
But the Covid-19 virus is not "too harmful" and spreads readily at present, so there is no evolutionary pressure to favor a less harmful version appearing and dominating. This is just wishful thinking by people who should know better.

The coronavirus is an RNA rather than DNA virus. Skipping the underlying medical theory, this means it can mutate more rapidly, but in practice, it seems to be less volatile than some other RNA viruses.[397]

Will such changes as do occur invalidate your immunity? We're told not to worry by articles such as this one.[398] A more neutral treatment is here.[399]

Should we worry, or should we trust the articles reassuring us? I don't know enough to say at this stage, and probably neither does anyone else, either. The virus is still too new for us to have an extended time series of data on how it mutates and changes and what the implications of those changes are.

There has been considerable concern that because this coronavirus is similar to the coronaviruses causing the common cold, immunity may not be very strong or very long-lived. As you surely know, there's no vaccine for the common cold (although this is as much due to there being so many different but similar viruses that can create what is generically termed a "cold"), and a person can have colds several times a year.[400] Is there anyone who has read this far who wants to look forward to a future with several Covid-19 infections every year in their future!?

As mentioned above, the CDC seems to have some ambiguous degree of confidence that most recovered virus sufferers will probably have three months

---

[397] See https://medicalxpress.com/news/2020-06-sars-cov-mutating-slowly-good.html or https://cov.cx/a1c17 Apparently, RNA viruses can sometimes have an extra function that "checks" the accuracy of its replication. The SARS-Covid-19 virus has this extra function which is why it evolves at a medium speed rather than high speed.

[398] See https://www.livescience.com/coronavirus-mutations.html or https://cov.cx/a1c18

[399] See https://www.sciencemag.org/news/2020/07/pandemic-virus-slowly-mutating-it-getting-more-dangerous or https://cov.cx/a1c20

[400] To be more exact, it is probable that having multiple colds in a year is likely to be due to many different virus strains out there, all of which result in what we vaguely call a cold. So rather than being infected multiple times in quick succession by the exact same virus, it is more likely we are being infected by several different viruses. See https://flucamp.com/catching-the-same-cold-twice-fact-or-myth/ or https://cov.cx/a1c22 But to continue that line of reasoning, there are already multiple strains of the Covid-19 causing virus out there. Will an infection caused by one of them, or a vaccine targeted at one of them, provide us immunity for others of them? This is not yet known. However, in that context, it is fair to say that as time passes and more Covid-19 virus strains mutate/evolve, it is likely the answer to this question, whatever it might be today, is likely to tend more to the "no" end of the range of answers than the "yes" end.

of immunity, and perhaps more.[401]   That's good, but..... Happily, as our understanding evolves, it seems that three months is more like a worst-case than a typical situation. Let's hope that immunity is much longer-lasting - I don't know about you, but to me, three months seems a tragically short period of "freedom" before starting to grow successively more anxious about repeating one's Covid-19 experience.

But there might still be outliers. Remember the young man in Nevada, coming down with the virus a second time after one month.

To me, Covid-19 is similar to a game of Russian roulette, although the one in six odds of losing are not quite so severe with the virus (unless you're over 80 and/or have other comorbidities – see "Your Risk of Dying" above on page 148).

No-one in their right mind would ever want to play Russian roulette, and doubly so, no-one would wish to play it repeatedly. So the thought of possibly getting infected multiple times – maybe even two or three times a year, every year, is most unwelcome.

Remember also that unlike winning a round of Russian roulette, the virus is not something you necessarily completely recover from, quickly and easily. Not only do some people have enduring symptoms for many months, but up to half of everyone who gets the virus end up with permanent harm – possibly to their lungs or heart or even brain, maybe permanent hearing loss, or any of way-too-many other possible negative outcomes.

The generally accepted answer to the question originally posed – can you get the virus a second time – seems now to have shifted more to a "yes" than "no", with the main uncertainty being how long before your immunity ends, either by the fading immune response in your body or the appearance of a new and "different" strain of Covid-19.[402]

---

[401] Hmmm – here's an amusing thought – "Covid-19, now with guaranteed immunity for three months – a free re-infection for anyone who doesn't get the full guaranteed three months"!

[402] For example, this interesting article published on 22 September about herd immunity possibly having been achieved in Manaus, Brazil, matter of factly refers to "The blood survey clearly showed that with time, people's antibodies become harder to detect. That could mean individual immunity to the virus is not permanent." See https://www.technologyreview.com/2020/09/22/1008709/brazil-manaus-covid-coronavirus-herd-immunity-pandemic or https://cov.cx/a1c23

Are Vaccines the Same as Immunity from Having the Disease?

We've mainly looked at the issue of immunity as a result of having been infected by the virus in the preceding sections.

From the point of view of the herd immunity function, it makes no difference how you are immune – whether it be as a result of a past infection, a natural immunity, wearing a mask, or as a result of a vaccine. The only thing that matters is that you are immune and won't get the disease a second time, and won't pass the disease on to other people because of your immunity.

To date, all the immunity research so far has been on recovered patients. That is necessarily so, because there are no approved vaccines out there, yet.[403]

In theory, immunity will work the same, wherever and however it is obtained. But after having said that, we need to move again from the black and white certainty we all prefer and turn to the many shades of gray.

The reality is that immunity is not a yes or no thing. There are a growing number of ways in which immunity can now be triggered/created. There can be degrees of immunity. And vaccines do not give absolute protection to everyone who is vaccinated.[404] Many of the current vaccine candidates for Covid-19 are expected to be weak and may need to be given in two doses rather than one to create a worthwhile level of protection.

Most vaccines are effective for about 85% - 95% of the people who are given them. One of the requirements for a vaccine to be approved is that it can demonstrate a high level of effectiveness.

But in this case, the FDA has clearly decided to lower the bar for what it takes to be approved, in their desire to get a vaccine deployed as urgently soon as possible, and so have said they'll approve vaccines that are as little as 50% effective.[405]   Unfortunately and inevitably, that may mean some of the

---

[403] Well, yes and no. On about 14 August Russia announced it had approved a vaccine and was proceeding to mass-produce it. That statement was greeted by incredulity both within and outside of Russia, because the vaccine is being approved prior to even starting its Phase Three trial. It was approved based on the results of a limited short trial of 76 people, and the results of that trial have not been publicly released for evaluation and discussion.

[404] Another consideration is that not all the 150 or so vaccines being developed work in the same way of creating immunity. There are some quite novel and innovative techniques being trialed, and which may provide different degrees of future immunity for differing lengths of time.

[405] See https://www.biospace.com/article/fda-s-guidance-on-a-covid-19-vaccine-must-be-at-least-50-percent-effective/ or https://cov.cx/a1c24

pharmaceutical companies developing vaccines might choose to come up with the first/fastest vaccine they can develop that will show a 50% effectiveness, rather than aiming for a higher degree of effectiveness, even if it takes longer to develop. There will be an enormous "first-mover advantage" – the first company to get their vaccine approved will be able to sell as many doses of it, and pretty much at any price, as it can manufacture, and to anyone, anywhere in the world.

Vaccines also last for varying amounts of time. Some vaccines can indeed last a lifetime – the Measles vaccine in particular gives about 96% of people a lifetime of protection. Other vaccines last for shorter periods – you might be familiar with the need to get occasional booster shots of the tetanus vaccine for example (recommended every ten years). At the short end of the scale is the tradition of an annual 'flu vaccine, although the largest part of the reason for annual 'flu shots is the evolution of the 'flu virus such that last year's vaccine often doesn't work with this year's virus.[406]

There are now reports that a new virus strain has been detected, mainly in minks, in Denmark, although it has also been passed to at least a dozen people that we know of so far. The big concern about this is that this new virus strain might not be blocked by the current vaccines under development. As a result, Denmark has slaughtered their entire 15 million herd of mink, hoping to prevent further spread of this new virus strain.[407] Even if this measure is effective in blocking the spread of this new strain, how long will it be before another new strain appears somewhere else and is not contained?

In other words, even if a vaccine might give us more than six months of immunity from present known strains, perhaps that period of immunity will be invalidated by the appearance of a new virus strain, the same as happens with the annual 'flu, and the same as prevents creating an effective vaccine for the common cold?

It is also probable that immunity from having had an infection will also be specific to a particular strain or family of virus strains.

So, which will be better – immunity after having the disease, or immunity via a vaccine? Unfortunately, we don't know at present, because we don't have much information on the degree of immunity obtained after having had the disease, and we don't yet know what vaccines will be approved or what their claimed effectiveness may be.

---

[406] Interesting data on vaccine longevity here
https://www.immune.org.nz/vaccines/efficiency-effectiveness or https://cov.cx/a1c25
[407] See https://www.theguardian.com/environment/2020/nov/04/denmark-announces-cull-of-15-million-mink-over-covid-mutation-fears or https://cov.cx/a1c26

One thing is hopefully certain, however. Being vaccinated will be a less risky procedure than having the disease, and certainly would be the desirable option! We discuss this further in the sub-section "Should You Take a Vaccine" on page 346.

The Three Main Infection Routes

In understanding how to avoid becoming infected, the first thing to understand is of course how it is that someone can get infected.

There are three main ways you can become infected

- By touching a surface with virus particles on them and then transferring the virus particles to your mouth, nose, or possibly eyes
- By breathing in (or having them land on your eyes, possibly) droplets contaminated with virus particles that were recently breathed out by a nearby infected person
- By breathing in tiny aerosol droplets, (or possibly having them get into your eyes) contaminated with virus particles that had been breathed out by an infected person and which hung suspended in the air for up to several hours

Our understanding of how one gets infected by Covid-19 has evolved over time, and even now, there is far from a unanimity of thought as to the relative risk factors of these three forms of infection.[408]

This uncertainty is understandable. To give an example, you go to an office for a business meeting. You meet three other people, shake hands, spend time around a conference table, coffee and cookies are served during the meeting, you end your meeting, and leave.

Some days later, you find you've come down with Covid-19. You then discover that two of the other people at your meeting also have the virus now, and decide you must have caught the virus from them at the meeting.

But – and here is the challenge. In what way did you catch the virus?

If you believe that shaking hands and other direct person-to-person contact is what causes the virus to be transmitted, you now have the "proof" you need to confirm that. You shook their hands. End of story.

But wait. What say that instead, you believe the biggest risk is by touching an exposed surface, then transferring an infection from there to your mouth/etc, by hand? You touched your chair, the door, the table, and then when you were having coffee and cookies, you touched the cookie that you ate and possibly

---

[408] There are even occasional but unpersuasive suggestions of other possible infection mechanisms such as via fecal contamination.

touched your mouth directly, too. Case closed – it was the exposed surface that you got the infection from and you transferred it, via your hands and possibly cookie, to your mouth. An open and shut case, right?

Or, maybe not right. Perhaps you think that the true method of transmission is via respiratory droplets. There you were, seated opposite the other people at the conference table, and they were talking to you, looking you directly in the face as they did so. Clearly, their respiratory droplets were spreading straight from them to you, and the conference table was only 5 ft wide – less than six feet, so that has to be how you became infected. It is obvious and logical, isn't it?

Or is it? Perhaps in this case the method of infection is via aerosol. The people you met had been in the conference room before you joining them, and it was a bit stuffy in there, not much air circulating. You remember wishing someone would open a window or turn on the a/c. Clearly, for some time prior to your arrival, and all the time you were there, the infected people were filling the air with an invisible cloud of aerosol particles, and everywhere in the conference room was dangerous.

So, it could have been any of these different pathways. Not only that, it might have been a combination of several or even all the pathways!

This is the problem. Most of the situations in which people get the virus provide multiple pathways for the virus to get from infected people to you. If you're looking, single-mindedly, for proof of one method of transmission, you'll find what you're looking for, especially if you close your mind to the possibility of other methods.

It seems a certain measure of this type of analysis has gone on, particularly by people who have influenced their analysis by their certain belief[409] of how other respiratory viruses have been transmitted. However, there is a more rigorous way of approaching the question as well.

What researchers can/could do is look for methods of transmission that were *absent* when an infection occurs. For example, if in the meeting, you didn't shake hands or have any direct person-to-person contact, then that would eliminate that possibility. And so on, trying to find scenarios where other elements were missing but the disease was passed on.

This is more difficult than it seems, which is why there ends up being some subjective elements and risks of "confirmation bias".

---

[409] I'm using the word "belief" rather than "knowledge" advisedly. As you'll shortly see, much of the body of work on how respiratory diseases are transmitted is based on a single very old study and somehow has never been challenged or reviewed in over 100 years.

What is clear however is that somehow, virus particles need to get into your eyes, nose, or mouth, and in sufficient quantity to be able to create a self-sustaining and growing infection. You can't get the virus through your skin or an exposed wound. Happily, you aren't at risk of getting the virus via sexual intercourse either.[410]

Some diseases do transfer via the so-called "oral-fecal" route, and there's been a lot of discussion about concepts such as "fecal plumes" of virus particles being created when one flushes the toilet. Studies have detected traces of the virus RNA in feces, and it is known that any time you flush a toilet, the rush of water creates a plume of aerosolized particles from the water and, ahem, whatever else was in the toilet bowl.[411]

That makes for a great headline, but the thing is, there is a difference between detecting traces of the virus and knowing for sure that what you have detected is a live virus particle capable of infecting you. Strangely, there's been little research on that point,[412] but the general conclusion seems to be that the fecal plumes – while sometimes malodorous – are probably not too harmful.

Nonetheless, for all reasons, we'd not linger in public toilets; neither at present nor normally. And whenever flushing a toilet, put the lid down first. If your toilets don't have lids, buying new toilet seats are inexpensive and easy to fit.

---

[410] Well, yes and no in that case. The "exchange of bodily fluids" is safe, but the act of being very close to another person, and breathing heavily close to them, gives plenty of opportunities for virus particles to be exchanged in the "normal" ways.

[411] This article has great pictures of plumes https://www.studyfinds.org/what-happens-when-you-flush-with-toilet-lid-up/ or https://cov.cx/a1c27

[412] Here's an article that is a subtle example of that. It is all about the theory and the potential, but is totally silent on the reality. The study it refers to was conducted in 2012, and while it shows the potential for whatever is in the toilet bowl to rise up into the air, it of course says nothing at all as to the most important point – are the viral fragments of Covid-19 found in feces actually dangerous? https://whdh.com/news/study-suggests-coronavirus-can-be-spread-through-toilet-plume/ or https://cov.cx/a1c28

This is a similar article that adds how viral RNA has been found in public toilets in China. https://www.nytimes.com/2020/06/16/health/coronavirus-toilets-flushing.html or https://cov.cx/a1c29 But the NY Times' own reporting of the viral RNA find - https://www.nytimes.com/2020/04/28/health/coronavirus-hospital-aerosols.html or https://cov.cx/a1c30 - says "scientists do not know yet whether the viruses remain infectious or whether the tests just detected harmless virus fragments".

So let's now look at the three ways that the Covid-19 virus is probably passed from person to person.

- *Strategies to Counter These Three Risks*

This table summarizes the information in the three sections that follow.

Route	Risk Mitigation Strategy
Surfaces (Fomites)	• Avoid touching at-risk surfaces • Regular hand washing • Hand sanitizer if needed
Respiratory Droplets	• Six-foot (or greater) distancing • Masks • Avoid Indoors • Avoid noisy speakers • Fresh air flows
Aerosols	• Masks • Avoid areas with lots of people or where lots of people have recently been • Avoid indoors • Avoid noisy speakers • Fresh air flows

Figure 52 Risk Mitigation Strategy table

Please don't skip the detailed content in the three next sections, though!

- *Surfaces*

The first transmission pathway is when you touch something that has virus particles on it, and then place your hand in your mouth, or up your nose, or in your eyes.

This assumes that the virus particles on the exposed surface are still viable and haven't "died", and further assumes you get sufficient virus particles on your hand and transfer enough of them to your mouth/etc for the virus to be able to viably get established.

There is a special medical term for the surface you touch that might be infected – it is called a fomite. You can probably live your entire life without ever saying "fomite" and if you ever should use the word, there's a good chance the person you're talking to will be puzzled!

Initially, the risk of getting infected via a fomite was the main focus of public health messages. At the same time, we were being told not to bother with masks, we were also being urged to obsessively wash our hands or coat them with hand sanitizer all the time. The mail was a threat – leave it outside for a few days, disinfect it if you could, and the same for food you bought at the supermarket, and pretty much anything/everything else.

There does not seem to have ever been any evidence suggesting this form of disease transmission was a major risk or major factor, and indeed, subsequently, there are very few – if any – known cases where the disease was acquired that way.[413]

Even WHO, after holding out for the longest time against the possibility of aerosol transmission and advocating fomite transmission as a major way the

---

[413] I don't know why this is. There was a rush of studies to test how long the virus could stay viable on all sorts of different surfaces – hard or soft/absorbent, and at different temperatures and humidities – see, for example, https://www.webmd.com/lung/how-long-covid-19-lives-on-surfaces or https://cov.cx/a1c31 . My guess (and, don't forget, I'm not a doctor) is that while it is possible to pick up some virus particles onto your hands this way, and even to then transfer them to your eyes/nose/mouth, the number of virus particles is generally too low to then create a viable infection.

An added guess, and this is a real reach, is that the main pathway into the body may be via the nose rather than the mouth. Here's a brand new study (as of 19 Aug) on this currently speculative point - https://www.marketwatch.com/story/johns-hopkins-scientists-examining-weird-side-effects-of-covid-19-say-this-could-be-how-virus-gains-a-foothold-in-the-body-2020-08-19 or https://cov.cx/a1c32

An alternate explanation is that there has been such efficient/effective cleaning, and people have been so great at washing their hands, that this theoretically very dangerous risk has been mitigated by good practices. Call me cynical if you must, but I'd rate this as low in terms of possible explanations.

virus was passed has finally been forced to change its official statement on how
the virus is transmitted.[414] It now says :[415]

> Despite consistent evidence as to SARS-CoV-2
> contamination of surfaces and the survival of the virus on
> certain surfaces, there are no specific reports which have
> directly demonstrated fomite transmission.

This article makes the point that an early focus on fomite transmission and
handwashing as a precautionary measure blindsided us to the importance of
mask-wearing and may have encouraged the spread of the virus.[416] That's an
interesting point, and we don't disagree with it at all.

But we do disagree with the article where it says

> The advice was informed by mountains of research into the
> transmission of other respiratory viruses: it was the best
> scientists could do with such a new pathogen.

As far as we can tell, the "mountains of research" *don't exist at all*, in any
context, for *any* respiratory virus! We discuss this further in the following
section on aerosols.

Airlines were plaintively saying "Don't worry, no-one has ever caught the
virus from one of our tray tables", and most of us ignored such statements,
pointing to people who seemed to have indeed become infected on a plane,
assuming that the infection would have been via touching a contaminated
surface.

We are still being urged to wash our hands a lot and use copious quantities of
hand sanitizer, but probably such admonitions are now more "out of an

---

[414] When WHO was still obdurately refusing to acknowledge the risk of aerosol
transmission in early July, 239 scientists and medical researchers wrote WHO a letter
demanding it changes its official position. WHO's earlier position remains prominently
on its website https://www.who.int/news-room/commentaries/detail/modes-of-
transmission-of-virus-causing-covid-19-implications-for-ipc-precaution-
recommendations or https://cov.cx/a1c33 with a focus on surface/fomite transmission
and secondarily droplet transmission, and a negation about the potential for aerosol
transmission. Its new supplementary statement grudgingly admits this possibility while
downgrading the importance it had earlier given to fomite transmission :
https://www.who.int/news-room/commentaries/detail/transmission-of-sars-cov-2-
implications-for-infection-prevention-precautions or https://cov.cx/a1c34

[415] See https://www.who.int/news-room/commentaries/detail/transmission-of-sars-cov-
2-implications-for-infection-prevention-precautions or https://cov.cx/a1c34

[416] See https://www.theguardian.com/world/2020/oct/05/did-early-focus-on-hand-
washing-and-not-masks-aid-spread-of-covid-19-coronavirus or https://cov.cx/a1c35

abundance of caution"[417] or out of a sense of giving us a sense of control over a virus that largely is out of control.

There is an understandable institutional reluctance to admit that the earlier focus on the danger of infection via touching a contaminated surface was over-hyped. But if you read between the lines, you'll see that it is generally acknowledged as such.[418] [419]

Don't stop washing your hands, etc. But don't be terrified of touching a can of baked beans in the supermarket, either.

Some surfaces are touched a lot more by a lot more people and might pose higher risks. Door handles, for example. Elevator buttons. You can probably think of more "high touch" items too. We'd be warier of the consequences after touching those sorts of surfaces. We still travel everywhere outside the house with hand sanitizer and use it regularly.

Our approach to hand sanitizer is several-fold :

(a) We use it to clean the handles of any trolley or basket we are using while shopping. We know these may have already been (in theory) cleaned by the stores, but we'd rather be safe than sorry, and we trust the adequacy of our own cleansing actions more than the half-hearted squirts of unknown liquids that partially cover a contact surface that we've seen store employees apply.

---

[417] Have you ever noticed how whenever this phrase is used, it is usually code for "this is really stupid and we can't justify it, but we're doing it anyway"?

[418] When my home county of New Zealand ended its 102 day stretch free of any virus outbreaks with a new mysterious outbreak that the public health authorities couldn't trace to any previous infection, there was thought the virus might have re-entered New Zealand on the surface of frozen food packages that had been shipped to the country from Melbourne, Australia, which was in the throes of a flare-up of virus numbers. The public health authorities then let slip a few unguarded comments about how unlikely any type of surface transmission of the virus was, and after testing both the frozen food storage depot in NZ and in Australia, found no sign of any possible contamination.

I've tried to find a good quote, but the best I can find now is rather weak, "The medical advice we have received indicates that the transferal of COVID-19 through mail and parcels is low risk. Respiratory droplets largely transmit Covid-19, and there is no good evidence that surface transmission is occurring in operational environments such as ours".

[419] This is a good article that tracks the evolving view from first "surfaces are dangerous" to now "surfaces are not a key risk factor" https://www.wired.com/story/its-time-to-talk-about-covid-19-and-surfaces-again/ or https://cov.cx/a1c36

(b)   If we're in a store for an extended time and touching many things, we try to remember to clean our hands at some point while in the store.

(c)   After we've got back in the car and removed our mask, we then give our hands another good washing with hand sanitizer.

We also generally give hand-delivered packages a quick squirt of disinfectant and leave them out for a while before bringing them inside. Better safe than sorry, right?

And that final comment – "better safe than sorry" seems to be about the sum total of the "science" that supports handwashing as a virus precaution.

We discuss how to evaluate hand sanitizer choices and disinfectants in the chapter "17. Medical Equipment & Supplies You Should Have", starting on page 398.

As you'll also see in that chapter, we don't advocate using gloves as necessary or beneficial further protection.

- ● *Respiratory Droplets*

We were all originally told this was the big "number two" method of the virus being passed from person to person, and was the rationale behind the six-foot distancing rule.[420] Now it seems that respiratory droplets and aerosols between them are the primary and possibly the only form of disease transfer and infection.

What are respiratory droplets? When a person coughs or sneezes, they project these tiny drops of virus-containing moisture. If you are nearby, then you might then breathe those droplets in, and become infected. That's fairly obvious and easy to understand. You can see them if you cough or sneeze onto a mirror. If you hold your hand in front of your mouth, you might feel little bits of moisture landing on it.

This is definitely a valid concern and a risk, and distancing can help. We discuss this in more detail in the section below, "How Close is Too Close", on page 249.

The other thing that can also help reduce your risk of infection from droplets is wearing a mask. Masks are a double-sided benefit – they cut down on the

---

[420] Just as a comment about this, there is nothing magic about the six-foot rule. Some countries have 1½ meters (5 ft), some have 1 meter (3 ft 3 in) as their versions of our 6′ rule. It is primarily a "nice round number" that compromises between "dangerously close" and "impractically far away".

spread of virus particles to other people when you exhale, and they cut down on you breathing in virus particles from others when you inhale.[421]

The key defining property of droplets is they are of sufficient size to make them heavy enough to fairly quickly fall to the floor. Yes, they can be projected some distance to start with, but they are only a short-lived risk, because they either then land on a surface or object, or quickly fall to the floor. They don't hang suspended in the air for hours.

More recently there has been a slow acceptance that another important transmission method – possibly even the most important – is via a very similar methodology, but with some very different properties - aerosolized particles.

We'll explain the difference between droplets and aerosols next.

- *Aerosols*

Regrettably, the major health authorities such as the CDC and WHO have been bizarrely reluctant to acknowledge the importance and risk of aerosol transmission of the virus. This is an excellent article,[422] appearing in an unlikely publication (Time), that clearly and convincingly explains how *aerosol transmission is the primary method by which the virus is spread.*

Even more astonishing is how the under-rating of aerosol transmission risks has been the case for 110 years since an ambivalent study in 1910.[423]

In our Covid-19 context, aerosols are essentially smaller droplets of moisture with virus particles within them. In other contexts, they are any sufficiently small-sized piece of liquid or solid. Whether liquid or solid, an aerosol is something so small that it remains suspended in the air for an extended time.

---

[421] This duality of benefit is one of the reasons why you should be wearing a mask, even if you don't like it (no-one likes wearing a mask) and are willing to take the risk of being infected as a result of being maskless. If you have no mask, you are also gratuitously increasing the risk of the people around you – both now and subsequently – who are now being "gifted" with more of your breathed-out air and possibly virus particles. By all means engage in risky behaviors yourself, but once you start risking harm to other people, please be considerate and moderate such actions.

[422] See https://time.com/5883081/covid-19-transmitted-aerosols/ or https://cov.cx/a1c37

[423] This is touched on in the Time article above and further discussed in greater detail in this excellent document, section 1.4, "When you say that the resistance to aerosol transmission is rooted in history, what do you mean?". See https://docs.google.com/document/d/1fB5pysccOHvxphpTmCG_TGdytavMmc1cUumn 8m0pwzo/edit#heading=h.n29zu41x8ctd or https://cov.cx/a1c38

With Covid-19, an aerosol can more readily be breathed out in normal breathing than droplets. They also are emitted in other exhalation events like laughing and singing and talking.

You know that your breath contains moisture because if you breathe on a glass surface, you can often fog it up, depending on relative temperatures and humidity.

Respiratory droplets are distinguished from aerosols in two ways. The first is in terms of size. A respiratory droplet is a very small drop of water, ranging in size from about 5 μ m (micrometers or microns) and upwards.

Aerosol droplets are smaller in size than respiratory droplets, and for definitional purposes are simply described as being smaller than 5 μ m. To put that number in perspective, a coronavirus particle, itself, is about 0.125 μ m.

The key difference however is not the size, but the way they behave (which is in part a function of their size). Droplets are affected by gravity and fairly quickly fall to the floor. Aerosols are much less affected by gravity, and hang, suspended in the air, for extended periods of time – hours, in some cases, more than one day, possibly much longer still.[424]

Think for example of smoke from a forest fire. It hangs in the air for a long time, indeed, it can travel hundreds, even thousands of miles, while suspended in the air, blown from one side of the country to the other. Aerosolized smog has traveled all the way from China, more than 6,000 miles across the Pacific, to the US.

One other point to note – droplets can become aerosolized – typically, if on a hot day, they start to shrink in size due to evaporation, and might end up becoming aerosol particles before landing on a surface/the ground.[425]

The infection danger of an aerosol is less than of a droplet because an aerosol particle has fewer viruses on it – if it had many more, it would grow in size/weight, becoming a droplet and fall down more quickly.

---

[424] You might be wondering how it is that an aerosol droplet is not affected by gravity. Does it have some magical anti-gravity property? Alas, no. There's a much simpler explanation. An aerosol droplet is so light that it is buoyed up in the air by colliding with air molecules, sort of a bit like a game of volleyball, with each air molecule bouncing the aerosol particle up again, until eventually, an air molecule "misses" the "ball" and it falls to earth. Yes, this is a massive over-simplification, but hopefully it provides an understanding. More information can be found here and elsewhere https://en.wikipedia.org/wiki/Deposition_(aerosol_physics) or https://cov.cx/a1c39 .

[425] Sort of the opposite of the story (of uncertain validity) of "It was so cold my urine froze before it hit the ground".

But, there might be many more aerosol particles than droplets, so the risk is sort of balanced out.

The amount of aerosol breathed out varies depending on how loudly a person is talking or shouting or singing or laughing. It is easy to understand that the greater the volume, the more forcefully a person is expelling air from their lungs, past their vocal cords, and out into the air. And in that expelled air may be some droplets and/or aerosolized particles.

The action item here is to avoid noisy people, and to avoid places where it is necessary to be noisy to be heard. This can have a major difference in the amount of aerosol being exhales.

The big factor is that respiratory droplets can be exhaled with great force and travel long distances – sometimes, but not often, as much as twenty, thirty, even more feet. [426] That's the bad news. The good news is they quickly fall to the ground, within a few minutes.[427] Think of them like a stone – you can throw it a distance, but it quickly falls.

An aerosol is more like a feather or a balloon. They don't travel very far, but they can stay suspended in the air for many hours.

How long can aerosols hang, suspended, in the air? The answer to that is "it depends". Different types of aerosols – different sizes and different densities – have different properties. But typical water-based aerosols might have a "half-life"[428] of about 1.1 hours according to one study.[429] Other studies have suggested longer times, or have simply said "detectable traces remain after x hours".[430]

---

[426] See https://www.nationalgeographic.com/science/2020/04/coronavirus-covid-sneeze-fluid-dynamics-in-photos/ or https://cov.cx/a1c40

[427] See https://www.nejm.org/doi/full/10.1056/NEJMicm1501197 or https://cov.cx/a1c41

[428] A half-life means that half of the aerosol falls to the ground in the first half-life measure of time. Half of the remaining half falls in the next half-life. Half of the remainder falls in the next half-life, and so on.

[429] See https://www.statnews.com/2020/03/16/coronavirus-can-become-aerosol-doesnt-mean-doomed/ or https://cov.cx/a1c42

[430] This study says that the virus remained viable for up to three hours, although we don't know if "up to" also means "at least", which it possibly may. See https://theconversation.com/coronavirus-drifts-through-the-air-in-microscopic-droplets-heres-the-science-of-infectious-aerosols-136663 or https://cov.cx/a1c43

A key limiting factor might also be not just how long the virus remains suspended in the air in aerosolized form, but how long it remains active and viable and capable of creating a sustainable infection within you. This is still being evaluated, and for now, the previous linked study and its claim of three hours seems like a good measure to consider.

Aerosol properties depend very much on the air within which they are suspended. In particular, if the air is moving, then the aerosol will tend to move in the stream of air. If there are semi-random gusts and currents, then the aerosol will be blown every which way, tend to disperse, and so the concentration of aerosolized particles around you will diminish.

Aerosolized virus particles are harder to protect against than respiratory droplets because they hang about in the air for longer, and are smaller. The best protection is to be somewhere with a good steady flow of *fresh* air blowing air onto you and blowing potentially infected air away from you.[431]

Masks are also very helpful, of course.

Note in the preceding paragraph we spoke about *fresh* air. Just blowing the same stale air around a room or suite of offices or home does little good. It just makes everywhere equally contaminated by the aerosol.

If you are recirculating air, you should make certain you have adequate filters to trap the virus particles before they are recirculated. Please see our chapter, above, "9. Self Quarantining" on page 206 where we explain the ratings used on air filters and recommend appropriately rated filters to use.

Of course, change the filters as per their guidelines, and even with the filters, try to exhaust as much air and bring in as much fresh air for each cycle as possible.

If you don't have a central air system, be careful if you just open a window to "let some fresh air in". You don't so much want to let fresh air in as you want to exhaust stale/contaminated air. Whenever air comes into a space, it also has to go out of the space again, at the same time, too. If it is coming in through the window, maybe it is going out through the doorway, and so on.

If the window and airflow cause air to come in, you are now moving the aerosol into the rest of the shared area of your home or office. Be sure to understand the airflow and if necessary, help it with fans.

If you live in an apartment block, there is a possibility that the building is designed with a pressurized central air column that then feeds air through the

---

[431] Perhaps surprisingly, one of the best examples of a good airflow set up is on a plane, with the air streaming from the top of the cabin down to the bottom. This blows fresh air onto your face, and takes your exhaled air down to the ground and out rather than to other passengers.

corridors and under the gaps in doors into each unit, and then from the unit and outside.[432] This is not ideal, and opening a window would serve to accelerate the flow of air from the corridor into your unit (because the air now has an easy way to leave the building). The concern of course is how safe the central air now entering into your apartment/condo may be.

With aerosolized virus, you are not just at risk of people within six feet of you. You are also at the risk of unknown unseen people who were in the same area, an hour, or two, or three (and possibly even longer) too. And people who were nearby, an hour ago, with their aerosolized particles now having wafted into the area you are now located within.

To summarize this section, the action item is to manage the flow of air in your environment. Have fresh air blowing on you, and stale air leaving the environment and venting to the outside. Do not have air from other people then blowing on to you.

The best airflow is vertically down from ceiling to floor (rather than up or horizontally), because it encourages the precipitation of both droplets and aerosols quickly rather than carrying them across a room and all around a set of offices or home.

My personal feeling is that airflow is an essential factor to manage and optimize.

Temperature and Humidity as Factors

Temperature and humidity both have impacts on the ability of the virus to spread. The impacts relate to how the virus spreads and the longevity of the period during which virus particles remain viable and able to start an infection.

In the case of temperature, there was a long-held hope that when we moved into our summer, the warmer temperatures would see the virus decline, much the same as happens with the annual 'flu virus. This was supported by maps claiming to show that the virus was most active, back in March/April, in cooler parts of the world.

The maps were ridiculous because they failed to consider that most of the world's population also lives in the latitude bands they were showing as being cooler, and there were also notable exceptions with both unusually low rates in some "cool" countries and unusually high rates in some "hot" countries.

---

[432] See https://www.buildingscience.com/sites/default/files/01.03_2015-08-03_ventilation_multifamily_ricketts.pdf or https://cov.cx/a1c44 - discussion starting on slide 16

It was also slightly over-estimating the effects of outside temperature (in my opinion) because we live most of our lives in temperature-controlled indoor spaces that remain much the same temperature in summer as in winter.[433]

The early studies were also conducted before aerosol transmission was acknowledged as a major factor, and so my sense is a lot of the researchers managed to see what they wanted/expected to see.

There's one more measure of the impact of temperature on the virus. It takes 50 minutes of 212°F/100°C heat to sterilize a face mask.[434] If it takes almost an hour at boiling point to inactivate the virus, it is reasonably stable for significant periods at temperatures half that level![435]

Now that the virus has been a major factor, everywhere in the world, for half a year, we've had a chance to see what happens when countries switch from winter to summer (and vice versa) and it seems clear that normal temperature ranges have very little impact on virus activity. Let's look at two severely affected countries, one in the northern hemisphere and one in the southern.[436]

---

[433] This sort of begs the question, "Why is the annual 'flu virus seasonal?". The short answer is "We don't know". There are a number of different theories, and some studies supporting one or other of the studies. I personally think the change in lifestyle from "being cooped up in winter with more people close by" to "being outside in the fresh air in the summer" is a major part of the issue, and particularly because the 'flu is generally less infectious than Covid-19, maybe that is enough of a variance as to make all the difference.

This is a good explainer. https://www.popsci.com/science/article/2013-01/fyi-why-winter-flu-season/ or https://cov.cx/a1c45

[434] See https://www.wsbtv.com/news/local/atlanta/need-sanitize-your-n95-face-mask-try-your-instapot/YCDAGFMEYJCKHNAMYFKX5IFKPQ/ or https://cov.cx/a1c46

[435] An interesting rule of thumb that gives a great insight into the impact of temperature on chemical reactions is that an increase of 10°C (18°F) will double the speed of the reaction. Does it therefore follow "If I increase the temperature by 65°C, I will double reaction speed by 6 ½ doublings (ie about 100-fold)?" More or less, yes, although other factors could come into play.

The point of this is to wonder if the breakdown of the virus works on a similar basis. If it does, then it allows us to work back from one hour at 100°C to 100 hours of longevity at 35°C (95°F) or 200 hours at 25°/77° and so on. With such longevity, a few degrees of ambient temperature change isn't very profoundly impactful.

[436] Any impact as a result of outdoor temperatures is minor compared to other impacts such as social distancing and mask-wearing and so is almost impossible to separate out of the overall trends. Data from Worldometers.

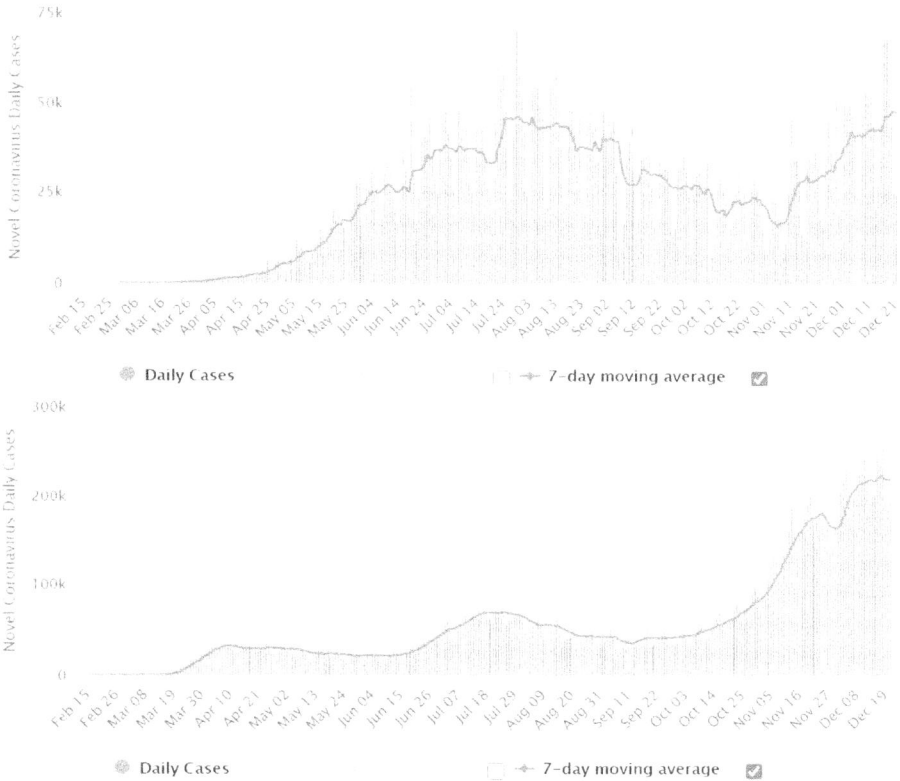

Figure 53 Daily New Cases – Brazil (top) & USA (bottom)

As can be seen, both the US in the northern hemisphere (moving toward its hottest months – July and August) and Brazil in the southern hemisphere (moving toward its coldest months, also July and August) had similar rises in cases in June, and tapering off again in late July.

And then, both the US and Brazil had rises in cases again in November, with Brazil moving to spring and summer, and the US doing the opposite, moving to fall and winter.

Although we don't think outside ambient temperatures are a major factor, for the sake of completeness, we should at least acknowledge there are probably three or four temperature-related issues that might impact on the virus.

The **first** is the potential for warmer temperatures to "melt" the outside coating of the virus, exposing its internal RNA and causing it to become inactive.

This has only a minor impact. The time it takes for 85°F (30°C) ambient temperatures to have a significant effect on the virus through this process is some/many hours. In this respect, higher temperatures are good, but normal ranges of temperatures don't make huge differences to the virus viability.

The **second** is related to the first – how long virus particles can remain on exposed surfaces. Higher temperatures mean shorter lives. Cooler temperatures mean longer lives, and if you freeze something, it seems you freeze the virus too, and it will happily reactivate again when you thaw the product.

There has been some unproven speculation recently that maybe the virus has been passed from country to country via frozen food. This might either be in the form of virus particles on the outside of packages, or on the food itself.

Tests have shown that virus particles can survive for up to three weeks at freezer temperatures.[437] The testing does not seem to have determined how viable the virus particles might be after three weeks of being frozen, and this method of passing the infection on remains theoretical and unproven, but of slight concern all the same.

I hasten to add – you've almost definitely got a much greater chance of getting the virus on an unfrozen package than on a frozen one, and either which way, the chance of an infection is very low.

With WHO going as far as to suggest that no-one has yet caught a case of the virus from touching something, this is clearly a very minor factor, too.

The **third** issue is that warmer weather causes the moisture in a respiratory droplet to evaporate. But as the respiratory droplet gets smaller, it becomes an aerosolized particle instead.

Unfortunately, that is bad, because instead of the respiratory droplet quickly falling to the ground, the aerosolized particle can hang, suspended in the air, for some hours. But the transition from droplet to aerosol particle does not seem to be very impactful, either.

One other (**fourth**) issue might also have some effect, especially outdoors – summer weather is distinguished by more hours of stronger sun each day, and with that comes more UV exposure.

The UV rays are harmful not just to us (in the form of sunburn and ultimately skin cancer) but also to the virus too.[438] This factor would reduce the longevity of virus particles, no matter in what form they were present.

---

[437] See the first part of this article https://www.mirror.co.uk/news/world-news/coronavirus-survives-frozen-meat-fish-22564733 or https://cov.cx/a1c47

[438] See https://www.accuweather.com/en/health-wellness/uv-radiation-from-the-sun-increases-by-a-factor-of-10-by-summer-and-could-be-key-in-slowing-covid-19/703393 or https://cov.cx/a1c48

So there are pluses and minuses to warmer weather, and it seems on balance, the "minus" effect of converting droplets to aerosols and the significance of that as a way of getting infected balances the plus of a shorter life, especially because there is little or no danger of getting infected by touching a surface.[439]

There is however **one other factor** we've not yet mentioned, and we'll agree this last factor may be impactful on how readily the virus spreads. It is our own behavior. In the winter, we are indoors together more, in groups in bars, restaurants, people's homes, concerts, or whatever – all great environments to spread the virus via droplets and aerosols.

In the summer, we are outside more – in the great outdoors, at the beach, or, if at a restaurant or bar or friend's home, outside on a verandah in a person's yard, rather than indoors. A much less "helpful" environment for the virus.

The good news part of that is we can (at least in theory) adjust our behavior more readily than we can the weather, so if social separation is an underlying factor (as we believe it is) then it is possible to optimize that in winter.

The other major weather factor[440] which impacts on the virus and varies both outdoors and also, to a much greater extent than temperature, is humidity. A rather puzzling study ended up advocating ideal humidity to minimize virus risk as coincidentally being that which is best for people – ie, 40% - 60%. The study said that in low humidity conditions, droplets lose some water and become aerosols, staying in the air for longer, whereas in high humidity conditions, droplets get larger and drop out of the air more quickly. This means higher humidity is better than lower humidity.

It is unclear exactly why the optimum humidity is recommended as being 40% - 60%. Different issues come into play with lower and higher humidities, so that some things become relevant at low humidities and neutral at high ones, and vice versa for the other issues. But I think the decision to feature 40% - 60% was made slightly independently of the virus, as it seems from some studies, there is

---

[439] Here's a roundup of various factors and theories, albeit published on 13 March before a lot was known. See https://www.accuweather.com/en/health-wellness/higher-temperatures-affect-survival-of-new-coronavirus-pathologist-says/700800 or https://cov.cx/a1c49

[440] Ignoring rain and wind, which perhaps should be considered, at least for that portion of our lives spent outside. Wind simultaneously spreads and disperses the virus, with the dispersal being good and the spread being bad. However, on balance, the dispersal factor probably outweighs the spread factor, because the number of virus particles per cubic unit of air rapidly dwindles down to a too-low number to be a substantive risk. Rain is generally good because it "washes" any aerosol particles out of the air.

continued reduction in virus threat if the humidity increases over 60% to 70% or so.[441]

When determining ideal humidity, there are many different factors to also keep in mind, as is shown in this chart :[442]

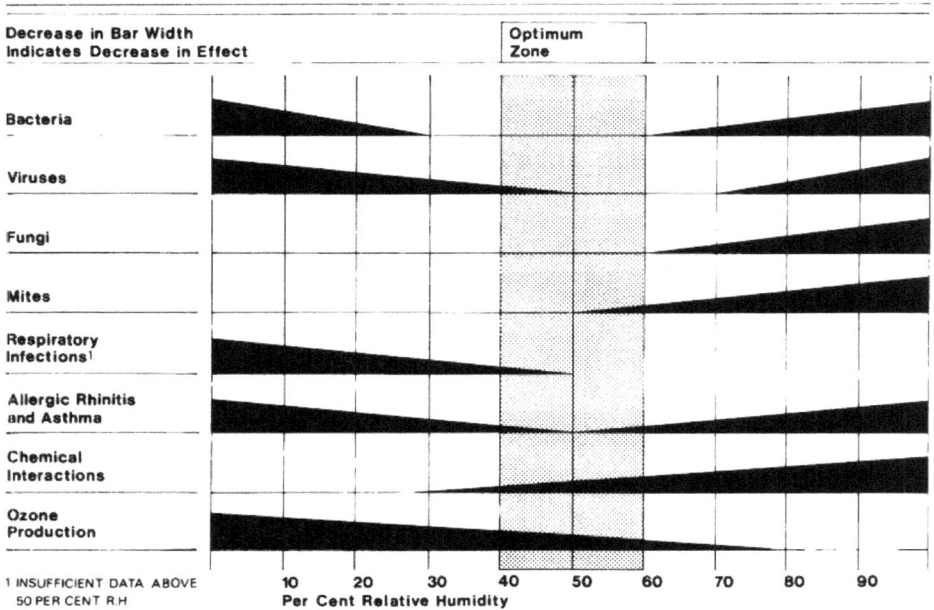

Figure 54 Impact of humidity on various factors

For whatever reason, and without focusing on ideal numbers, it seems clear that lower humidity does help the virus. An Australian study suggested that a 1% decrease in humidity could increase the number of Covid-19 cases by 6%.[443]

---

[441] The study, which analyses other studies, is fairly short and can be seen here : https://www.dw.com/en/coronavirus-transmission-humidity-aerosols/a-54639765 or https://cov.cx/a1c50

[442] Source - https://www.ncbi.nlm.nih.gov/pmc/articles/PMC1474709/pdf/envhper00436-0331.pdf or https://cov.cx/a1c51

[443] See https://medicalxpress.com/news/2020-06-humidity-linked-covid-.html or https://cov.cx/a1c52

That seems astonishing to me – 1% is within the margin of error for most general humidity readings, and it is unclear how the study was able to get such accurate measures or adjust for the humidity exactly where each infection occurred. The precision of tying 1% differences in presumably public published regional outdoor humidity levels with a change in virus cases of 6% beggars the imagination, and may be a classic example of trying to correlate two factors without allowing for other factors that might also be impacting on the observations and perceived outcomes.

Can we just say "humidity affects new virus case numbers" and agree that we should all try and keep the humidity as high as comfortable and convenient.

The action item is to keep an eye on the humidity in the environments you live and work in. Come winter, when the heating systems in many homes and offices dry out the air, you absolutely should invest in a humidifier and some hygrometers so you can monitor the humidity and boost it up from whatever it might be, and up into the higher part of the 40% - 60% range – say 50% - 60%.

We discuss hygrometers (often unreliable) and humidifiers in the chapter "17. Medical Equipment & Supplies You Should Have", starting on page 398.

How Close is Too Close

This is an important question – at what point does it become unacceptably dangerous to be close to another person?

Unfortunately, like most things to do with this virus, the answer is unclear rather than exact. You can think of a diminishing element of risk, the further you go away from another person, ranging from maximum risk if you, ahem, have "locked lips" at zero inches, and less risk as you successively move further away from that point.

We find it interesting that while the issue of mask-wearing continues to be subject to surprising controversy, there has been much less controversy about social distancing. This is all the more surprising because there is no clear agreement that our distancing rule/guideline should be six feet. Some countries say three feet, some say four and a half. Metric nations variously say 1/1½/2 meters (3¼/5/6½ ft).

Although some bar and restaurant owners have grumbled a little bit, we think they've generally understood it better to "give in gracefully", because if they were to demand scientific "proof" of the need for six feet of separation, there's a great likelihood that the proof might end up justifying an *increase* rather than decrease in the six-foot distance.

Some studies, dating way back to the 1930s, and even further back to 1897, suggested that *most* respiratory droplets would fall within six feet of the person breathing them out. For a long time, those have been regarded unquestioningly as the definitive answer, but now we have better measurement tools to "see" and track the flow of exhaled respiratory droplets, it is clear that while "normal" droplets may generally fall within six feet, some can travel massively further – especially if they've been given an extra "push" to start with in the form of a cough or sneeze or shout.

Note also that these studies were in the context of respiratory droplets. They ignored aerosol clouds. Now that there is greater acceptance of aerosol clouds as being a primary potential means of becoming infected, the six-foot rule needs to be adapted to recognize the longer distance aerosol clouds can travel.

One interesting point is immediately apparent. The concern about droplets is why some supermarkets have made their aisles one-way.[444] The idea is that the person in front of you is shooting their droplets ahead of them, and they quickly then fall to the floor, so it is safe for you to be behind them. That's a moderately sensible concept, but what about aerosols?

The one-way concept now means you're following the person/people in front and walking straight into their fresh aerosol clouds. From that point of view, walking toward a person and then quickly past them (in a two-way aisle) is probably at least as safe and may be safer than an extended time walking behind them.[445]

An interesting article provides a great rule of thumb.[446] It says that if you can smell smoke from a smoker's cigarette, you are probably also breathing in any virus particles they might be exhaling along with the smoke. Both smoke and the virus can be in aerosol form, so it is a good rule of thumb to consider. It does rather graphically show how aerosols can easily travel more than six feet.

So, the six-foot rule. If you consider the three forms of infection discussed above, it has no relevance for touching, definitely helps and reduces but doesn't eliminate the risk for people coughing/sneezing, and doesn't help so much for aerosolized particles just hanging in the air.

---

[444] I don't know about where you live, but where I live, in a suburb of Seattle, I'd say at least half the people I encounter in supermarket aisles are going the wrong way – including, sometimes, me (not deliberately, but accidentally).

[445] A good way to think about aerosols is to imagine the other person is smoking a cigarette. You know that if you are walking behind a person who is smoking (smoke is an aerosol), you're all the time smelling their smoke. But if you're walking towards a smoker, you only notice the smell when you are close, and it quickly recedes behind you once you've passed the smoker.

[446] See https://www.chron.com/news/article/Can-you-get-coronavirus-via-secondhand-smoke-The-15504536.php or https://cov.cx/a1c53

Why was it decided to set the distance at six feet? Why not more? Why not less? It is nothing more than a round number that is easy to visualize and easy to explain.

The airlines have tried to distort this and have risibly suggested that if six feet is the necessary distance, then anything less than that is a fail, and (they say) in such a case, a fail is a fail, and there's no difference then as between 5 feet and 4 feet, and so on down to the 18 inches that separates people in adjacent coach seats[447]. Some airlines have used this to justify why they are not blocking out middle seats, and allowing passengers to be boxed in, with people in front and behind (typically with about 2'4" spacing – the "seat pitch") and passengers on either side (typically with about 1'5" spacing – the seat width).

This is **totally incorrect**. Six feet is not a magic distance, but the closer you are, the more your risk increases. Three feet is more risky than six feet – especially for an extended period of proximity such as on a flight, but it is still very much better than 1 1/2 feet, which is what the airlines are trying to now tell us is perfectly fine.[448]

This also raises another point. The risk of infection is a combination of both distance and time. A brief close encounter when passing someone in the opposite direction on a narrow sidewalk (especially if outside) is much less risky than being seated next to someone on a plane, at "danger close" distance, for many hours.

It is also not just being seated next to one other person. With three people in the row ahead, two alongside you in your row, and three more in the row behind, that is eight people who are all way too close, plus more in the rows on the other side of the aisle and the rows two ahead and two behind.

------

[447] Well, it depends on how you measure distance, doesn't it. As you surely know, we are uncomfortably squashed up against each other in airplane seats with zero separation at all between the part of us closest to our neighbor and the part of them closest to us. But if you measure from center to center, or if you just note the width of each airplane seat, you're at about 17" – 18" of separation. Way too close, however it is measured!

[448] An average airline seat in coach class is about 17" wide. Even business class and first class seats aren't all that wonderfully better, but you are then getting the benefit of greater "pitch" – the distance between rows as well as the distance between seats. Business class seats are about 20" – 21", first class seats are 22" – 23" wide.

But, back to the six-foot rule again. Here's an article now questioning the six-foot rule (or, as it is in metric countries, 2 meters which is actually 6'7"), from the perspective of wondering if it is unnecessarily too much distance.[449]

It is very foreseeable that businesses that are currently being inconvenienced by the six-foot rule would be happy to see it dropped to something smaller. It is also true that wearing a decent mask – one that actually works, rather than one that just looks good – can compensate for some of the increased risks with closer distancing,[450] but we think particularly in environments where we are eating and drinking, at least six feet should remain the absolute minimum.

In a restaurant or bar, we of course can't wear a mask while eating and drinking, and we have a terrible combination of proximity, extended time while close to other people, a larger number of other people passing close to us (meaning more risk that at least one of the many other people passing by might be infected), people speaking louder than normal (and expelling more virus particles as a result) and an entirely new way of becoming infected – virus droplets can land on our food or in our drink and be ingested that way. That's a whole bunch of reasons to be very much more cautious.

Distance is important, and while six feet doesn't guarantee our safety, it is very much better than three feet or any other lesser distance. This is admitted in the article linked to above, although only when/if you read down to the bottom. It then reveals that some experts equate just a few seconds of interaction at 3 ft (1m) as being the same as an hour or two at 6 ft (2m).

This points to an important added factor. Being twice as close does not simply double your risk, it multiplies it by more than this – perhaps the risk is four-fold rather than two-fold, although in the cited example, it was much more.

Let's be sure to insist on, and observe ourselves, six feet of distancing, and discourage any attempts to reduce that down.

A new paper published in The BMJ[451] on 25 August provides an excellent collation of various studies and findings. It is well written, easy to understand, and not unduly lengthy.[452] It has a nice summary table showing relative risk but

---

[449] See https://www.dailymail.co.uk/news/article-8339837/Government-scientist-says-2m-social-distancing-rule-based-fragile-evidence.html or https://cov.cx/a1c54

[450] The concept of masks is not to make other risky behaviors now slightly less risky. Masks are supposed to make current behavior safer, not to enable riskier behaviors.

[451] Formerly known as The British Medical Journal before it puzzlingly wished to turn its back on its illustrious past and "modernize" itself

[452] See https://www.bmj.com/content/370/bmj.m3223 or https://cov.cx/a1c55

is silent on the distancing other than distinguishing between low and high occupancy, or time exposure. Nonetheless, it provides a great illustration of what are more or less risky activities and environments, and shows the impact of mask-wearing.[453]

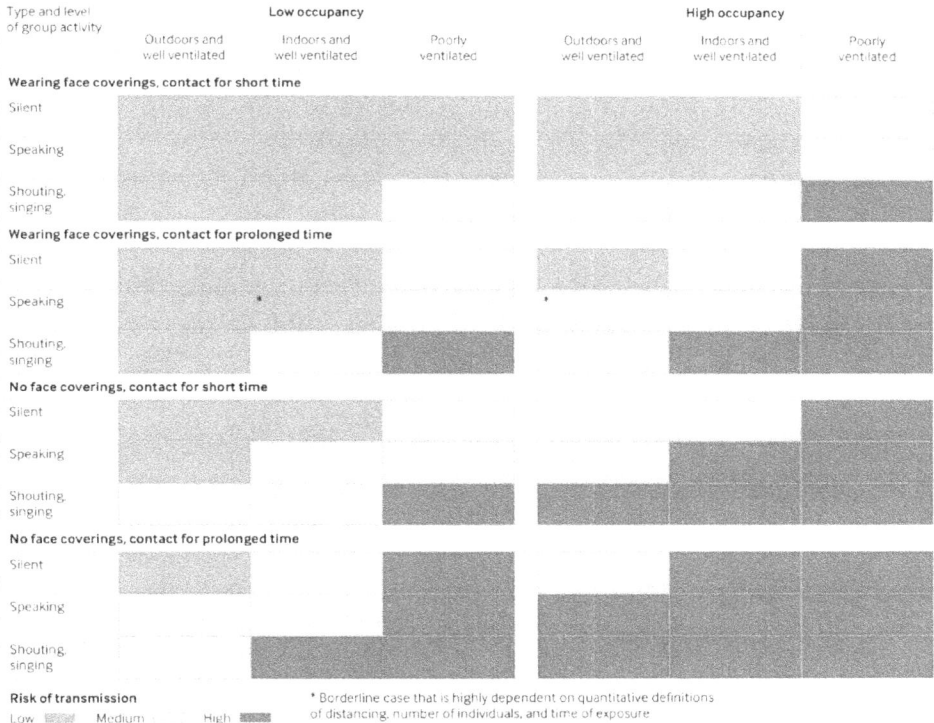

Figure 55 Relative risks of activities and settings

The higher the risk, the more you want to compensate by increasing the distancing, being sure to wear a mask, and minimizing the time in such a situation.

The Second Factor – Time

A good way of thinking of the risk of catching the virus is to think of the virus as having similar properties and threats to our health as does radiation.

---

[453] ibid

Many of us are familiar with, from movies or real life, the staccato sound of Geiger counters and understand how radiation risk is a function of both the strength of the radiation and how long we're exposed to it. It is almost exactly the same with the virus.

The preceding section was all about the "strength" or concentration of the virus (as a function of distance). The other part of understanding your risk is the time you're exposed to it.

This doesn't require a lot more explanation. Simply stated, any time you're in a place of elevated risk, try and spend as little time there as possible. Be quick when you go shopping. Have a shopping list, know where you need to go in the store as best you can, and don't linger. If you need to converse with someone else, as well as keeping your distance, be brief. If you're told something will be ready in five or ten minutes, wait outside not inside. And so on.

Each extra breath you take in a higher-risk environment is more opportunity for more virus particles to be inhaled. Ultimately, catching the virus is all about inhaling sufficient virus particles to allow the virus to establish itself. That either means inhaling a few breaths of unusually contaminated air or spending more time inhaling not quite so severely contaminated air.

Additionally, the sooner you leave a risky environment, the more immediate is the end of the virus being given more "reinforcements" with each successive breath you take.

The CDC Guideline on When Risk Becomes Significant

The CDC updated its guidelines for determining if a person may have had a significantly risky contact with another person, in mid-October.

Previously their guideline was that contact between two people involved a significant chance of passing the virus from one person to the other if it was for at least 15 consecutive minutes.

Now, perhaps as part of their slow and seemingly grudging acceptance of the risk of aerosol spread, they are saying that the 15 minutes need not be a single period of continuous contact, but could be a series of shorter exposures that in total come to 15 minutes within any 24 hours.

This is an easier risk factor to trigger. You can probably think of people in your work environment who you interact with regularly during a day, but with each interaction being no more than a minute or two. Previously, that was officially deemed to be safe. Now the CDC says it is dangerous. we agree with them, although there are some simplifications – 15 one minute exposures, evenly spaced over 24 hours, is not nearly as impactful as one single 15-minute exposure, but to keep the calculations simple, it is probably acceptable to have the "total of 15 minutes made up of any number of any length contacts" apply because it is more strict than the earlier rule.[454]

Disinfectant – Helpful or Harmful?

When does clean become too clean? Businesses and public venues in general have been boasting about how they are constantly cleaning all their surfaces to keep us safe. The airlines in particular love to tell us – reassure us – about how they are cleaning their planes much more than ever before, even between every flight. You've probably seen the pictures of people in white coveralls, masks, and goggles, spraying some type of liquid in an airplane cabin.

But there's a possible flipside to this much-publicized temporary obsession with cleanliness. Is it possible that disinfectants that kill viruses and bacteria might also be harmful to larger organisms, such as, for example, people? Unsurprisingly, the answer to that is emphatically yes. There's a reason the cleaners wear their coveralls, masks, and goggles - because breathing the disinfectant is harmful.

Reading the label on my bottle of Virex II disinfectant concentrate not only has the usual warning about not getting the product in your eyes and not swallowing any but has an astonishing line that if you get any on you, you should urgently wash your skin for 15-20 minutes. I've never seen any other chemical that requires 20 minutes of washing if it makes contact with your skin. Clearly, it is powerful stuff, and not in an altogether good way.

So, is there a problem with these disinfectants? There are two considerations.

The **first** is if there is any of the disinfectant in the air or still evaporating off absorbent rather than hard surfaces – things such as seat cushions, carpets, drapes, and other such surfaces when you enter the area. If you can smell disinfectant, then it is probably not a good thing. That "clean" smell is not a desirable smell.

It is also worth noting that after a plane takes off and the cabin pressure drops at altitude, that encourages additional off-gassing of any remaining chemicals that might be remaining, still drying off on plane surfaces.

The **second** is there might be a build-up of the poisonous products from the disinfectant on the surfaces you then touch. Remember the warning on my Virex II label? Do you really want to be touching the chemicals directly?

---

[454] The rule change is discussed here https://www.msn.com/en-us/health/medical/the-cdc-now-says-you-can-catch-covid-from-someone-in-exactly-this-long/ss-BB1agYdC or https://cov.cx/a1c56 and the exact rule is here https://www.msn.com/en-us/health/medical/the-cdc-now-says-you-can-catch-covid-from-someone-in-exactly-this-long/ss-BB1agYdC or https://cov.cx/a1c57

When we consider also that virus transmission by touching contaminated surfaces is the least likely method of becoming infected, is this a case where the cure is worse than the problem? Do we need every surface in a space to be regularly sprayed with noxious poisons? Couldn't we simply use a wipe or a bit of hand sanitizer on the surfaces we are going to directly touch, and not bother about the parts of a room we're not going to touch, but which can soak up and then slowly release poisons for some time after they've been sprayed?

There's also the issue of the range of possible viricides that can be used. The most common ones use the most noxious chemicals - a family of chemicals known as "quaternary ammonium compounds". But simpler and safer chemicals such as citric acid (found in lemon juice) or hydrogen peroxide (you probably have a bottle of that in your medicine cabinet already) might do just as good a job, without the noxious consequences.

The airlines assure us there's no need to worry, but what is the scientific basis for their assurance? They can't cite any. This article in the WSJ[455] provides interesting additional information about disinfectants used on airplanes.

Nine General Strategies to Avoid the Virus

In general, there are a number of things to do.

1.   Try and stay in a safe controlled environment as much as possible. A safe and controlled environment is one with no strangers in it and no contamination from outside sources. It is hopefully your personal residence, but that too is under threat if you're sharing it with someone who has a high-risk job or lifestyle.

Even if the other person (people) has/have their own bedroom(s), the aerosolized virus particles they could be breathing out in your shared kitchen, dining, living, and bathroom areas are a risk. Try and avoid your roommates as much as possible. Don't have them cook for you, and don't have them offer to do the cleaning up, either.

2.   When you have to go to an area of higher risk, wear a mask and steer well clear of anyone who doesn't wear a mask (or is not wearing a "good" mask, or is not wearing a mask correctly).[456]

---

[455] See https://www.wsj.com/articles/to-battle-covid-airlines-bet-on-disinfectants-that-come-with-questions-11601474460?mod=djemHL_t or https://cov.cx/a1c58

[456] I'm becoming a bit obsessive about this, and am avoiding not only unmasked people, but also people with useless masks that don't really protect either the wearer or the people around them. It dismays me greatly that there aren't any standards or controls on mask quality/performance.

3.   Keep your distance from everyone else (to avoid short-term droplets), and also try to avoid enclosed areas where other people have been (to avoid aerosol clouds).

4.   Yes, even though it is of very little value, you should continue to practice excellent hygiene and wash your hands or use sanitizer regularly while in higher-risk areas.

5.   Spend as little time as possible in higher-risk areas.

6.   Meet people outdoors, not indoors.

7.   Try and plan the times you need to be in public to avoid crowds of people. Don't go to special events, and shop in "off-hours".

Google can give you very helpful information about the relative number of people in a store by the hour of each day of the week.

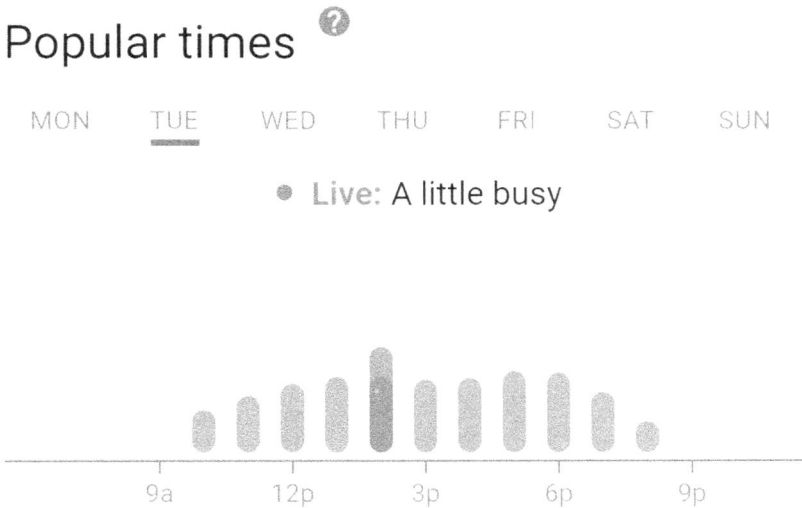

Popular times ②

MON   TUE   WED   THU   FRI   SAT   SUN

● Live: A little busy

9a   12p   3p   6p   9p

① People typically spend **20 min to 1 hr** here

Figure 56 Google's information about busy times at a store

Search for the store you are planning on visiting and in the information panel about the store that Google shows you, look at the popular times and choose the day you are planning to go, and/or look day by day throughout the week to get a sense of both the busiest days and the busiest times of each day.

8. Keep the humidity above 50%, and ideally close to (or even above) 60%, especially in communal areas. Use HEPA filtered air purifiers to keep a flow of clean/safe air on you, and avoid indoor spaces in general as much as possible.

9. Please also see our chapter on "15. Non-official Treatments to Consider" - below, starting on page 320, for comments on other strategies.

11. Avoiding Infection at Work and Home

Note – this is the second of four chapters on how to avoid or minimize your risk of catching the virus. We've tried to split the topic into four helpful pieces, but we urge you to read all four chapters as an entirety, because elements of each chapter and the recommendations within it apply to the other three chapters, too.

I t is a regrettable outcome of a virus that "came from nowhere" and so suddenly that there isn't yet any clear regulatory consensus as to what should be fairly required of businesses in terms of providing a safe workplace for their staff.[457]

There is also clearly a hope that the Covid problem will go away "any day now", with the current "*deus ex machina*" being the increasingly strident claims of a vaccine coming out very soon. There was almost irrational exuberance after Pfizer issued a press release on 9 November pointing to the possibility of a high effectiveness rate of their virus – phrases such as "Covid Miracle" and "The end

---

[457] Not only are the obligations of an employer to maintain a safe (from the virus) workplace unclear, and the obligations of a retailer to provide a safe environment for customers also unclear, but some employers are seeking liability waivers so they won't be liable and can't be sued if they don't do whatever is needed and appropriate to make their work environment as safe as prudent/possible!

of the virus" and "Return to Normalcy by Spring" appeared in the press. Even the staid WHO managed to enthuse that the vaccine "could fundamentally change the course of the pandemic".[458]

We discuss when the virus might finally go away in the chapter of that name, starting on page 102.

A cynic would also observe that some of the compliance and best-practice measures can be potentially disruptive and definitely costly, meaning there is very little groundswell of desire for strong biosafety measures by businesses and their lobbying groups. While the coronavirus and its Covid-19 disease are new, respiratory infections are not at all new, and neither is the seasonal/annual 'flu that kills tens of thousands of people every year. Society seems to have a selective blind spot when it comes to respiratory illnesses – "Oh, it's just a passing cough and cold". Is it time to revisit that blind spot and come up with more general guidelines and requirements for workplace safety?[459]

These broader implications require broader responses – social acknowledgment and agreement on what is a new definition of "appropriate" steps, and probably legislation/regulation/case law to specify what such obligations actually are. I'm all in favor of such a discussion, but it will take months/years of lobbying and evaluation for any new and beneficial measures to become mandatory. For now, and for you, it is necessary to focus on the immediate threats and issues as they confront you, at work, at home, and when traveling, to encourage better standards and practices by your employer and other companies you interact with, and to adopt the best personal practices yourself in the environments you can control.

So, unfortunately, creating an optimized and safe workplace may be a difficult issue to finesse and optimize. The best improvements to your work environment may be perceived as being overly costly or disruptive to your work environment or in some other way intrusive and unwelcome. You can act unilaterally in your home, but at work, whether you're the manager – even owner – or the lowliest staff member, you're constrained in what you can do.

Anything that requires modifications to personal behavior will be challenging, due to needing to get your fellow workers on board with your recommendations/requests, too. If it is a struggle to get people to wear masks

---

[458] For more hype and hope, see this collection of British newspaper front pages https://www.bbc.com/news/blogs-the-papers-54882074 or https://cov.cx/a1c59

[459] It is, of course, a much wider issue than just workplace safety. The same considerations apply to transportation, entertainment, social groups, and any other type of activity that involves people more or less in close proximity to other people.

and keep 6' apart in other settings, there's little reason for optimism that such people will suddenly become paragons of excellent behavior in their workplaces.

I'm having to write this section half for managers and half for employees. But that is easier than you might think, because the underlying truth that needs to be recognized and accepted by both workers and bosses is this is a win-win (or, lose-lose) situation. Companies are as harmed (well, almost) as people when there is increased absenteeism due to preventable illnesses, and the corporate cost of replacing lost workers, while nowhere near the personal cost of "replacing" a lost loved one, is also an impactful factor that *should* encourage companies to act positively and responsively in terms of the safety modifications they add to their workplaces.[460]

There should be another corporate incentive to "do the right thing". Many of the changes instituted now in response to the Covid crisis will continue to be beneficial into the future, resulting in fewer people catching coughs and colds and the seasonal 'flu each year, too. A general improvement in workplace hygiene is of permanent benefit, so there's no reason to think "there is no point in spending this money for just a few months" (always assuming, of course, that the virus will only be with us for just a few months more – see our chapter "3. When Will the Virus Finally Go Away?" on that point, starting on page 102.)[461]

This might be an area where trade unions can help. Rather than you, as one single worker, approaching "the big boss" alone, you can go to your union representatives, discuss the matter with them in a possibly more sympathetic environment, and have them make representations on behalf of the entire staff, with a more persuasive "voice" that is more likely to be heard (and which won't result in recriminations focused at specific individuals).

Companies should create "safety committees" – there's probably a better name – that have a mix of people on it at all levels, from front-line staff to senior executives. I've found, as both a front-line junior staff member, and as a top-level executive, that the two perspectives are often very different. Sometimes the

---

[460] A problem is that these employee loss costs are obscured, making no manager clearly responsible for them, whereas the safety costs are obvious and required "upfront". In our culture of short-term profit measurement and fast ROI requirements, it can be hard to justify expenditures that in the longer term and when judged on humanitarian grounds make splendid sense.

[461] Companies have slowly come to realize the costs of poor health and bad lifestyles when it comes to smoking, so there is a precedent to cite and reason for hope – maybe that same awareness can flow to respiratory diseases in general, rather than just smoking-related, and to at-work measures as well as advocating employee lifestyle choices.

best solutions – and the best-accepted solutions – are developed when all perspectives in a company come together to solve a shared problem.

Front-line staff see operational issues and challenges because they are hands-on; senior executives are aware of the broader strategy, issues, capabilities, and constraints within which solutions can be implemented; front-line staff can ensure the details of theoretical fixes mesh with the reality of actual operations. This safety committee group should of course convene to develop solutions, and meet regularly to monitor their implementation, and to resolve arising issues and challenges. An important part of such a group is to have an open and easy (and possibly anonymous) method for all staff to provide feedback and ideas.

Some people have discovered, to their embarrassment, that if they complain to the local Health Department about workplace issues, their complaints may become public record and their employer will know who made the complaint. Be careful if you're considering this approach.

When we talk about workplaces, there is of course a huge range of possible workplaces, from production lines in factories, to retailing, to office work, to outdoors work, and everything else imaginable. This requires some generalizations as to how to optimize a workplace environment, but happily, most of the issues are similar, no matter the workplace environment.

In general, in a workplace, the strategy should be to cut down on the number of physical interactions people need to have with other people; to have necessary interactions with as few other people present as is possible, conducted as briefly as possible, and in as safe an environment as possible (particularly from the perspective of airflow).

There are also some possible modifications to the workplace itself that will keep its environment as safe as possible.

Minimizing Time Actually at Work

You should minimize the number of other people each employee has to interact with in-person. There are many ways to do that. The obvious one, which many people have come to embrace, is remote working from home. Anyone who can realistically work from home should be encouraged to do so – even if only for one day a week, that's comparable to a 36% reduction in contacts (each person is now at work for only 80% of the time, and while they're at work, there are only 80% of their colleagues present).

There quite likely will be some people who have to have direct in-person contact with customers, suppliers, contractors, and others, and there may be some people who should split their time, working some days from home and other days at the company's offices.

In addition to reducing the number of people working at the business location each day, there is a second strategy to further reduce the number of people simultaneously on-site. Maybe it is possible to change the company's working hours, and have half the people working one set of hours and the other half working the other half. This can be made into a major benefit for staff, too – for example, how about a schedule where people swap between working 12 hours a day for three days, then four days off, and the other week, working four 11 hour days, and then three days off.

Another approach is to have staff working four ten-hour days then three days off. Most studies suggest that staff love having a third day off each week, and will happily add a couple of hours a day to four days of work in exchange for three day weekends, and end up being more productive too.

Yet another option could be maybe half the staff arrive very early in the morning and leave mid-afternoon after the usual eight hours, and the other half arrive at mid-day and stay until evening.

Or any other arrangement that allows for fewer people together at the same time.

Another thing to do is to stagger the break times. Retailers necessarily do this already, other businesses should do it too, to keep as few people in the office at the same time during the day.

Staggered break times (and also staggered working hours) avoids rushes on and crowds in common areas, restrooms, and other facilities.

It also reduces the stress on elevators in large office buildings – with reductions in how many people should all crowd into an elevator at the same time, some buildings are reporting long waiting times and lines for people wishing to take an elevator. Interestingly, the busiest times are not when people arrive at the beginning of the day or leave at the end of the day, but during the lunch period.[462] All the more reason to stagger lunch breaks.

Limiting Personal Interactions While at Work

After a company has optimized its staffing schedule and moved as many people to work from home for as much of each week as possible, the next point of focus is to consider how to minimize staff interactions while people are present.

This requires a reversal of much of what we've taken for granted to date. Certainly there are benefits from having informal as well as formal

---

[462] See https://www.wired.co.uk/article/lifts-coronavirus-logistics-return-to-office or https://cov.cx/a1c60

communication lines, and the concept of "management by walking around" has long been espoused as a great idea. More interactions, and casually rather than formally, tend to encourage a friendly happy workplace environment, but it is possible to find a middle ground between a glorified social club at one extreme, and a wordless sterile environment at the other extreme.

The movement of people around the business premises should be minimized as much as possible. People should use the phone to talk to each other, or an instant messaging program for office workers. If you feel you need to "eyeball" the other person, call them on a video messaging program. Offices should fully implement corporate accounts with Zoom or other video messaging services to make it instant and easy to video message anyone (and everyone) at any time.[463] [464]

---

[463] A related suggestion – when using any sort of instant messaging service, all participants should use headphones, even if they are in private offices. It keeps noise levels down in the office space, and makes it easier to manage the audio in a group meeting.

Noise rises or falls in a feedback loop. In a noisy environment, people speak louder to be heard, which increases the noise, requiring other people to speak louder, which increases the noise, requiring the first people to speak louder, and so on. Or, hopefully, the opposite. If one person is quiet, the next person doesn't need to be so loud either, and so on.

Keeping ambient noise down means people don't have to shout, and if people speak quietly, they don't emit as many aerosol particles and respiratory droplets.

We urge you to keep your work environment as library-like as possible in terms of sound levels.

[464] It is important that any form of instant messaging be as convenient as possible.

I remember working in a company, decades ago, that had both regular phones for everyone on their desks, and also semi-hands-free intercom type sets as well. Not everyone was privileged to have an intercom set, and – not having one myself – I didn't see any benefit in them. "Who needs an intercom unit when you already have a phone, and when you can get up and walk to see them too."

But when I eventually got one of the units myself, I was astonished at how convenient it proved to be, and how it resulted in much more efficient communication, both from me to other people and from other people to me.

The moral of this story is to choose some type of instant communication system that is indeed close to instantaneous, and then *make sure everyone is trained in how to use it*. Even now we cringe when we see people with only one screen rather than two or more connected to their computer, and painfully closing one program window before opening another, and only having one browser tab active. If you and/or your coworkers

(continued on next page)

Possible changes to office layouts are likely to be beneficial. All that open-plan office space with direct sight-lines isn't looking quite so appealing now. You can still preserve much of that ambiance if it is desirable and part of your corporate ethos/culture, but clear Perspex barriers should be added between work stations as much as possible, and desks should be shifted to have people working side by side or back to back rather than facing each other directly.

Minimize Meetings

One of the banes of office/administrative life are meetings. Just about every regular meeting attendant acknowledges that many meetings are only marginally necessary, and when held, have too many attendees and go on for too long.

So, Covid or not, it may be beneficial to cut back on meetings, and for the meetings that must continue, reduce the number of attendees, and set firm deadlines on their duration.

Another strategy could be to have a "rolling meeting" where people join and leave for specific parts of a meeting, rather than having everyone present from start to finish.

Whenever possible, meet via video-conferencing rather than in-person.

I don't know what to suggest about a company lunch-room, if such an amenity is presently offered, or what to suggest as an alternate approach, other than the suggestion already offered about staggering lunch and break times so as not to overload any such space.

---

don't know about Alt-Tab (in Windows) it is well past time to learn what a powerful friend it is.

Computers have become such a commonplace accepted thing these days that there is less perceived need to teach people how to use them most efficiently. Something as simple as adding a second screen to a computer can make a person 25% more productive, and some studies go further to point to even more efficiency with a third monitor. See https://www.inc.com/tim-crino/careacademy-ankur-jain-kairos-health-care.html or https://cov.cx/a1c61 . Now consider this :. Generally, a company expects to get more than three times the benefit from an employee compared to their cost. So even a $20/hr office worker is expected to be making $60+/hr for the company. If that $20/hr worker is made 25% more productive, that means they are now making $75/hr for the company. A second computer screen probably costs less than $300. That means in half a week, the cost of the monitor has been returned in productive benefits. In a year, the $300 monitor has resulted in $3000 worth of extra productivity.

Yes, this is nothing to do with Covid-19, but it is all to do with common sense and overlooked business improvement. To turn it back to Covid-19, maybe by making the worker 25% more productive, you can now reduce their hours each week with no negative impact to the company, and making both that worker and everyone else safer as a result.

Intuitively it feels very risky having a concentration of people all eating food, necessarily without masks, and with probably much less than 6' distancing between each person.

Splitting/Separating Different Parts of the Company

The more people you interact with, the greater the risk that one of them might be infected and will pass their infection on to you. Another way of reducing the number of people you physically interact with is trying to split your company into independent units with no physical interactions between each unit.

For example, if your company occupies multiple floors in a building, is it possible to limit or even eliminate all physical travel between floors?

If you are all in one single working space, is it possible to create some new partitioning that separates accounting from sales from purchasing from customer service, and so on?

While traditional corporate practice favors mixing and matching people so there are fewer "silos" and more interaction and understanding, these are not traditional times, and perhaps this will help reduce the number of risky interactions in a company still further.

Elevators vs Stairs

We mentioned above how, in high-rise buildings, elevators are becoming a bottle-neck, and cited an article that reported in some cases, as much as a 20-minute wait for an elevator.

Elevators are problematic in all situations, because they seldom have much airflow in them, and so it is best to keep people out of them whenever possible. A policy encouraging taking the stairs when going up only one floor, or down one or two floors, is a good policy to have all the time – it saves a bit of energy and gives people a bit of exercise, and this is something to stress more strongly at present. Not only does it keep some people out of the elevators, but it also reduces the loads on the elevators and therefore helps if there are growing delays waiting for an elevator.

If your company is having problems with elevator bottlenecks, it is a good idea to speak to your elevator maintenance company. We know hoteliers who have massively reduced the waits for elevators in their hotels by speeding up the elevators – not in the sense of making them go up and down more quickly,[465]

---

[465] It would certainly be good if you can speed up the elevator travel speed, but that is more likely to be a more costly enhancement, and – surprisingly – with less impact on total time and capacity.

but in the sense of door opening/closing routines. If it is possible to speed up the open/close movements, and to reduce the time the elevator waits before closing its doors at a floor, and also to ensure that the "Door Close" button actually does work (some are deliberately disconnected) and that the elevator immediately responds to a door close request, that can speed up the overall throughput of the elevator greatly. A typical elevator journey spends more time during the door opening/closing time than it does through the actual traveling between floors.

Air Flow

Managing the airflow in your environment is one of the very most important things you can do – at work, at home, and everywhere.

Some of our other recommendations are not feasible for all workplaces, or unevenly apply to some workers but not others.[466] Improving the airflow is something that everyone will benefit from, and there is seldom a reason why a company can't improve the quality of the air within its premises (other than the cost, and even that doesn't have to be prohibitive).

The thinking about how people catch the Covid-19 disease has slowly evolved over the months. Now it seems the greatest risk of infection comes from contaminated air – air that either has respiratory droplets or aerosols exhaled by an infected person, that you in turn breathe in. This is now understood to be how the vast majority of people become infected. We discuss air quality in other parts of this book as well, most notably in the chapter "9. Self Quarantining" starting on page 206 above, because it is so important, and a relatively easily improved factor.

Several essential things really must be done, and probably the first essential thing is to get a well-qualified HVAC engineer or consultant – probably a member

---

[466] Don't get hung up on the concept of "fairness" in the sense of "It isn't fair that this would benefit some people rather than others". That's a classic glass-half-empty attitude, and also overlooks an important consequential benefit to everyone else.

First, the glass-half-full perception – why should people who can benefit from a workplace change not be allowed to benefit from that workplace change? A benefit to any employees flows through to a benefit for the company as a whole. Alternatively, how are the people who didn't get the benefit of a workplace change harmed? They're not harmed at all, their life continues as before.

Actually, their life changes too, which brings us to our second point. Every person you can either take out of the workplace or improve medical safety for, is a benefit for everyone else, too, because it reduces the number of potentially risky contacts and interactions in the workplace for everyone else. Taking one person out of an office or off a shop floor means one less person for everyone else to brush shoulders with and risk getting infected from.

of ASHRAE – to help your company in its analysis and to work with the company to come up with a priority list of the most beneficial, least costly and most readily implemented enhancements to the current airflow system.

The chances are no-one in your company even knows how many changes of air your premises get currently, what type of filtration the air goes through, and how much of the air is fresh and how much is recycled.[467] You might know what the ambient temperature is, but how about the humidity?

Almost certainly, most commercial building space has been designed to meet the barest minimum of requirements, and equally almost certainly, some upgrades will profoundly improve the quality of air and reduce the level of contaminants and virus particles within it.

I'd point out, also – in case this is necessary – that air quality is something that affects the "man in the corner office" just as much as it does the most humble worker. So everyone in the company should be equally keen to improve air quality.[468]

Because most of us know so little about the quality of the air in our work environments – it has not been a factor to consider for most work situations and workers – perhaps the first thing to do is to establish some air quality monitoring within your work environment.

---

[467] I've been involved in numerous building projects, both commercial and residential; both new construction and fitting out existing space, and of sizes up to, I think, about 50,000 sq ft. While I've been involved in every last detail down to the number of power outlets per foot of wall space, carpet weights, lighting temperatures, and so on, the HVAC has never been something I – or any of the other people working on the projects – have ever stopped to question or ask about beyond confirming it will be adequate to keep us warm in winter and cool in summer and will have enough zones to maintain even temperatures throughout the space. We've never thought to ask any more about it. Filter changes? Maybe the landlord did it, but I'd never thought to ask. And so on. Chances are that lack of focus is true of most other businesses and their managers, too.

[468] Air quality is another feature with permanently lasting benefits. It is astonishing to see how poor the air quality is in some buildings currently – but not in obvious ways. Instead, there are insidious and subtle problems, commonly in the form of higher than optimum percentages of carbon dioxide that can interfere with concentration and energy levels. Cleaner fresher air might boost a company's productivity, reduce its error rates, and make its staff happier and more cheerful. That's a huge return on a few pennies more of electricity an hour, and changing better filters more often.

A low-cost approach would be to get one or several of the Purple Air or other similar air sensors[469] and to consider the particulate density of PM2.5 matter to be an approximation of risk/concentration of airborne virus particles.

A more sophisticated solution would be to monitor carbon dioxide levels, considering that to be an approximation of air that has been breathed out by people and not replaced with fresh/clean air as well as still tracking PM2.5 density too.[470]

Needless to say, in the likely event that the company doesn't own its premises, it may be able to get its landlord to either do the work for free or to have the landlord capitalize the costs and reflect it in future rent increases.[471]

In terms of specific measures to consider that are easy and quick to implement, here are some, slightly modified from the ASHRAE guidelines[472]

- Increase outdoor air ventilation (use caution in highly polluted areas); with a lower population in the building, this increases the effective dilution ventilation per person.
- Disable demand-controlled ventilation (DCV).
- Further open minimum outdoor air dampers, as high as 100%, thus eliminating recirculation (in the mild weather season, this need not affect thermal comfort or humidity, but becomes more difficult in extreme weather).

---

[469] See https://www2.purpleair.com/collections/air-quality-sensors or https://cov.cx/a1c62

[470] This article discusses the issue and suggests some equipment https://spectrum.ieee.org/tech-talk/telecom/wireless/indoor-airquality-monitoring-can-allow-anxious-office-workers-to-breathe-easier or https://cov.cx/a1c63

[471] Every situation is different, but if you have an engineer's report showing elevated levels of CO_2, or other air quality issues, you may be able to get the landlord to do most of the upgrading at their cost. If not, the landlord might agree to spend money on upgrades in terms for the company extending its lease for another some years – the landlord probably saves on a realtor fee for re-leasing the space, and the hassle of doing so, plus if releasing the space, they'd be up for some build-out costs anyway, and possibly some free rent.

Especially at present, with all the future uncertainty hanging over all our heads, in most parts of the country, landlords are desperate to keep good tenants.

[472] See https://www.ashrae.org/file%20library/technical%20resources/ashrae%20journal/2020journaldocuments/72-74_ieq_schoen.pdf or https://cov.cx/a1c64

- Improve central air filtration to the MERV-13 rating or the highest compatible with the filter rack, and seal edges of the filter to limit bypass.
- Keep systems running longer hours, if possible 24/7, to enhance the two actions above.
- Monitor humidity levels and keep them at the high end of the optimum range (about 50% - 60% is ideal).
- Consider UVGI (ultraviolet germicidal irradiation), protecting occupants from radiation, particularly in high-risk spaces such as waiting rooms. Be sure any such devices don't generate measurable ozone.
- Add portable room air cleaners with HEPA filters in the most challenging areas.

All these suggestions are great, and the three which can most readily be done without needing to call in a tradesman or secure a new bank loan are

- Adding portable room air cleaners and UVGI units (certified as ozone free)
- Monitoring and probably boosting humidity
- Not turning off the a/c at night. Sure, set the temperatures back, so you're not actively heating/cooling the space so much, but keep the air circulating and going through the filters (by switching the fan mode from "Auto" to "On" on most thermostats).

A specialist HVAC engineer will doubtless have other and excellent suggestions.

Mandatory Effective Mask-Wearing

I hate wearing a mask as much as anyone (and probably more than many!). I similarly feel awkward and uncomfortable with the loss of non-verbal feedback when interacting with someone else wearing a mask. I'm seen all the many reasons people cite for why masks should not be work.

But.

Much as I hate mask-wearing, I hate the thought of death or permanent disability much more. So anytime I'm in public, I've a mask on, and now I find I feel much more uncomfortable when close to anyone not wearing a mask.

It seems to have been proven every which way, repeatedly, that wearing an appropriate mask cuts down on the transmission of virus particles.[473] When you

---

[473] Here are two excellent articles. There are dozens more.
https://fastlifehacks.com/n95-vs-ffp/ or https://cov.cx/a1c65 and
(continued on next page)

breathe out, any infection you might have and virus particles you are breathing out are reduced in number, with the vast majority being trapped in the mask. When you breathe in, most of any virus particles in the air that are drawn into your breath are trapped by the mask and don't go into your nose or down your throat.

You shouldn't care what your state's policy is, and neither should you care what the preference of other people is. You should always wear a mask, yourself, and you should do everything you can to ensure that everyone else around you does too. If you're in a position to do so, please make it a mandatory company policy.

Sadly, it is necessary to go beyond the simple statement "Everyone must wear masks". It is necessary to stress the "must" by adding words like "at all times". And, most regrettably of all, it is necessary to specify what are and are not acceptable types and styles of masks.

Masks should completely cover the face from underneath the chin to some point part-way up the nose (ones that barely reach to the tip of one's nose are not good enough). They should seal, more or less, at the bottom, and on the sides, and conform reasonably to shape around the nose. Elastic straps that loop over the ears are good, straps you tie behind you can be better if you get the tension right, but tying them can be inconvenient. Fixed-size/loop straps with no elasticity are bad.

Masks should not have vents in them. Why do I even have to say this? A vent that allows air to freely bypass the mask in either direction defeats the entire purpose of the mask.[474]

Bandanas are not as good as real masks. Washable masks wear out after a limited number of washes – you know that from your clothing already. The more you wash a mask, the more the fibers lose their bulk and effectiveness. Face shields are of very little value – they can be allowed together with a mask to provide a small amount of additional protection, but are totally not a suitable substitute.

Companies might want to consider giving their staff a surgical mask every day. These are now commonly available, and cost as little as 20c – 25c when bought in quantities of 50 or more at Costco, Walmart, Amazon, and elsewhere.

---

https://www.thedailybeast.com/5-myths-on-face-masks-amid-the-coronavirus-pandemic or https://cov.cx/a1c66

[474] So why do some masks have vents? Because they have been designed for purposes where the mask only needs to provide one-way filtering. For example, if you are a painter, you want the mask to block paint being breathed in, but there is no need to filter the air you breathe out.

Make sure the masks have three layers, and the middle layer is not woven. Instead, it should be a sort of fibrous mat of material.

The same requirements should be imposed on visitors, customers, suppliers, contractors, and everyone else that comes to the company's premises. It is not possible to have one law for some people, and a different law for others. Everyone needs to accept this essential safety measure.

Other Policies

Here's a grab bag of some other thoughts for companies to adopt and encourage.

The first point is that **managers must model good behavior** for their employees to emulate. If mask-wearing is mandated (and hopefully it is) then the managers must of course conspicuously over-comply with that policy themselves.

Staff should be encouraged to stay home if they feel unwell. That policy should be extended in cases where staff have sick family members too.

We all know staff members who feel they're doing their company a favor by coming in when they're sick – the problem is they then boast about it to everyone, and cough/sneeze everywhere, meaning that instead of one person off work, the company ends up with half a dozen off work.

An adjustment to whatever sick pay policies apply might need to be made so there are no penalties for employees when they choose to responsibly keep themselves away from the workplace. sick – no exceptions, liberal sick pay policy; also allow people to stay home to care for sick family members.

We don't like **temperature testing** in cases where organizations boast they temperature test everyone entering an area, but do nothing more, and feel that temperature tests then guarantee everyone who passes the test is safe.

That is totally wrong. Many infected people never get a fever, and most people who do get a fever are infectious before they have a fever, and once they do have a fever, don't need to be told to stay away, because they're truly feeling unwell.

But, as an "extra string to the bow", it does no harm to add temperature testing as one of the many elements of risk minimization. People could be temperature tested (the usual cut-off point is 100.4°F or 38°C) and at the same time quizzed "Are you coughing or suffering from shortness of breath, or have any other people close to you reported similar symptoms?".

I suggest companies consider having dispensers that squirt out measures of **hand sanitizer** at the entrances to their premises, and strategically elsewhere on-site as well. Make sure the sanitizer has at least 60% alcohol content, and very preferably 70% or slightly higher.

In November, we are finally starting to see the deployment of **low-cost instant virus test kits**. These have their limitations, but if every employee is tested every day, the frequency of testing compensates for the test weaknesses and can be enormously helpful in reducing the risk of bringing the virus into your organization. We strongly advocate your company considers deploying these types of instant testing products as soon as they are readily available.

Something to consider is **how employees travel to and from work**. In pre-virus times, some companies have subsidized and encouraged the use of public transportation services or car-pooling. Those are commendable policies in normal times, but maybe not quite so wise at present. There's no safer way to travel than in one's own car, alone. Personal transportation of course becomes more convenient if you have employees traveling outside of the usual morning and after peak commute hours, when it is harder to find convenient transport options.

There is a direct correlation between how loudly someone speaks and the distance and amount of virus they project. I noticed, just today, two employees at a local supermarket carrying on a conversation, being at opposite ends of the fruit and vegetable department. One of the two men was staring directly at me while shouting to his colleague. That is so rude on so many levels, but rather than create a fuss, I simply moved away.

Companies should have a policy that **people must only speak in quiet voices**. If people are far apart, they should move closer together (but not too close!) to converse.

Normally, in places where I work, some of the business equipment is "communal" that everyone shares and some is "individual" (that is often shared, too!). There should be a **"no-sharing" rule** for anything other than things that are unavoidably shared (photocopiers, for example). But staplers, pens, rulers, scissors – everyone should have their own set of such essentials, and if someone loses/breaks/forgets their own, they should ask for a replacement, rather than randomly sharing others.[475]

Companies should try and come up with new strategies to **restrict and minimize personal contact** with customers, suppliers, and contractors.

A low-cost enhancement, if applicable, is to make sure **all toilets have lids, and to encourage people to lower the lids before flushing**. Covid particles can be found in feces, and the water flow when you flush a toilet causes

---

[475] This is not a major threat, because there is an increasing downplaying of the threat of catching the virus after touching something infected. But it remains a small threat and is easy to minimize.

a plume of aerosol and droplet particles to rise from the toilet bowl if there is no lid, or the lid is up.

Restricting customer contact in particular is something that needs to be delicately optimized. You don't want to lose your customers – but hopefully there's a positive way you can explain your changed procedures as being for the customers' safety and convenience – "We have altered things to make it easier for you to continue to deal with us without requiring you to have as much direct personal exposure to us as is normal. We love to see you and spend time with you, but feel you'll appreciate these measures." Make more use of email, voicemail, video calls, video messages, and other modern technologies to keep in touch with customers, just go easy on personal visits.

It might go without saying that companies should **limit and restrict their employees' business-related travel** as much as possible. Most companies are doing this at present, and the chances are that just as your company is keen to reduce its contacts with customers, suppliers, and others, so too are the companies and people that you and your colleagues would otherwise be visiting also keen to minimize their contacts with you!

Trade shows – once a potentially very valuable way to meet many people in a short period of time – are of course terribly risky at present. Many have been canceled, or somehow changed to some type of online experience instead. Those that continue to be held have unknown levels of participation, making them no longer as valuable as they normally are, and making it easier for you too to skip them.

If you and other company members unavoidable need to travel, consider the best way to travel. Depending on distance, this might mean driving by car. If flying, be sure to choose an airline that promises to keep the middle seats blocked out. When staying in overnight accommodation, the best choice at present is to stay in an "external corridor" type motel/hotel.

Personal Steps

If the company you work for doesn't do everything we suggest above (and probably few will implement every point suggested) then you can still attempt to modify your own behavior, actions, and environment to minimize your personal risk.

One overriding comment. If your employer is failing to require some very basic and very obvious safety measures, you could try **complaining to your city/county/state department responsible for workplace safety** (and to all three if there are multiple such organizations). Beware of the risk of having your complaints shared with your employer though – it might be best to anonymously complain using a made-up email address/identity, or to arrange for a friend who is not obviously connected to you to complain on behalf of you and everyone else at your company.

If there is not much response, you should add to the pressure with **letters to your state representatives and senator, and to the governor too**, and see if you can get some **media attention** too. The media attention is more likely if/when people at your company become ill from the virus, and particularly if someone is seriously ill or suffers a fatal attack.

So, what can you do, yourself, while at work? Of course, as long as the social pressures against this are not too overwhelming, you should **wear a mask**, even if those around you are not.

You should have **hand sanitizer** where you work. We'd suggest having it conspicuously on display and available for others to use as well. Helping boost the health of the people around you directly benefits you – if the people you come in contact with are less likely to be infected, then your risk is lowered, too.

Try **not to share items** that would normally be shared. If you have desirable things, keep them out of view. If someone asks for your (whatever), explain your concern that you don't want to risk passing any infection you might have to them, and then add that the vice versa risk is also present too. Remind them that in normal times you've been happy to help/share, but at present, you don't think it is appropriate.

If that becomes a big problem, consider taking the desired object home so you can truthfully say "I no longer have it". Or, if the item is inexpensive, get a sharing one as well as your own one.

If you still do share objects, clean them with hand sanitizer when they are returned.

If you work primarily in one particular area, consider getting a **personal air purifier** (see the chapter on "17. Medical Equipment & Supplies You Should Have", starting on page 398) that blows air through a HEPA filter, creating a stream of cleaner air, and having it in your workplace blowing cleaner/safer air at you.

This is a slightly ambiguous benefit. While the unit is hopefully blowing cleaner air toward you, you are also increasing the volume of air that passes by you, with a slight increase in risk that some of that air will still have virus particles within it. On the other hand, you're not increasing the volume of air you breathe in and out, and even a fairly low, say, 97% filtration rate means as long as you have less than 33 times more air blowing past you, you're overall better off, so probably on balance a personal air purifier is more beneficial than harmful.

As part of managing the air quality in your own space, if you have a physical office or small contained work area, and if the building HVAC system doesn't have high-grade filters and a high percentage of fresh rather than recycled air, see if you can **reduce the flow of air from the HVAC** into that area. That way your personal air cleaner, and its small volume of cleaned safe air isn't having to do battle with the duct in the ceiling that is flooding your space with untreated air.

You have to be careful when adjusting dampers in the ducting because the entire air distribution system is balanced based on overall damper settings. If you change your damper setting, and other people do the same, then the entire airflow will be changed with possibly negative consequences.

Try and keep your **contacts with your coworkers to a minimum**, and use phone/texting/instant messaging/emailing rather than personal interaction whenever possible. Beg out of attending meetings where you're not needed.

Try **not to roam around the premises any more than necessary**, and when doing so, choose routes that are less trafficked.

And maybe now is the time to recommit to a personal fitness regime and spend more time **using the stairs than elevators** to go up and down a reasonable number of floors.

What If Someone at Work Becomes Infected

With over 100,000 people known to be getting infected every day at present, it seems inevitable that sooner or later, someone in your workplace will get infected.

Slightly more subtly, even if a coworker isn't directly infected, maybe someone in their family or close circle of contacts has become infected, which increases the chances that your coworker may be or soon become infected, too.

How to respond to such events is something the company needs to determine, rather than you individually, of course, and this is something the company's newly constituted safety committee should consider and have a policy for.

The three essential elements are :
(a)   Finding out, as early as possible, that a coworker is infected
(b)   Taking that person out of the workforce and having them stay at home until cleared and no longer unwell or infectious
(c)   Identifying who might have been infected by the coworker, and having them be more cautious in their interactions (ideally also isolated) until they have been tested and cleared.

Now that test kits are finally becoming more readily available, with test results available in minutes rather than hours or days, and with reducing costs of testing, we'd urge all employers to institute an employee testing program that has all employees regularly being tested.

How regularly? The greater the degree of contact with others, the more regular the testing. Ideally, as mentioned above, everyone should be tested upon arriving at work, every day.[476] But anything is better than nothing.

Testing should be supplemented by fever (ie temperature) checks and simple questioning – do you have a cough? Are you feeling unwell?

As soon as a person gets advice of a positive test result (positive in the sense of "you have an infection"), they should immediately drop everything and leave the workplace. Don't even pause to tell a supervisor they are going. Leave the building, even with their computer still turned on, and wait until they are well clear of the premises before then phoning in to explain why they suddenly left.

They should isolate themselves from their coworkers (and everyone else) until their infection is over. See our two chapters, "7. How Long Does an Infection Last", starting on page 195, and "8. How to Know if You are Cured", below on page 204.

One point to consider. There may be a high incidence of false-positive results when randomly testing everyone, whether they feel well or unwell (we discuss this, above, in the section "Test Accuracy" starting on page 184). People with positive tests should be retested to confirm the positive result.

The third part of this process is the contact tracing to find out who the infected person might have already infected. Depending on the frequency of testing and how the infection was finally detected, there might be anywhere from a day to a week of "at-risk" contacts who should be advised they might have been infected.

Some states provide formal contact tracing services, although their efficacy seems to vary enormously from barely satisfactory to very unsatisfactory.

---

[476] Well, even that is somewhat of a compromise. If one wished to be obsessive, particularly in very high-risk environments, one might require testing more than once a day. Remember the big weakness with all tests is that it requires several days – at least two, possibly three, maybe even four or more – between when a person gets infected and when a test will correctly report the infection.

So a test at 9am doesn't mean "this person absolutely has no infection"; it means "two or three days ago, this person was not infected, but we don't know what happened to them since then".

This means it is possible that a person could test negative at 9am but positive at 1pm – not because they became infected during that morning, but because an infection they acquired two or three days ago finally became of sufficient strength to register on the test.

The really big issue is whether a person is infectious before or after a test detects their infection. In some cases, particularly with non-PCR testing, it is possible there is a day or two of infectiousness before a test registers an infection.

What your company should do is immediately announce, to everyone, who it is that has tested positive and gone into self-isolation, and ask everyone to examine their movements and interactions over the last several days, and if they've had any close contact with the person, voluntarily leave and self-isolate and get tested to establish their status.

Such departures from the workplace of course should be on a paid absence basis. Otherwise, many people might choose not to disclose their contact.

What is a risky contact that could trigger self-isolation? There is no one thing and no exact point where a contact shifts from safe to dangerous.

But here are a series of factors. The more negatively a person scores their contact with the infected person, the greater their risk.

Factor	Comment
Indoors or outdoors	Indoors is very much riskier, depending also on the quality of the air supply/purification/recycling/filtering/etc.
Distance	Within six feet is much riskier than further apart, beyond twelve feet starts to become a trivial risk factor.
Contact duration	The longer you are together, the greater the risk becomes. Each minute gives you more chance of breathing in more virus particles. A total of 15 minutes of contact in a single day is considered to significantly push the risk factor up to high.
Mask-wearing	Best-case scenario both people wear masks, second-best-case the infected person wore a mask, least good case the other person wore a mask, worst case neither person did.
Whispered or shouted	The louder a person talks, the more virus they exhale and the further it travels. Coughing and sneezing is very bad, but so too is laughing, shouting and singing. A quiet voice is best.
Frequency of contact	Interacting with the contact once is better than interacting many times. On the other hand, multiple

> brief contacts totaling the same number of minutes are better than fewer lengthy contacts.
>
> *Figure 57 Assessing risk of infection*

Hopefully, a risk analysis on factors like this helps people to strategize their risk level and know if they should self-isolate and test themselves or not.

How Safe is Your Home

You might think that some of the protective measures discussed in this chapter are not needed for your residence. At work, yes, and in public, definitely, but not at home. After all, when you're at home, surely the only person you're protecting against is yourself, right?

Well, that's only true if you live alone and are observing perfect social distancing with no-one ever visiting you and coming inside your residence, and with your own fresh air flow, uncontaminated by other people in their homes.

If you are living by yourself, then you don't need to worry too much about temperature and humidity. But keep in mind if you're in a block of apartments, then airflow considerations and minimizing your risk of getting contaminated air from another part of the block of apartments remains a concern.

If you're living with a partner or roommate, you need to realize that any time the other person leaves the house – *even if accompanied by you* – they may possibly become infected, as much by bad luck as by bad social distancing and imperfect other measures,[477] and so they may be introducing a threat to you upon their/your joint return back to your home.[478] Short of living life in a "spacesuit" type decontamination suit, everything we do outside our residence is

---

[477] This is an important point to appreciate. Nothing is black and white. Everything is a case of greater or lesser risk/odds. Even the most cautious and fastidious person can get unlucky (and similarly, even the most careless of people can sometimes seem to lead a charmed life free of consequence!). So don't think "I completely trust my partner to be careful, so I don't need to worry about what they're doing". It isn't a case of trust, and tragically, sometimes all the care in the world can be negated by a very unlucky event.

[478] In case it isn't obvious, the opposite applies, too. Every time you go out, you return back home as a potential threat to anyone/everyone else in your home, too. It may be easier to delicately raise issues of at-home protocols on the basis of volunteering that you don't want to risk giving an infection you might acquire to the other people, rather than accusing them of being risks to you!

a compromise between safety and convenience. If done well, the compromise is more balanced to safety than risk, but there remains an element of risk.

And so, while your home hopefully has fewer threats within it than an uncontrolled space elsewhere, remember that all threats are judged not only by their innate level of danger, but also by the time you are exposed to them, and for sure, on the time scale, you're spending a great deal of time at home, and so want to ensure it is as safe as possible for you and everyone else with you.

If you find yourself in a situation where you're obliged to host visitors, you might want to consider things like airflow and humidity, to make the environment as hostile to the virus as possible. Get the humidity cranked up high before your guest arrives, and have plenty of air flowing through the room they're in (and flowing on out of your residence) while they are present – and also for a few hours after they leave, to flush out any aerosols they've emitted.

If it is not practical to have all the windows open – maybe it is too hot or cold outside – then you should consider deploying some HEPA filtering air purifiers in the parts of your home that visitors will be in, and in that case, you want to cut down on airflow rates so the possibly contaminated air where your visitors are, does not get circulated through the rest of your home, and making it easier for air purifiers in the rooms where your visitors will be to do an efficient job of processing the air. See our discussion on air purifiers in the chapter "17. Medical Equipment & Supplies You Should Have", starting on page 398.

Another thing to consider is upgrading the filters in your home furnace. This can be an impactful and relatively inexpensive way of treating the air in your entire home environment. We suggest choosing air filters with a MERV rating of 13 or more (see Figure 50 MERV filter ratings on page 210).

We've been asked about the value of adding plants as a natural way of purifying the air. We like plants too, and they certainly can make a house seem more like a home, "softening" the artificiality of a space and making it more natural. There are benefits in having plants in your living environment, and it is true they do play a role in converting carbon dioxide into oxygen and even remove some types of chemicals from the air.

But how useful are plants as a natural air filter? The widely held and repeated belief about the ability of plants to act as a natural air filter seems to all trace back to a single source – a NASA study in the late 1990s headed by a Dr Bill Wolverton. His study concluded that plants could help maintain the air quality on the International Space Station.

But the ISS is a closed-system. At least in theory, there is no outside air coming in (other than replacement oxygen generated by electrolysis of water) and no air leaking out, so it is easy to treat the finite air within the small ISS. Compare that to a house, with significant quantities of air blowing in and out all the time. The volume of air to be treated in a house overwhelms the very minor air treatment capabilities of plants.[479]

Additionally, there are no studies suggesting plants will filter out viruses.

So by all means, have plants in your home because they look nice and create a nice ambiance, but don't expect them to give you any material improvement in your air quality and safety.

In addition to implementing such of our suggestions as you feel appropriate, you also might like to give some advance thought as to how you'll respond if one of the people in your household does come down with an infection, so that if/when it happens, you can quickly create an isolation area for that person with the minimum of spill-over of air and contact between that area and the rest of your residence.

Our chapter, "9. Self Quarantining", discusses those issues further, starting on page 206.

---

[479] This is a good article that sadly debunks the wish/belief that having a few plants improve our air quality. They say you'd need one plant per square foot of space to have a notable impact on air quality, and that by doing so, you'd end up with too much humidity. https://www.theatlantic.com/science/archive/2019/03/indoor-plants-clean-air-best-none-them/584509/ or https://cov.cx/a1c67

12. Avoiding Infection on Planes, etc

Note – this is the third of four chapters on how to avoid or at least minimize your risk of catching the virus. We've tried to split the topic into four helpful pieces, but we urge you to read all four chapters as an entirety, because elements of each chapter and the recommendations within it apply to the other three chapters, too.

In the preceding chapters, we've shown that your risk of becoming infected increases, the closer you are to people, and the longer you are together. Surely an airplane scores close to max on both those scales – very close to many other people, and even with middle seats empty, you're still only 3 ft away from the next passenger on your side, plus under 3 ft away from the next passenger in front, and 3 ft from the next passenger behind. So much for the 6 ft distancing guideline.

Instead of being in the same environment as someone else for only a few minutes, you might all be on the plane for many hours. Don't think things get better before and after a flight – the boarding and deplaning is usually crowded, and the air terminals have plenty of too-close experiences also.[480]

For a while, almost every flight in the US was empty. Passenger numbers crashed in March, and by early April, there was barely one person in 20 still flying (ie about 5% of the 2019 passenger numbers).

---

[480] Social distancing around a luggage carousel? .Good luck with that!

This is vividly illustrated in this chart showing the number of people going through TSA checkpoints each day, which also shows the slow but steady return of people to planes since that time.[481]

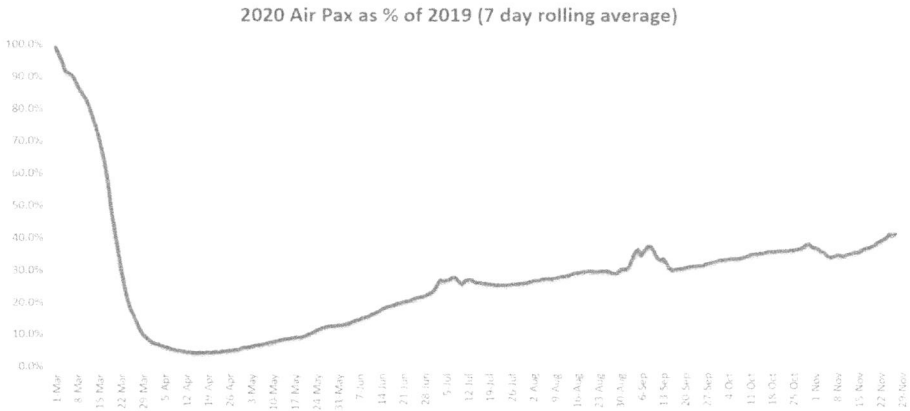

Figure 58 2020 US Air passengers as a percent of 2019

At first, the airlines were caught unawares, and it took them time to reduce their flight numbers to reflect the diminished passenger numbers, meaning most flights were ridiculously and wonderfully almost empty. But now, because the airlines have reduced flights to compensate for reduces passenger numbers, flights are filling up again. Confident of continued growth, Southwest says it expects to be back to operating its full schedule by the end of the year once more.

Some countries have been relaxing their travel bans and quarantine requirements. It may be possible, in the next month or two, to start to travel to many/most other countries, although who only knows what type of vacation experience would await you after getting there.

The safety of air travel is increasingly a consideration (and possibly a concern). Just because we can travel doesn't mean we should. How safe is it to fly, and how can we shift the odds in our favor?

In June the International Civil Aviation Organization issued a series of guidelines on how flights should be operated to minimize the risk of Covid-19 infection.[482] We noticed the guidelines were very weak on any type of assurance

---

[481] Taken from the data at https://www.tsa.gov/coronavirus/passenger-throughput or https://cov.cx/tsa-c

[482] See https://www.icao.int/covid/cart/Pages/default.aspx or https://cov.cx/a1c68

of safety, and with most of the input coming from industry organizations such as IATA (the international airline lobbying group) we were not surprised by the weak and vague guidelines issued.

The guidelines contain an abundance of vague terms rather than hard specific requirements – phrases such as "wherever possible" betray the reality of these guidelines – they are a compromise between absolute safety and essential commercial requirements to profitably and efficiently provide air travel services. Call us cynical, but we fear the "wherever possible" escape clause means that commercial rather than public health issues will generally be in the ascendancy.

There's a focus on cheap easily implemented measures – requiring passengers to wear masks,[483] more cabin cleaning (whatever that means – and in early August, Southwest stunned the nation by announcing it was reducing the amount of cabin cleaning it was doing between flights because it was slowing down their turnaround times), and advocating the almost entirely useless temperature checks of passengers before boarding.[484] Expensive but proven to be effective measures like keeping middle seats free were not recommended, clearly on grounds of profit/cost rather than for public health reasons.

Unfortunately, the virus doesn't give a free pass to the need for airlines to be profitable and just as relentlessly hunts down its victims in a commercial environment as it does anywhere else.

Some airlines have been quite strident in their assurances that it is safe to travel, even on full planes with every middle seat taken. "There have been no proven cases of Covid-19 infections being acquired on planes" is a statement that has been offered up in the earlier days of the virus pandemic, and maybe it might have been true then, but probably not so much now. Indeed, here's a write-up of a situation where perhaps a dozen people caught the virus on a nearly empty (only 49 people on board) 7½ hour flight to Ireland.[485]

We note that a medical advisor for IATA is now saying[486]

---

[483] After a slow start, the airlines have been eager to embrace this. It shifts a lot of the hassle factor for ensuring safe flights from them and to us, and also provides a visible indication of "doing something" to reassure would-be passengers.

[484] See https://blog.thetravelinsider.info/2020/04/checking-your-temperature-for-covid-19-is-meaningless-and-even-dangerous.html or https://cov.cx/a1c69

[485] See https://www.dw.com/en/how-safe-is-air-travel-during-covid-19/a-55435284 or https://cov.cx/a1c70

[486] See https://www.businessinsider.com/is-flying-safe-right-now-coronavirus or https://cov.cx/a1c71

> "The risk of transmission of COVID-19 from passenger-to-passenger onboard an aircraft appears already to be very low, based on our communications with a large number of major airlines during January through March 2020, and a more detailed IATA examination of contact tracing of 1,100 passengers [during the same period] who were confirmed for COVID-19 after air travel."

One has to wonder, of course, what "very low" actually means. Back in January – March the incidence of the virus was very low, everywhere, in all circumstances and situations. Maybe the risk was "very low" on planes and "extremely incredibly low" everywhere else!

Since that time there has also been research published that suggests your chance of getting an infection on a flight almost doubles if the seat next to you is filled.[487] Guaranteeing you an empty middle seat is probably the most valuable thing an airline can offer at present. Some do, and some don't. We recommend you should check your airline's policy and choose your airline based on that.

In October results of a new study were published that suggested the chance of getting a virus infection on a flight was very low. The study was conducted by the Department of Defense, Boeing, and United Airlines – and at least two of those three organizations can hardly be considered as neutral parties.

While the testing they did seemed correct, they *did not test all scenarios*. Not all possible risks were considered. That's a bit like testing your chances of getting in a car crash – but while the car remains safely parked in your garage at home!

In this article, one comment offered is that if real-life conditions had been considered, the results would show 10 to 100 times greater risks of catching the virus on board.[488] Here's further commentary critical of the research.[489]

A credible analysis of real-world risk while flying was published in November by a group of New Zealand researchers. They looked at an 18-hour flight from Dubai to Auckland in late September. It had 86 passengers on board, and seven of them subsequently tested positive for the virus. Five of the seven infected passengers said they wore a mask on the flight, and the passengers were up to four rows apart from each other.

---

[487] See https://www.medrxiv.org/content/10.1101/2020.07.02.20143826v3 or https://cov.cx/a1c72

[488] See https://finance.yahoo.com/news/covid-19-risk-airplanes-really-120021101.html or https://cov.cx/a1c73

[489] See https://danto.info/Not_Traveling_4th_Week_October-2020-JSM.htm or https://cov.cx/a1c74

By comparing the virus strains of the infected passengers, the researchers were able to determine that one of the passengers – someone who had shown a negative test before boarding the plane – actually was infected, and proceeded to pass his infection on to at least four of the other passengers.[490]

Other credible studies also point to the reality of people getting infected on flights.[491] It is very hard to know if the danger of becoming infected on a flight is therefore higher, lower, or about the same as it is in other everyday tasks, but certainly, there is a risk present when flying and to suggest otherwise or to excessively downplay that reality does no-one any good (except the airlines).

We also note that while the risk of getting the virus from touching a contaminated surface is generally considered very low, there seems to be clear evidence of this happening on a flight that was carefully monitored to see what happened to the passengers.[492]

It is of course very difficult to be able to exactly establish where one gets an infection. But we know four things :

1. In general, we have noticed ourselves, and many other people we know have experienced the same, that whenever we go on a long-haul flight, no matter what the time of year, there's probably one chance in two that within a week or so we'll have come down with a cough or cold. Was that acquired as a result of a 10+ hour flight? We can't "prove" it was, but statistically, after hundreds of such flights over the years, we notice the clear correlation between "long flight" and "catching a cough/cold".

If we're at risk of catching a cough or cold after a flight, it seems likely we'd also be at risk of catching other respiratory type viral infections such as Covid-19.

2. We were speaking with a physician who is also a professor at the leading teaching hospital in Singapore about this matter, and she has personal knowledge of a person who did catch the Covid-19 virus, almost certainly on a flight from Europe to Singapore. This was established through Singapore's contact tracing program – one person was discovered to have the virus on the

---

[490] See https://research.esr.cri.nz/articles/preprint/A_case_study_of_extended_in-flight_transmission_of_SARS-CoV-2_en_route_to_Aotearoa_New_Zealand/13257914 or https://cov.cx/a1c75

[491] See two more studies cited in this article https://www.forbes.com/sites/suzannerowankelleher/2020/09/19/covid-19-can-spread-on-long-airline-flights-per-two-new-studies/?sh=6caf176476a9 or https://cov.cx/a1c76

[492] See https://wwwnc.cdc.gov/eid/article/26/11/20-3353_article or https://cov.cx/a1c77 and the apparent acquisition of infection via an airplane toilet

flight, and the contact tracing program checked with people on the same flight and one of the people was a relative of a colleague of hers and he was found to have the virus too.

3. Several studies are suggesting what seems to be an elevated level of virus infections among flight attendants. This probably points to an increased risk of infection in their workplace – ie, on planes.

On 10 April, a story circulated about 100 American Airlines flight attendants having tested positive for the disease.[493] At the time, there were 510,000 cases in total in the country, a rate of 1544 per million. AA has just over 26,000 flight attendants, and so this represents an infection rate 2 1/2 times greater than the general population. Considering also that probably not all flight attendants were tested, and not all flight attendants would be actively working as flight numbers shrank down, and some flight attendants might have already had the disease and recovered, the real rate is probably even higher again.

But keeping it simply to the 2 1/2 times greater than normal number, that seems to be **a strong indicator of elevated risk of catching the virus on a flight**.

Sure, flight attendants fly a lot more than we do, and by moving around during a flight, have a higher risk of catching the virus. We accept all those points, however, we'd ask the airline executives who say "there have been no proven examples of people catching the virus on a plane" to take back their statements.

4. There have been a number of studies, over the years, of the risk of catching an airborne infection on a plane. The conclusions have varied, but they all show there is some element of elevated risk, with the risk level dropping off rapidly with the distance between the infected person and other people on the flight. You're not likely to catch an infection from someone ten or twenty rows away from you. This 2018 study[494] concluded that the most significant increase in risk was associated with people one or two seats on either side, and one row ahead or behind. That could potentially be eight people. Other studies have shown a greater virus spread.

---

[493] See https://www.webmd.com/lung/news/20200410/100-american-flight-attendants-have-covid-19 or https://cov.cx/a1c78

[494] See http://news.emory.edu/stories/2018/03/airline_disease_transmission_study/ or https://cov.cx/a1c79

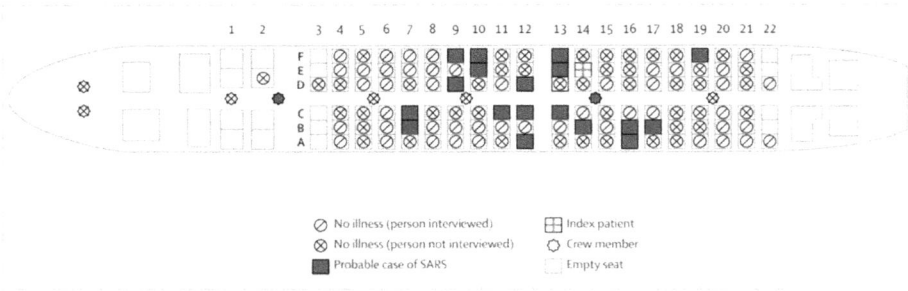

Figure 2: Schematic diagram of SARS outbreak aboard Hong Kong to Beijing flight

Figure 59 Spread of infections on a flight

The above image, taken from this study,[495] shows how one person infected 20 others with SARS during a relatively short three-hour flight from Hong Kong to Beijing. This was an outlier outcome, but just because it is rare does not mean it does not exist. It has been speculated that maybe there was an air circulation problem on that particular plane – perhaps there was. But that is not altogether reassuring – what is to say there mightn't be a similar problem on your next flight?

The major reason for citing this is to show a proven "worst-case" scenario to keep in mind when airline executives try and assure you there is no measurable risk at all.

The Risk of Flying Depends on Several Things

Not all flights have the same risk associated with them. There are some obvious and subtle considerations and factors. To start with, here are some obvious issues :

- ◆ Longer flights have slightly more risk than shorter flights.
- ◆ Crowded flights have more risk than less-full flights.
- ◆ Planes with adjustable overhead air vents (called "gaspers" in the trade) that you can angle to blow air on your face are safer than planes that don't have these.
- ◆ The airport is just as (or possibly even more) risky an environment as the airplane.

There's also a harder-to-quantify unknown factor. **Your fellow passengers** and the possibility you're seated close to someone with the Covid-19 infection at present. At one extreme, if you're flying on a domestic flight

---

[495] See https://www.ncbi.nlm.nih.gov/pmc/articles/PMC7134995/pdf/main.pdf or https://cov.cx/a1c80

between two cities in New Zealand, a country that went without new infections for 102 days before possibly having new infections originating from imported food items. Until that time, it seemed to have eliminated the virus presence entirely.[496] It requires international arriving visitors to quarantine for 14 days. In NZ, you're probably under very low threat from your fellow passengers. At the other extreme, if you're flying in Chile at present (a country with a very high rate/million (about 250) of new cases being reported every day at present), then you'd be understandably anxious as each additional person boarded the plane.

It becomes harder to guess the risk from other passengers when you're on an international flight, particularly to or from a hub, meaning there are lots of people from many different countries/cities funneling through the hub and your flight. This was vividly demonstrated when a Qatar Airways flight from Doha to Athens landed in Athens and 12 of its 91 passengers tested positive for the virus.[497] Note – these 12 people who tested positive are not people who contracted the virus during the flight – they are people who boarded the plane in Doha already with the virus. It is not yet known how many of the other 79 passengers will end up with the virus, too.

There are two other considerations as well. Your **own susceptibility to the virus** and risk level, plus **your tolerance for accepting risk**.

If you're in a higher risk category – older, overweight, diabetic, heart/lung problems – then you are more likely to get a viable infection from a smaller number of virus particles, and the infection is more likely to be severe rather than mild. There is a lot of difference between one chance in ten of getting an extremely mild infection that you don't even notice, and one chance in ten of getting a severe infection you will probably die from.

A younger person in good health living on their own can also decisions about the risks they accept, with little impact elsewhere, but if you are living with your parents and grandparents in a higher density home environment, you need to consider not just your personal risk but the risk of infecting others around you.

---

[496] It took NZ over a month, but in October they returned back to zero cases again, other than among arrivals from other countries during their period of mandatory, Army-supervised, quarantine, and occasionally a "leaked" case thought to be from a quarantined person to one of the people working in the quarantine facility.

[497] See https://airwaysmag.com/airports/breaking-greece-suspens-qatar-flights/ or https://cov.cx/a1c81

The Risk of Travel in General

It is important to understand that the risk of flying is only one part of a broader picture – the risk of an overall travel experience.

When you travel, you unavoidably tend to find yourself needing to accept less social distancing and greater risks – on all forms of transport, not just planes, when checking in and out of hotels, eating meals, attending functions or meetings, or visiting leisure attractions.

To be clear, there are risks on trains and long-distance buses as well, although the risk on trains is probably lower due to them typically having a lower density of passengers on board.

Perhaps the riskiest type of travel of all is on local public transport within your city, particularly during rush-hour when many people are squeezed tightly into buses and subway/metro carriages. The only modest saving grace is that such journeys are sometimes short, and with buses in particular, there's a lot of fresh air with the bus starting and stopping, opening its doors at each stop along the way. That is very different in a subway/underground transportation system – you're in an enclosed environment from when you first go down to a station until when you finally emerge out again at your destination, and even though the metro train might be making frequent stops, it is merely exchanging the stale and possibly dangerous air in the carriage for more stale and possible dangerous air at each station.

Avoiding peak public transport experiences is definitely beneficial if at all possible.

You need to consider all these different risk factors, and the level of virus activity in the places you're visiting – and recheck virus activity numbers immediately before travel because numbers can suddenly start climbing with no warning.

The Riskiest Time on Your Flight

When the plane is calmly cruising along for however much time it takes, things are fairly stable in the plane, and there are nice protective airflows going from the cabin ceiling to the cabin floor, helping to minimize virus transmission. Plus you've hopefully cleaned your immediate touch surfaces and environment. This is a relatively low-risk time.

Risks increase when people walk past your seat, especially if you have an aisle seat, and when flight attendants do their food and drink services.

The riskiest time of all is during the boarding and disembarking, before and after the flight. There are two reasons for this. The first is that the cabin airflow changes. Instead of a nice controlled environment with relatively high rates of directed airflow, the airflow rates massively reduce (you've probably noticed how, on almost every flight, shortly after engine start the air flows out of the "gasper" vents suddenly increases). Making this worse is the second reason – you've people moving around everywhere, messing up the airflow further, and, quite literally, "getting in your face".

Board your flight as late as possible. Remember, while you are not supposed to board before your boarding group/row number is called, you don't have to board at the time your row is called. Wait until pretty much everyone is on board, and the gate staff are starting to say things like "this is a final call for anyone on flight —".

As for getting off the plane, if you're near the back of the plane, and especially if you're not in an aisle seat, we suggest you wait, seated, until the plane has largely emptied, then get up and leave. If you're near the front get off the plane as quickly as you can.

Don't Rely on the Airline to Help You

We read about airlines providing wipes and masks and perhaps other sanitary materials to their passengers. But we also see, in the tiny print, "while supplies last" and other disclaimers. For example "Guests are provided with a complimentary sanitizing wipe while supplies last" quoted in this article.[498]

So bring plenty of your own products with you. The TSA is now allowing people to have up to 12 ounces of sanitizer with them when going through security. There's no need to have a full 12-ounce bottle, but certainly have more than a tiny travel-sized one or two ounce bottle.

We also suggest you have a few spare disposable masks with you in case you encounter nearby passengers without masks (or, if you feel able to do so, to encourage passengers with inefficient masks to change to better masks), and to replace yours as needed.

We see a lot of people with some type of wipes, using them to clean surfaces. But we never really know exactly what type of wipes they are, or how well they might work. We've seen "anti-bacterial" wipes being used, but remember, Covid-19 is a virus, not a bacteria. What might be effective for controlling bacteria might not be effective for controlling viruses.

Our simple approach is to use hand sanitizer for everything. It seems to be more readily available again and more reasonably priced[499]. Simply slather

[498] See https://www.staradvertiser.com/2020/06/02/hawaii-news/hawaiian-airlines-adopts-virus-stopping-policies/ or https://cov.cx/a1c82

[499] See https://amzn.to/2XvHtRe or https://cov.cx/a1c83

hand sanitizer on all touch surfaces – you don't even need a cloth or tissue. Just squirt some onto your hand or the surface, and use your hand to wipe it over. Use a regular tissue if you wish.

Very important – do not wipe the sanitizer off. Depending on the alcohol concentration, the temperature, and the surface, it seems that generally, the sanitizer needs 30 – 60 seconds of contact to kill any virus particles. It is easiest and best to just leave the surface wet and allow it to slowly evaporate. The longer the surface has sanitizer on it, the more time for the sanitizer to kill the virus.

Using hand sanitizer also has the benefit of reducing the number of different cleaning products you need to travel with.

20 (!) Steps to Minimize Your Risk While Flying

Here are 20 things you can do to maximize your chance of stepping off a flight as healthy as when you arrived at the airport earlier in the day.

1.   Drive yourself to the airport, or have a family member living with you take you there. Buses seem to be a high-risk environment, and any other sort of public/shared with unknown others transport is similarly much riskier than using your own safe vehicle.

2.   Wear a mask from before entering the terminal building until back in a safe environment (whatever that might be – keep your mask on until outside the terminal) after arrival.

3.   Arrive as late as prudent to the airport terminal, do not do any shopping or eating/drinking, and keep as far away from other people as possible.

Try to do all parts of the check-in process electronically rather than interacting with people, and use the electronic boarding pass app on your phone rather than printing out a boarding pass.

We'd recommend using the toilet facilities at the airport so as not to need to move about the airplane cabin if your flight is going to be sufficiently short. But don't linger. Public toilets are probably the highest risk area of an airport (or plane), not just from contact surfaces but from "viral plumes" possibly emerging from toilets when flushed.

When going to your gate, it is better to keep your distance from all your fellow passengers – as long as you can hear the boarding announcements and see what is happening, that is fine. You can probably do that from an adjacent empty gate, or the other side of the corridor.

4.   Upgrade from Coach Class if you can afford it, or if you have frequent flier miles. The lower seat density and passenger numbers in Premium

Economy, Business, or First Class mean lower risk and better social distancing.

In a premium cabin, try to be at the opposite end of the cabin to where the toilets are. For example, in First Class, if the toilets are at the front of the cabin, try to get a seat near the back.

5. If you're in Coach class, pay extra for a seat as close as possible to the front of the plane. This means you'll have less distance to travel on the plane to and from your seat. More than that, it means you'll be one of the first people to leave the plane upon arrival.

Alternatively, take a seat in the very back of the plane (unless there are toilets next to or behind you). The very back of the plane can be a "refuge" with little traffic, but of course, if there are toilets in the back, you'll have a steady stream of people moving past you all flight long.

I have a vague sense that the airflow in a plane, while predominantly from ceiling to floor, also might be from the back of the cabin to the front. This article[500] suggests there is some airflow from the rear to the front of an airplane cabin, and I know from personal experience that usually the temperatures at the rear of a plane are cooler than at the front, which might imply the air being introduced, cool, at the rear, and warming up as it moves forward and is heated by all the bodies it passes.[501]

The SARS study (see Figure 59 Spread of infections on a flight) also shows a clear skew of infections to people ahead of rather than behind the unwell passenger, which might point to air flowing from the rear to the front as well as from top to bottom.

If this is so, then **sitting in the very back of the plane might be the safest place** – as long as you're not next to toilets. It is also usually the least comfortable, though – my sense is the plane moves about a lot more at the rear, which is logical if you consider the wings as the "pivot" on which the plane moves. Even if not the wings, an airplane's center of gravity is close to the wings.

If the very first row of Coach Class is a bulkhead row, and if there are toilets nearby, it might be preferable to sit one row back from the bulkhead. Passengers sometimes spill into the bulkhead area a bit while waiting for their toilet turn. In theory, airlines are seeking to limit the

---

[500] See https://www.travelandleisure.com/airlines-airports/how-airplane-cabin-air-works or https://cov.cx/a1c84

[501] The average human radiates 100 – 120 watts of heat while sitting at rest. So every ten people are giving off as much heat as a one-bar electric heater.

number of people now standing around waiting for toilets, but what the reality of this will be is probably very variable.

6. Break the habit of a lifetime and be the last to board the plane rather than the first (unless you have priority boarding and truly will be one of the first, and are seated at the very rear of the plane). The time of greatest risk is during the boarding and deplaning process. Get on last and you'll avoid most of that risk.

7. If you're in Coach Class and it is a relatively short flight such that you probably won't need to use the bathroom during the flight, take a window seat. That gives you one relatively safe side, and also more protection from the uncontrolled environment in the aisle and the air currents caused by people moving up and down the aisle.

8. Once on board, get anything you might need out of your carry-on then stow the carry-on and try to leave it for the rest of the flight.

9. As soon as you arrive, clean your seat area and touch surfaces. We're not too worried about the seat surfaces, but the armrests, the tray table, the seat belt, and the air vent above you are all surfaces you are likely to be touching. If there's a seat-back video screen, and you plan to use it, be sure to wipe that down too. Use hand sanitizer (and tissues if needed) to wet all surfaces, and let them air dry – the longer the sanitizer stays on the surfaces, the more time it has to kill more virus particles.

10. Adjust the overhead air vent to blow air directly on your face. You may need to adjust the flow rate after the plane has started up and the pilots turn on the main cabin airflow.

   This means you're getting a steady stream of direct-from-the-filters-or-outside air blowing onto your face, and pushing the existing air around you away. It is thought – and intuitively it seems to make sense – this might blow away any viral particles that otherwise could end up in your face and being breathed in.

   We'd suggest you don't set the flow to maximum. If you do that, and if some virus particles end up getting "sucked" into the stream of air flowing at you, the force of the air makes it more likely the viral particles will enter your mouth or nose and travel on down to your lungs. A gentle breeze should be sufficient.

11. After you've cleaned your area, clean your hands.

At this point, you've optimized your environment and yourself, and there's little more you can do. Here are a few pointers for while you are in-flight, however :

12.   Do not speak to the passengers close to you (unless they are traveling with you). There is no risk in you speaking to them, but when they speak to you they will be looking at you and projecting virus particles directly at you.

13.   One exception to the "don't speak to the person next to you" suggestion. If you see they don't have a mask, cough a bit, then say to them "I'm sorry, I've a bit of a cough, I'm wearing a mask and I have some spares – can I give you one just to be certain I won't give you whatever it is I might have". [Update – in theory, all US airlines are now mandating mask-wearing. You can be more assertive and if necessary, complain to a flight attendant or at least ask to be moved. We'd also consider some sort of "intervention" if you see your adjacent fellow passengers have poorly designed masks – especially ones with vents or which barely cover the nose. You could now say "I'm sorry, I'm worried I might infect you because I see your mask isn't covering your nose fully", for example.]

       This is a much less confrontational way of handling the situation – of course, your main concern is they wear a mask to protect you, and the cough is merely an artifice to help encourage them to accept your offer of a mask.

14.   Unless the flight is "too long" try not to accept any food or drink from the flight attendants. It is best not to eat or drink at all, but if you must, it is better to eat your own food and drink your own water because you know its source, so if possible, bring your food and drink with you.

       Drinks in sealed bottles from the flight attendants are probably okay, and sealed food containers are okay too, although if it is a cold item like a sandwich, you have no way of knowing how sanitary the process and environment was when it was made.

       If you are going to eat, we recommend you use hand sanitizer again before eating. It is a good habit to get into – always wash your hand/use hand sanitizer before any eating, whether you "need to" or not (because, especially at present, you always need to).

15.   Don't handle any of the material that is in the seat-back pouch in front of you.

16.   Again, unless the flight is "too long", stay in your seat for the entire flight. Don't go to the toilet unless you must.

       If you need to use the toilet, there's no need to contort your body and do strange things to avoid touching surfaces in the toilet. Simply be sure to thoroughly hand sanitize after leaving the toilet and before returning to your seat, and then again once you are seated.

17.   If you're on a longer flight, the lack of humidity can have an impact. Consider having a small little misting/squirt bottle that you can use to create a very fine spray of water that you can breathe in through your nose and mouth occasionally. This helps keep your mucous membranes moist and therefore better able to trap viral particles before they go down to your lungs.

Once the plane lands :

18.   If you're near the front of the plane, get off the plane as quickly as you can. If you're near the back of the plane, wait in your seat until most other people have left the plane.
19.   Move efficiently through the airport, without doing any non-essential shopping, and leave it as soon as possible.
20.   Drive yourself from the airport to your final destination (rental car or your car) or have a family member you live with collect you.

Gloves, Goggles and Protective Clothing as well as Masks?

We occasionally see people who have taken a much more serious approach to keeping themselves safe from any possible virus infection.

There are two common extra steps that some people take. Gloves and goggles or a face shield.

We don't generally see any benefit in gloves whatsoever when it comes to protecting yourself from catching the Covid-19 infection. The virus is not thought to be able to seep in through your skin, or through any cuts/abrasions on your skin, so from that perspective, gloves add no extra value.

If you wear gloves, all you do is replace the ability of the virus to get onto your hand, and then be directly transferred from your hand to your mouth/nose/eyes, and instead, the virus can get onto the glove, and then transfer just as easily (maybe even more easily) from the glove to your mouth/nose/eyes, the same as before.

Gloves quickly get as dirty as your skin would. It is easier to not bother about gloves, and any time you're worried about touching an unclean surface, simply reach for the hand sanitizer.

On the other hand, goggles or a face shield might be helpful, because it seems the virus can enter your system via your eyes. The risk of this is low if you're in a risky environment for a short while, but if you're on a plane for half a dozen hours, then you've had a steady stream of air flowing onto your eyes, some of which may contain virus particles.

A pair of safety glasses might be a positive addition – they can deflect a stream of viral particles away from your eyes. The larger the safety glasses, the better. It is possible to wear some types of safety glasses and not have them look too unusual. Even a pair of large-framed sunglasses would be a help.

Goggles can also help because they make it harder for you to instinctively reach up and rub your eyes with your hands.

A pair of goggles can reduce your eyes' exposure to whatever is floating in the air around them, and especially on longer flights, this might become of value, although they are more "distinctive" and you might feel self-conscious wearing them.

A face shield seems to be about the same as glasses or goggles. If you prefer a shield to glasses/goggles, then there is no harm in choosing a shield instead of glasses/goggles, but probably no measurable benefit.

One point we must stress, though – neither a face shield, nor glasses, nor goggles, is a substitute for a mask. You should still wear a mask as well.

As for protective clothing, we don't think that necessary. It seems there is a reduced concern about catching an infection from touching something.

Summary

For sure, you've more chance of getting the virus on a flight than you do staying at home. But equally for sure, currently we've about 850,000 people flying every day in the US, and, as best we know, more than 99% of those fliers don't catch the virus.

So is your risk 1 in 100, or 1 in 1,000, or even 1 in 100,000 that you'll catch the virus if you fly somewhere? That depends on very many things, and – most of all – it depends on you and how careful you are to minimize the risks while traveling.

We're trying to avoid air travel whenever possible at present, but if it becomes necessary, we're reasonably confident we can fly without problems. If you follow our recommended strategies, you're most likely to complete your flights without any problems, too.

13. Avoiding Infection in Hotels, etc

Note – this is the last of four chapters on how to avoid or minimize your risk of catching the virus. We decided to split the topic into four helpful pieces, but we urge you to read all four chapters as an entirety, because elements of each chapter and the recommendations within it apply to the other three chapters, too.

You might think there is not a lot you can control when you're in a hotel, motel, or other type of accommodation, and in large part that is true.

However, that's no reason not to focus on the things you can optimize and control, but all the more reason to do so. Happily, you have one very important control point right from the start - you can choose the hotel you stay at. This can potentially make a huge difference to the risk you experience when overnighting away from home.

Choosing a Hotel

The very first thing to do when considering where you'll stay while traveling is to look at pictures of possible hotels/motels/etc. We suggest you give a strong priority to properties with external entrances to the rooms – the typical "old-fashioned" style motel type of building with external open to the element corridors and doors from the rooms that open directly to the outside, rather than to an enclosed internal corridor.

As we go on to discuss in other parts of this chapter, that not only makes it safer when getting to and from your room, it also probably helps greatly in terms of ensuring the air that comes into your room is fresh from outside rather than potentially contaminated and recycled air from inside the building.

We suggest, after provisionally selecting a hotel but before you book a stay, you telephone their front desk[502] and "interview" them to find out their current approach to minimizing virus risk for their guests.

Make your call a "neutral" call and don't disclose the types of answers you are expecting. That is more likely to elicit thoughtful and truthful answers.

You could ask questions such as "What is your face mask policy" – a nice open-ended neutral question that doesn't hint as to if you're hoping for a positive or negative answer; and then follow up with "So do you require guests to wear face masks when checking in and when going to and from their room" and "Do all your staff wear face masks all the time" and "What would you do if someone reported a guest – maybe even me – or staff member, to you who was not wearing a mask?".

You could also ask "When I check-in, will you be able to see when my room was last occupied and help me to select a room that has been vacant for several days", and of course, ask any other questions that might be of concern to you, maybe "How many people do you allow in an elevator at one time?".

You should also enquire about any new checking in and out procedures to minimize your time at the front desk. Hopefully they have express check-out already, maybe they have some new form of express check-in too.[503] If the property has your credit card on file, the only issue should be how you pick up your room key. Nothing else needs to involve in-person interaction – this is now termed "contactless checking in".

We don't suggest you necessarily ask technical questions about their a/c setup, because it is unlikely the person on the front desk will know the answers to such questions, and they're likely to give you incorrect answers as a result.

---

[502] Don't call the (800) reservations number, but the hotel's direct number, and when the phone is answered, make sure you are speaking to someone actually physically at the hotel, rather than in a central call center somewhere else.

[503] One of my pet peeves is being required to provide name/address/phone numbers/email/credit card number when booking a hotel, and then find, upon arriving at the home, that I have to write it all down again onto a reservation card that the computer has printed out, but only with my name at the top, none of the other details. Oh, and if you do have to do that, be sure to use your pen, not their pen, to ensure that there's no risk of catching the virus from a much-used pen!

One point about all of this. Don't think you're an outlier with your concerns. A mid-August survey conducted by the American Hotel & Lodging Association shows that most guests want face masks required, don't want daily room service, and want social distancing.[504]

Not only that, these measures are all being advocated/promoted by AHLA to their members.[505]

Once you've chosen your hotel, there are several aspects of your hotel stay to optimize.

Room Airflow

The first thing to consider is your room's airflow. The thing you most want to avoid is a hotel that has a central air system, such that air is pumped into your room via ducting from a central heating/cooling service somewhere.

If your air is coming from somewhere else, you get to share in everything and everywhere else in the hotel that is using the same common air system. An infected person three floors away could have their virus aerosol particles sucked into the central air system and then blown into your room.

While a hotel might claim to have air filters to protect against such things happening, we would view such claims extremely skeptically. Unless the hotel staff can advise the filter rating (see our discussion on MERV filter ratings in the section about "The Quarantine Period" on page 208), the frequency of filter changes, and the date of the last change, I'd totally not trust their claim of having adequate filtering, and – call me cynical but – I'd be hesitant to trust any other assurances they offered about adequate filter changing policies, too.

Shared air systems might have some sort of air outlet somewhere in a wall or more likely ceiling, and possibly have a return inlet for air to be taken back to the central unit, somewhere else. A temperature control/thermostat opens some louvers somewhere to allow for more or less airflow.

Our perception is that most hotels do not have common shared air systems in the rooms – they are more often found in office buildings and possibly in hotel

---

[504] See https://www.ahla.com/sites/default/files/Survey_Frequent%20Travelers%20View%20on%20Hotel%20Cleaning%20and%20Safety%20Initiatives.pdf or https://cov.cx/a1c85

[505] See https://www.ahla.com/sites/default/files/safestayguidelinesv3_081420_0.pdf or https://cov.cx/a1c86

public areas, than in hotel bedrooms.[506]   It is more likely that a hotel has a central air conditioning system that pipes either hot or cold water from the central system to heat exchangers in each room, or possibly "in-window" or "in-wall" or individual "split unit" a/c units for each room.   Lower quality accommodation might not have a/c of any sort, and just have in-room heating units.[507]

Piped systems are usually described as either two-pipe or three-pipe (although it is unlikely the staff at reception will be familiar with these terms). A two-pipe system can either have hot or cold water going through the pipes (one pipe to bring the hot or cold water into your room, the second pipe to take the water out again after going through your heat exchanger), but it can't have both. So the entire hotel is either set to heating or cooling – I know that many times I've asked a hotel if I could cool my room, but have been told the entire hotel is set to heating,[508] and all I can do is turn the air off and maybe – hopefully – open a window.

---

[506] There are two main reasons hotels don't commonly use these types of ducted air distribution systems. The first is noise – the systems provide an easy route for noise from one room to impact on others nearby. The second is security – while not all ducted systems feature the large size rectangular ducting that people crawl through in action movies, some do and that is obviously not acceptable from a security point of view.

On the other hand, we were astonished to visit a 1960s vintage and low-quality motel in rural Montana, recently, that did have a central air system. So you can't take anything for granted!

[507] The nice thing about in-room heating units is that you know for sure you're not getting air from somewhere else, and you are free to then plan your airflow strategy more or less separate from your heating strategy.

[508] Actually, although sometimes I've been directly told that, but more often I've been outright lied to by staff who don't want to get in an argument about why they can't provide cooled air to my room, or who simply don't understand how their system works.

I'm the type of guy who travels with a temperature probe so when I'm told "just give it half an hour to equalize the temperature in your room, it takes time" I can reply "how can it equalize the temperature down to the level I'm asking for if the air that's coming out of the register is hotter than that at present?". It also gives one credibility when an engineer reluctantly appears in your room to wave your own temperature probe around and means you're more likely to hear the truth rather than more lies designed to shut you up and delay the ultimate argument until after the person in question has gone off shift.

A three-pipe system has two pipes into your room – one with hot water and one with cold – and one pipe out with whichever water went through your heat exchanger.[509]

In the case of these types of systems, there is typically a heat exchanger unit in the ceiling with an intake somewhere close to the door you enter the room, and an outtake directing the treated air into the main part of the room. The ceiling is often lower in that area to provide space for the heat exchanger.

The thermostat/control unit adjusts the water flow that either heats or cools the air and also adjusts the speed of a fan to circulate the air in your room.

These systems are okay, because you are recirculating your own air, rather than getting air from somewhere/someone else.

In-wall or in-window units (ie units that go through the wall or window) are often found in older type hotel rooms – I've memories of them in many a Holiday Inn, decades ago. Often they seem to have a noisy compressor with worn bearings and need to have their heat exchanger cleaned so it will work efficiently. They are simultaneously taking your room air and passing it through your side of the unit, while independently taking outside air and passing it through the other side of the unit, transferring the heat either into or out of the room in the process. Outside air may or may not be mixed in with the inside air being sucked in and blown out of your unit. Some units have a setting where you can choose between outside or inside air coming in.

If you have the choice, and assuming the temperature of the outside air isn't too extreme to make it difficult for the unit to keep the temperature in the range you want, you should usually set it for outside air to be admitted, assuming you feel that the outside air is likely to be safer than inside air, such as may come in from the corridor outside your room.

Split systems have a heat exchanger somewhere outside, then pipes transferring the heat or cold from the outside unit to the exchanger somewhere in your unit. There is no outside air that is brought in, you're just recirculating the air in your room. These are more modern and usually much quieter than the in-wall or in-window units of yesteryear.

---

[509] There are also four-pipe systems, with two completely independent water flows rather than a shared return water feed. These are more efficient than three pipe systems, but also more costly. For our purposes, the distinction is of course meaningless – the only thing that matters is that "your" air comes from your room and stays in your room.

Opening Windows

We also like to have a room with a window that can open to the outside, so some fresh air can be brought into the room. These are common in smaller hotels, but less common in large new hotels.

Totally sealed windows, from a hotel perspective, are usually cheaper and safer.[510] The last thing a hotel wants is for their guests to be "wasting" heating/cooling energy by opening a window direct to the outside air, and a solid slab of glass without any opening fittings is cheaper than a window that can partially or fully open.

You might wonder "How do I get fresh air and not suffocate if the windows don't open". There are several answers to that question,[511] ranging from "Well, actually, you can't" to "It's complicated".[512]

The simple answer is that fresher air comes into the room variously when you open the door, and through leaks and pressure differentials, clearly in sufficient quantities that you're not going to die from lack of oxygen.[513] Air might come in from the external walls of your room or from the building interior.

The following image is an interesting depiction of the three different factors that typically impact on air flows in a multi-story sealed hotel, using sample values for the model result displayed.[514]

---

[510] Apparently it really is a known "thing" that needs preventing - people will book a night in a hotel with a view to jumping out the window to commit suicide. Some hotels with windows that can open, but with stops/locks on them to prevent opening more than an inch or two, will agree to remove the stop/lock but only if you sign a form first promising to be careful and not jump/fall out the window.

[511] The "collective wisdom" of the internet is particularly disappointing on this issue. In researching this topic, we were appalled at how much nonsense was being offered as fact in authoritative seeming articles.

[512] Here's a great article looking at one element of sealed-window type hotels and their air flows https://www.energyvanguard.com/blog/adventures-in-hotel-bathroom-ventilation or https://cov.cx/a1c87

[513] In actual fact (in case you wondered) the big problem in sealed rooms is typically not too little oxygen but too much CO_2. Too much CO_2 will give you headaches and make you drowsy/inattentive long before the oxygen concentration drops to a dangerous level.

[514] Image from this excellent presentation https://www.buildingscience.com/sites/default/files/01.03_2015-08-03_ventilation_multifamily_ricketts.pdf or https://cov.cx/a1c88

Stack Effect, Wind, and Mechanical Ventilation

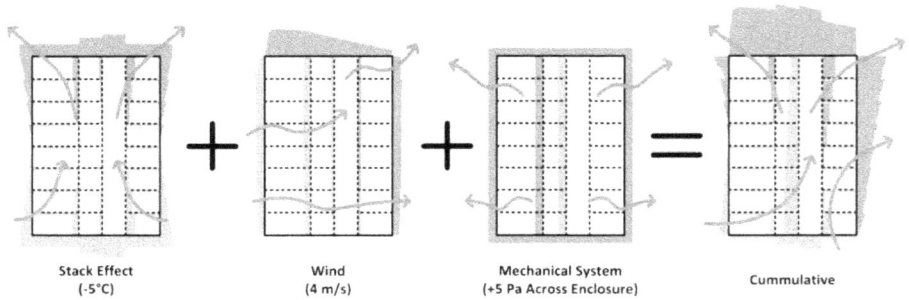

Stack Effect   Wind   Mechanical System   Cummulative
(-5°C)   (4 m/s)   (+5 Pa Across Enclosure)

Figure 60 Different forces influencing sealed hotel air flows

Our take on the above diagram is that it is preferable to be in a lower level room where at least you have the stack effect meaning that fresh air is more likely to be coming into your room from outside, rather than in an upper-level room where it is more probable that stale air from the rest of the hotel will be entering your room and then exiting through leaks around the sealed windows and external wall in general.

Unfortunately, other air quality issues complicate the matter.[515] Probably my choice would be to compromise and choose a room on a low but not ground floor.

Overall, it seems fair to say that many sealed hotel rooms have poor quality air that is insufficiently exchanged with truly fresh and truly clean air. Dust and CO_2 levels might be high but oxygen and humidity levels might be low.

Air quality in hotel rooms is an overlooked issue that deserves more attention all the time, not just during Covid-19 times.

Back to the windows, again. If you have windows that can open, that is potentially good, but not invariably.

The key issue is to understand the direction of airflow when you open your window. Is fresh air flowing in through the window, or is dirty air being taken out? In particular, if air is leaving your room, that means you are drawing air into your room, not from the outdoors, but (depending on room design) from the corridor that you came into the room from. That is less desirable, especially if it is an internal closed corridor rather than an external corridor, open to the outside

---

[515] Ibid, although this depends on the form of overall ventilation.

air. The diagram and our comments, immediately above, apply with only slightly less force if the windows are openable.

A second issue is - if you do have a window, is it likely to give you fresh air, or are you in a huge high-rise hotel with windows of other rooms everywhere above, below, and alongside your window? In that case, maybe you are having air from other rooms simply coming back into your room. Some people know this from their experience living in apartments – they open an outside window but instead of getting fresh air, they get the cooking smells and smoke from other adjacent apartments.

The best room of all has windows on two opposite sides, so you can have a draft of fresh air coming in one side and going out the other. That's rare in a regular hotel room, although sometimes you can get that with corner rooms or suites that have windows on two sides.

If you can't open any windows, you might want to consider bringing a portable air purifier with you.[516] As best we can tell, purifiers that add "ions" to the air actually make no real difference at all to the air quality, and purifiers that add ozone are a bad choice, because ozone is poisonous, even in very low quantities. You simply want a unit that blows air through a HEPA type filter (and make sure you understand how often the filter needs changing and comply with that recommendation).[517]

There is one more strategy you can consider when it comes to managing your air flows. You can turn on the bathroom fan and leave it running, and thereby sucking some air out of the bathroom and hotel room in general. Although bathroom fans often provide only very little airflow, they at least provide some, and perhaps that might help to bring fresh air in from outside (assuming you've managed to open a window) and going through your room and then out through the bathroom fan.

Common Areas

This brings us to another major consideration when choosing accommodation. Avoiding shared "common areas". If you're in a traditional hotel, you have a reception area, elevators, and corridors that you have to pass

---

[516] There are plenty to choose from on Amazon - https://amzn.to/2EEisvY or https://cov.cx/a1c89

[517] One more point about a portable air filter. Keep it sealed inside a zip-lock bag or some other sort of reasonably air-tight container when traveling with it. The last thing you want is the bumps and vibrations of traveling to knock the dirt and virus particles off its air filter and into your suitcase, onto your clothes, etc.

through every time you go to and from your room. You know that sometimes there's little or no airflow in some of those areas because the air in them is often much hotter than in your room, stuffy, and smelly. Those are all areas that it would be great to avoid at present.

Social distancing in an elevator, in particular, is close to impossible (assuming the hotel doesn't have a "no more than two people in the elevator" rule at present, and further assuming the rule is observed), although happily you are not in them for long.

It might seem counter-intuitive but ask for a room as far from the elevators as possible.[518] The reason for this is the further from the elevators, the fewer the number of people walking past your room's door and possibly breathing out virus particles that might then be sucked under the door and into your room by air flows.

Talking about elevators, if you're not too far up, consider at the very least walking down the stairs (particularly the emergency exit stairs if you have a choice between "official" internal stairs and the emergency exit stairs) rather than taking the elevator. Maybe even walk up the stairs to your room too on occasions when you're feeling particularly energetic.

If the hotel has both garage parking and outside parking, we'd probably choose the outside parking, especially if the "inside" parking is in a basement or a poorly vented building.

Your hotel might have all manner of enticing and appealing amenities and guest services/features, like a pool, a gym, a lounge, bar, and restaurant, a business center, and maybe other things as well. We'd recommend staying well clear of all such communal places at present.[519]

All these issues and considerations make the old-fashioned "external corridor" motel become more appealing. You can park your car close to the door to your unit, which you can walk directly to, or perhaps go up a flight of stairs and then walk to, and probably, the walkway is open-sided to the outdoor elements, assuring you of fresh air.

---

[518] Many people do this anyway, because such rooms are quieter, for the same reason – fewer people walking to/from their rooms and outside the door.

[519] As a related comment, if you're staying in a dishonest hotel that charges a dastardly Amenities or Resort Fee of some sort or another, and if the hotel has also closed its gym and/or pool, ask for that fee to be adjusted. The fee of course is nothing other than another way of charging you money, but play their own game back at them – "You are charging me $25/day for using your pool and gym, and both are closed at present, so you should cancel your fee".

The best possible solution is a separate free-standing cabin, of course, giving you maximum separation from other guests.

Often a motel unit will have openable windows on two sides, making it easier to get a fresh airflow through your room. Free-standing cabins might have windows on even more sides, and much less chance of contaminated air from an immediately adjacent cabin coming back into your cabin.

Apart from checking in and out, your entire stay can (and should) be conducted without needing to enter any enclosed areas or get close to anyone else.

As for checking in and out of a motel, that might be simultaneously less sophisticated but more flexible than in a larger hotel. Phone in advance and ask them how this can be arranged, and if they don't already have a good system, suggest you simply phone them from your car upon arrival and they bring the key out to your car for you.[520]

This gives you the best possible control over your environment while staying there.

There might be another benefit – and also cautionary note – to staying in a motel room. If the room has some cooking facilities – a fridge and microwave, possibly other cooking equipment too – then you can avoid the risk of eating in a hotel restaurant.

If there are cooking facilities, it might be prudent to disinfect them before using them – especially cutlery and crockery.[521] The pots and pans probably get hot enough while cooking food to kill any virus particles, but the plates, glasses, knives, and forks probably do not.

Is the Room Safe or Contaminated

There is one other consideration, too. And that is the biosafety of your room when you first get there, and maintaining it throughout your stay. Depending on your risk tolerance, you might content yourself with merely saying "there's very little chance of infection via an exposed surface/fomite, and any risks have been

---

[520] This can be offered on the basis of "It is safer for you as well as me".

[521] Keep in mind that disinfectant is a powerful poison. After disinfecting the cutlery and crockery, you then need to rinse the disinfectant off before using them.

Note also that with diminishing focus on surfaces as potential pathways for the virus to spread, this is optional, although if you had to choose one thing in particular to disinfect, we'd suggest cutlery that might be "fresh from their mouth to your mouth", then glassware second, then crockery third.

countered by the hotel's cleaning policies" or you might take a more proactive stance to this issue.[522]

If you wanted to be more proactive, we'd suggest bringing disinfectant with you, and spraying down the surfaces you're likely to come in contact with.

These surfaces also include the bedding. That might be the most significant risk of all. Imagine the guest before you, spending all night coughing and breathing into a pillow. Then the housemaid changes the pillowcase but leaves the pillow untouched. How safe is the pillow within the fresh pillowcase?[523]

I don't know the answer to that, but you might want to consider spray disinfecting the pillow as well as the pillowcase, and/or possibly traveling with your own pillow. You can get small-sized "travel pillows" that take up less space in a suitcase than a full-size pillow.[524]

If you wanted to go still further, perhaps you could consider spray disinfecting the top half of the top and bottom sheets/blankets/duvet on the bed – the parts that come in contact with your hands and face. We'd pull back the top sheet and covers and have them on the bottom half of the bed, then spray the top half of the bottom sheet and the top half of the bottom sheet accordingly. No need to soak the sheets in disinfectant, but applying a mist of spray will help shift the odds of avoiding the virus in your favor.

If you are certain the sheets are fresh/new, rather than just smoothed out and re-used, you could skip this step, or alternatively, replace it with a spray of the top of the mattress or mattress cover (whatever is immediately underneath the bottom sheet) and a spray of the blankets or the actual duvet filling inside the duvet cover.

---

[522] Can you really trust the same housemaids who are regularly observed and shown in YouTube videos from hidden cameras to clean drinking glasses with a cloth that they've just used to wipe the toilet with, to now do a better job of truly disinfecting and ensuring the hygiene of all the various surfaces in your room?

[523] That is also making an assumption that the pillowcase is changed. Probably it is, but for sure, not every hotel and housemaid changes every pillowcase after every stay.

[524] Amazon of course has plenty, but be sure to get a travel pillow for sleeping on a bed with, rather than a neck pillow for while you're in an airline seat! See https://amzn.to/34CF3UL or https://cov.cx/a1c90 We'd also suggest you try the travel pillow at home first, to make sure it is acceptably comfortable. Even two travel pillows are smaller (for travel purposes) than one single hotel pillow and might make a lot of difference to your sleeping comfort.

If you're in a hotel with many other decorative pillows, put them all in a corner of the wardrobe or somewhere and don't touch them for the duration of your stay.

One more point. If the bed has a bedspread, as it probably does, be careful how you move that. You don't want to shake a bunch of virus particles loose off the covers and throw them up into the air, where they might hang, suspended in the air like dust particles do, and wait for you to breathe them in. Fold the covers gently in on themselves, then move them to a corner of the room and carefully place them on the ground, and wear a mask during the process.

Towels are probably okay. They are almost surely fresh from the laundry and haven't been used by a prior guest after being laundered.

We're not sure about the status of bathrobes/dressing gowns if they are provided. In theory, you'd expect them to be freshly laundered; in practice, who only knows.

If you are spray disinfecting items, you should wear a mask while doing so then leave the room for a while to let the spray settle out of the air and dry. Wear the mask before moving sheets and bedding around, because the act of doing so could dislodge virus particles and get them back up into the air again. In addition, it is not good to breathe too much of the stronger disinfectants.

There's one other thought. When checking in, you should ask the front desk person helping you "Was there anyone in my room last night?". Most systems will allow the hotel to see the history of who was in the room in the past, and they should be able to tell you when it was last in use. The longer the period the room was vacant, the less you need to worry about these things, because any virus contamination will have naturally died out during the intervening time. Indeed, when checking in, see if it is possible to have a room that hasn't been slept in for the last three or four nights – many hotels have very low occupancies at present so this might be possible. The longer it has been empty, the less chance of any remaining viable virus particles.[525]

---

[525] I'd suggested, earlier, asking if this would be possible when you do your prior-to-booking phone "interview". If someone hopefully offers to make a note in your reservation of that request, I suggest you thank them, and ask what sort of occupancy level the hotel is expecting in the nights prior to your arrival. If it is under 90% and you're just asking for any regular/standard room, there's little to be gained by accepting this offer, because the reality is that room assignments are usually done by computer and there's no easy way, short of actually blocking the room off for the previous night, to ensure a room remains empty.

Certainly, don't rely on any such "notes on your reservation", which in my experience are often never looked at, or, if they are looked at, seem to be ignored. Ask as if you're asking for the first time when checking in.

There's an important related issue. Once you've gone to all the trouble to make your room safe, you now want to keep it safe if you're staying more than one night. We'd recommend not allowing the housemaids into the room during your stay.

Tell the front desk you don't want daily servicings, and hang a "Do Not Disturb" sign on your door. If you're obsessive about this, also carry a sign that says in big bold colored letters "Do not service my room" and leave it on your bed (yes, sometimes housemaids ignore the "Do Not Disturb" signs, especially if they know you are not in the room – they just think you forgot to take the sign off or consider there's no way they'll disturb you if you're not there).

Try to go without fresh towels, although they are probably low risk to exchange.

Things to Bring With You

If you want to understand and optimize your room environment as much as possible when traveling, you might want to think about bringing some items with you :

* An accurate hygrometer (ie ideally one that is accurate to about +/- 3%) to understand the humidity in your room – see https://amzn.to/2YyqkGA or https://cov.cx/a1g14
* A small portable humidifier if you might need to increase the room humidity (especially in the winter) – see https://amzn.to/3hyO6cT or https://cov.cx/a1g15
* Disinfectant and a spray bottle to apply it with – see our discussion in the chapter "17. Medical Equipment & Supplies You Should Have", starting on page 398
* Travel Pillow, as mentioned above, see https://amzn.to/34CF3UL or https://cov.cx/a1g16
* A portable air purifier – see https://amzn.to/2EEisvY or https://cov.cx/a1g17

PART FOUR : Treating the Virus

14. Include Your Doctor in Your Decision-Making

While I want to give you the information you need to intelligently participate in how you adjust your life to minimize the risk of getting a Covid-19 infection, and the information you need to similarly participate in any healthcare treatment decisions should you become infected, it is not my suggestion that this book replaces the need for normal consultations with your normal physician.

This document could be used as a discussion point to go through with your present doctor. Of course, I don't know who your doctor is, and even more so, he doesn't know me, and I think you and I both have to feel less than certain that any doctor has the time to read through over 400 pages of information, especially when written by a non-medical-professional!

Like the rest of us, doctors tend to have their preferred sources of information and choose to discount information that appears elsewhere.

There are of course valid reasons for being selective in how and where a physician obtains his information. We discuss that in some detail, way back near the beginning, see our section "Why Are So Many Doctors So Risk-Averse?" on page 24.

There is a problem with being too risk-averse and cautious when it comes to the virus. Keep in mind this virus is killing people, almost literally every minute, as you read this. It is a "clear and present danger" that we don't have the luxury of responding to in a leisurely measured manner.

Remember, it is only in March that we in the US officially started to pay attention to this (although, as my newsletter readers know, my first mention and warning was much earlier).

What that means is that some medical publications are still digesting and considering and preparing material for publication, but new information is emerging on an almost daily basis. Most medical issues these days are only slowly evolving, but our knowledge of the virus is changing almost daily.

The resources your doctor uses are almost certainly not updating and publishing new data on an accelerated daily/weekly schedule.

I have tried to keep on top of the deluge of data about the virus – although, perhaps I've also contributed to it! I've written over 160 articles on the virus since I started counting in February. I've written close to half a million words on the topic, so farm as well as this book which is on the high side of 140,000 words.[526] A busy physician has no time to spend trying to keep on top of all of this (it truly takes me an hour or two, every day, seven days a week, just to keep abreast of the latest news and developments).[527] The chances are your doctor is already overloaded with direct patient workload – for example, how many minutes do you have to chat with him when you meet?

While your doctor may not admit this (you want a doctor who does!) he is probably far from an expert on the virus, and has chosen to glance at headlines of articles, read the summaries of articles from trusted sources, and seldom/never gone into an article's tables and appendices and footnotes, and reviewed the sources used and critiqued the methodologies. Most of all, he's

---

[526] I am *not* suggesting that simply reading and writing a lot makes me an expert on the virus! And also, reading this book now doesn't make you an expert, either. But I do suggest it makes you more informed than 99%+ of the rest of the community, so all is not lost.

[527] This is an important point, too. The truth changes regularly in terms of what are considered good and not so good treatments for the virus.

Think of hydroxychloroquine – it started off with a burst of positive publicity, then got sandbagged by negative reports, but since that time, albeit unreported by most mainstream media, there was been a steady drip-feed of new studies being released, almost all positive. But now there's an automatic turning away from any mention of HCQ by people who have closed their mind to the topic – they'll say something like "the three leading studies all showed it to have no benefit and was dangerous to patients' hearts" (even though the studies have subsequently been convincingly criticized and the heart danger was theoretical rather than real, and what about the 90+ studies subsequently that have been positive), and their automatic dismissal is not the correct thing to do.

probably never ventured into the shadowy fringes of mainstream medicine to hunt out the advance hints of promising new treatments.

For all the understandable reasons discussed earlier, there is a sometimes unfortunate propensity to approach new and novel approaches dismissively and negatively. It is regrettably true that "non-traditional" and "non-mainstream" medicine is too-often ridden with nonsense, but that doesn't mean everything that hasn't been hallowed by decades of tradition should be rejected. Indeed, every current medical practice had to evolve from something different previously. Every new treatment was once non-mainstream and non-traditional. It is essential to keep an open mind on alternate approaches.

I'm not saying I know more about the virus than your doctor, but I am saying there is a very uneven distribution of knowledge out there at present, and that much to do with the virus does not require half a dozen years of medical school to understand.[528]

A normal and mainstream approach to medicines is "Do we know this medicine will help and are we certain it will do no harm?". If there is not positive proof that the medicine will help, or if there is doubt about the medicine's safety in use, then of course, it is seldom prescribed.

But there is another less cautious approach that some people advocate, in some cases. It still asks the second question - "Could this particular drug do the patient harm?"; and, in the interests of further caution, "Would this particular drug interact with any other drugs the patient is taking or any other conditions the patient suffers?"

But it doesn't mandate a certain definite proven answer to the first question. Instead of demanding the highest standard of proof of benefit, a lower degree of confidence of possible benefit is accepted.

In the case of a nasty disease such as Covid-19, which threatens death or lasting disabilities to a significant proportion of everyone who suffers it, you might feel – as I do – that this second approach has a lot to recommend itself.

To put it in non-medical terms, if a drug will definitely not cause any harm, and maybe might slightly provide some benefit, isn't that sufficient justification to risk it? There's no downside (other than possible disappointment) and potentially, a lot of upside.

---

[528] Indeed, much of the research into the virus is more based on statistics and data analysis than on the actual medical treatments – when it comes to evaluating outcomes and determining their significance, the medical side of evaluating "did the patient live or not" and "how many days in hospital before discharge" is totally trivial, but the analytical side of "is this a significant or insignificant difference" is key.

This is at the heart of any discussion you need to have with your doctor, and with yourself. Where on this scale do you place yourself? Where does your doctor stand, and will he respect and honor your decisions and requests for your personal care regimen?

One of the adages and golden rules of the medical profession is "First, do no harm". So it is natural and normal for all doctors to view any type of medical intervention with caution and concern. But – here's the important thing :

"Do no harm" *is not the same as* **"do nothing"!**

Indeed, doing nothing obviously can be harmful. All infections are easiest to treat and clear when the intervention is early rather than delayed.[529] The current official US approach of doing nothing when people are first discovered with an infection and waiting to see if it gets worse is not the best approach, as the analogy explains. Contrast that approach with the method adopted in Hong Kong, where anyone who tests positive is immediately given a cocktail of antiviral drugs, designed to halt the infection in its tracks before it becomes too substantial to easily stop.[530]

My personal feeling is the standard of proof required to support any type of drug-taking in the context of this virus should not be "is this drug 110% guaranteed to work against the virus" but rather "is this drug (100%) guaranteed to be safe to take".[531] If the drug is *acceptably* safe to take and will do no harm,

---

[529] An infection is like a forest fire. To start with, you light a match, and can blow it out with a small breath. It sets fire to a piece of paper. You can stamp that out. The paper starts a small piece of wood burning. You can throw a jug of water on it. The piece of wood sets other pieces of wood on fire. Your garden hose will see to that. But leave it much longer, and you're going to need a fire truck, and leave it longer still, and you'll need helicopters with monsoon buckets, hundreds of fire-fighters, and so on.

It is exactly the same with a virus, and for the same reasons. Time is essential when fighting a viral infection with weak anti-viral drugs that work in the early stages of an infection but not later on.

[530] See https://www.bloomberg.com/amp/news/articles/2020-10-17/treat-covid-19-early-to-save-patients-lives-sars-veteran-urges or https://cov.cx/a1c91 Hong Kong has a very low infection rate (710 per million, as of early November) and a 2% case fatality rate (14 per million). The world average is a 2.5% CFR, which is also the US rate. So the Hong Kong approach isn't transformative, but it does seem to be beneficial.

[531] Of course, the reality is there is no such thing as a 100% safe drug. Every drug known to man, and even every natural product, starting with oxygen and water, can be harmful in some ways and forms, depending on how it is applied or taken. Every drug has side effects (but not every person gets every side effect). The universality of side

(continued on next page)

isn't it better to take the drug based on "Heads, it might help, tails, it won't hurt"? That policy, while open to criticism as being too simplistic, can be expressed as a situation with very little downside, and a ton of possible upside.

Of course, there have to be some realistic limits on how far you take that. The concept could conceivably have you swallowing everything in your medicine cabinet "just in case" it helps. That's not a good idea, either. But there is a point where some medicines and other substances reach a measurable level of "possibly might help" such that, as long as there is no downside, the question shifts from "Why should I take this" to "Why should I not take this".

That's a personal value and risk decision you should be allowed to participate in. It is your life, and your health, that is at issue here. I am absolutely not trying to persuade you to accept my opinion, but doctors too should be diffident at unilaterally imposing their values and morality on their patients. "I know best, I'm a doctor" and not even telling patients what is wrong with them and what the prognosis is, was formerly a normal state of affairs, 50 and more years ago, but we've moved past that point. These days, it is never a valid statement to make when it comes to balancing risks and outcomes. The patient – you – must be involved as much as is possible. Doctors should advise and counsel, but you must participate in the decisions ultimately taken.

Considering treatment options and choices is something you should think about now, *before* you come down with the virus. As you can see, there are some things you can be taking now to possibly reduce your risk of infection, as well as other things that should be taken at the first sign of an infection.

It might be awkward to phone your doctor now and say "Hey, doc, if I get sick, will you prescribe me XYZ?",[532] but for sure, you need to know what some of these treatment options are – treatment options which, as you'll see, some doctors advocate and use – and be ready to discuss them with your doctor if/when the time comes. Early intervention and treatment can be very beneficial (remember the footnoted fire analogy) – so if you become infected, you don't want to then get locked into a series of delays while trying to find an open-minded physician who will work with you to explore the best possible treatments.

---

effects gives doctors an automatic justification for refusing any treatment they may wish to reject.

Everything in life, including medicine, is always a case of balancing, minimizing, and optimizing risk; we can never eliminate it. "First, do no harm", while appealingly simple, is also unhelpfully simplistic.

[532] You know your doctor and the relationship you have with him. Maybe this is something you can discuss upfront, and surely, if you're seeing him for some other reason, maybe it can be worked into the conversation.

Doctors are also usually more conservative at how they respond to new patients than how they respond to existing patients – there is more mutual trust after a developed relationship. The last thing a doctor wants is to be unfairly trapped and then misquoted in some unfair piece of "investigative journalism", and so new patients tend to be treated more formally than existing ones.[533]

The further reality is that if you become infected, and if the infection becomes serious, you become less and less an active participant in your care program. When you're sedated and intubated on a ventilator, you're obviously no longer participating in much at all. Even before then, you may be dealing with emergency room/ICU type people who have no time for a careful discussion about treatment options, and who are unfamiliar with your medical history in general and any other issues that should be considered.

This is why discussing these concepts with your family physician/GP now, when there is no time pressure or urgency, and you're healthy and fully able to participate in the discussion and decisions made, would be a good thing if convenient for you and him.

With so much unknown, and with the virus so new, it is not realistic to expect there to be already existing ultra-rigorous proofs of new (and repurposed existing) medicines to guarantee they reduce the impact of a Covid-19 infection. There just hasn't been the time for that, yet. But if there is encouraging evidence of benefit to some patients in some cases, and an assurance of no harm attached with taking the drug, well, what is sensible in that case?

Many of the drugs mentioned in the following chapters have been in widespread use with extremely low levels of dangerous side-effects, and some of the drugs are even available, "over-the-counter", to anyone, without a prescription. Those are things I'm happy to take, as long as they don't interact with each other or with other medications. As for you, it is up to you; or hopefully is up to you, if your doctor will let you.

Drug Interactions

There's another reason not to just take one of everything you have in your medicine cabinet. The thing about anything you ingest – anything you breathe in, drink, or eat, is that it may interact with other things you are also ingesting.

This type of interaction is of little concern for "normal" things, but when you start taking medicinal products that are designed to change the way your body works and responds, there is every possibility that the way these medicines

---

[533] We have a link to a list of doctors known to be open to the concept of "early treatment" in our Reference section in the appendixes.

interact with you might be influenced by any other medicines you are taking as well.

Even some ordinary, apparently safe, and natural-seeming things can interact – for example, you might know that grapefruit can affect how some medications work.[534]

Safe and ordinary medications can change to potentially dangerous and harmful due to these types of interactions.

So if you're adding some new types of medications and supplements to your daily intake of such things, you need to consider not only the individual safety of each product, but also the potential for interactions between each and all of them. This is one of the reasons why so many medicines are only dispensed via prescription – the concern that a medicine, while ostensibly safe, in the correct dose and by itself, might either be taken in too large a dose, or in conjunction with other medicines and in combination, cause an unexpected negative outcome.

There are several ways to manage the risk of drug interactions. Asking your doctor is for sure the "gold standard" to aim for always.

Another is to ask a pharmacist, especially if you're taking a mix of "over-the-counter" type non-prescription medicines as well as (or instead of) prescription drugs.

And then there is the "self-help" method, using Google to do some online research. We don't encourage you to in effect become your own doctor. But we do encourage you to be an active and "value-adding" participant in your health-care regimen, and so it is fair and appropriate for you to back-stop your healthcare professionals' actions on your behalf with your own research, too.

You can look up detailed information on specific drugs using the same sites that doctors and pharmacists use. The Medscape website is excellent, but only allows you a limited number of page views before requiring you to join their service, so use it sparingly.

https://reference.medscape.com/ or https://cov.cx/a1f74

Another site is https://www.healthline.com/ or https://cov.cx/a1f75 and still another is https://www.rxlist.com/script/main/hp.asp or https://cov.cx/a1f76

We also like this site https://medlineplus.gov/ or https://cov.cx/a1f77

These sites don't necessarily spell things out in clear layman terms. Cryptic references need to be fully "decoded" – for example, "Not to be taken with

---

[534] This is because there is an enzyme in the grapefruit that can impact how quickly your body eliminates some types of drugs. See https://www.fda.gov/consumers/consumer-updates/grapefruit-juice-and-some-drugs-dont-mix or https://cov.cx/a1c92

macrolides" – don't just let your eyes glaze over the unfamiliar term. You need to know what a macrolide is.[535] Maybe that is another term for a drug or category of drugs, one of which you are also taking.

This is important. If you don't think you can do this adequately, you need to stay "plugged in" to the traditional healthcare system and use their tried and true support resources.

More consumer-friendly sites explain things in less technical terms, and in particular, this is a good site where you simply add a list of drugs and supplements you are taking and are then told of any possible interactions.

https://www.webmd.com/interaction-checker/default.htm   or https://cov.cx/a1f78

One more thing to be aware of – any allergies you could have to the various medicines you might be considering. Again, this is something best discussed with your doctor, or failing that, a pharmacist.

There are other types of interaction type issues to consider as well. For example, if you are pregnant, you have an entirely new series of issues to consider.

One more comment to keep in mind. We suggest you keep it simple. For example, if you decide you want a Vitamin D supplement, don't get something that also includes some other supplement in the pills/capsules too. That way you never risk "doubling up" on something, or if you need to boost one of your supplements, you can do so without risking an unwanted over-boost of other supplements that might also be present in the pills you are taking.

---

[535] Simply asking Google exactly that question – "What is a macrolide" will quickly take you to a page such as this one with a helpful answer - https://www.rxlist.com/script/main/art.asp?articlekey=11422 or https://cov.cx/a1c93

15. Non-official Treatments to Consider

I was listening to a podcast by a physician about the virus the other day and he made an excellent point. While there has been endless coverage in the press about contagion control – wearing masks, washing hands, social distancing, and so on, there has been almost no coverage or discussion about treatments (other than negatively in the case of, eg, HCQ).

The cost to our societies and economies from all the contagion control measures, closures, and so on, has been and continues to be measured in the trillions of dollars. But it is, at best, only partially working. We don't know how much worse things would be if we abandoned these measures, but we can clearly see that the measures we have in place at present are not helping us to get ahead of the virus. This chart shows which states have reducing numbers of new cases every day compared to which states have increasing numbers, as of 5 November 2020.[536]

---

[536] See https://rt.live/ for the latest update.

Figure 61 Current Rt rates for the US, 5 Nov 2020

We discussed what the R number is way back in the chapter "4. How the Number of Infections Increased So Quickly"; the relevant section being "The Virus Reproduction Rate" that starts on page 136. All the states (49 plus DC) with red circles above the 1.0 line have growing daily cases, only one state – Mississippi – has a green circle and reducing new daily cases, with a current Rt value of 0.83. The vertical bars are the error ranges – the actual values are somewhere on those bars, most likely where the circles are, but could be higher or lower.

We're not going to say that the contagion controls have been wrong – if anything, we might say we needed more not less of them. But we do want to acknowledge the curious contradiction between an obsession with a failed effort to control the virus spread, and a relative silence on what we do when each of the (currently 100,000+) new cases occurs.

Sure, we're encouraging investments of billions of dollars in new vaccines, which may or may not ever give us much benefit or control over the virus at some unknown future point. But what about the person – maybe you or a loved one – who gets the virus, today? What are we doing for them?

Isn't that sort of important, too?

So, what are we doing for people when they come down with a disease that is killing more than one in every hundred people who catch it? The official line on treatments for Covid-19 can be seen on the FDA and CDC websites, and probably many other places too. On the FDA site,[537] you'll see this question/answer

> Q : What treatments are available for Covid-19
>
> A : Currently there are no FDA-approved medicines specifically for COVID-19. However, the FDA has granted

---

[537] See https://www.fda.gov/emergency-preparedness-and-response/coronavirus-disease-2019-covid-19/covid-19-frequently-asked-questions or https://cov.cx/a1c94

Emergency Use Authorizations for some medicines to be used for certain patients hospitalized with COVID-19. The National Institutes of Health provides more information about treatment options.

People with COVID-19 should receive supportive care to help relieve symptoms. People with mild symptoms are able to recover at home. If you experience a medical emergency such as trouble breathing, call 911 and let the operator know you may have COVID-19. Never take a prescription medicine or drug if it is not prescribed for you by your doctor for your health condition.

The CDC site has a similar shorter statement.

The understated and dismaying reality of the present situation is there are, indeed, no *officially approved* medicines to take upfront, either to reduce your chance of becoming infected or, if an infection has been acquired, to quickly cure it or at the very least reduce your chance of the infection becoming severe.[538] That makes for a very helpless feeling, with the totality of official medical advice in the US for people in the early stages of an infection being to take it easy and get plenty of sleep, to drink lots of fluids, and do nothing else except hope things don't get worse and require hospitalization.

It seems astonishing that in this day and age and state of medical knowledge, this is the best response that can be offered. Unsurprisingly, that has caused some people to go exploring possible non-traditional solutions, and sometimes a bit too eagerly! Don't let desperation blind you to caution and common sense.

However, note the italicizing of the words "officially approved" above. There are lots of possible treatments being advocated by various physicians and researchers, and some of them may be perfectly sensible. But while everyone is doing everything possible to rush through new vaccines in scary-fast record times, the traditional snail-pace and (some might suggest) excessively cautious approach to considering new treatments remains unchanged.

Shouldn't the "Operation Warp Speed" concept to urgently develop a vaccine also apply to endorsing treatments? As of 6 December, the US has suffered 15.2 million cases and nearly 290,000 deaths, and many of the 14.9 million recovered sufferers have not and may never make a full recovery. Where is the sense of urgency – in any country – for identifying treatments?

---

[538] Remdesivir was approved as a Covid-19 treatment in late October, but we don't think a $3120 costing drug, plus the cost of the hospitalization required while being given it, is exactly a broad-based solution for most people and with early and mild infections.

The FDA is cutting every possible corner to rush out a vaccine that might be at little as 50% effective for only a short period – for example, reducing a six-month observation of test subjects in the Phase 3 trial down to only two months. Instead of running a full six-month trial,[539] after the shorter trial, people in "at-risk" groups will be given a smartphone app they can use to report any serious side-effects after being vaccinated. That's very cold comfort if you are one of the people who then get a serious side-effect after the accelerated approval of a new vaccine, isn't it.[540]

But at the same time that it is breaking many of its usual rules for vaccine evaluations, and rushing to get vaccines of unknown safety and functionality to market, it is taking its leisurely and slow path toward cures – cures that in some cases, such as early administering of HCQ, promise as high as 64% success rates[541] and using ivermectin as a prophylactic with apparently a 73% success rate[542] – much better than the vaccines of unknown safety.

Why this duality? Why not treat cures with the same enthusiasm and priority as vaccines?

We also note with interest the disclosures about the treatments President Trump was given as soon as he tested positive. There is also some doubt about when he was first shown as being infected, a doubt that is exacerbated by what seems like an astonishingly rapid onset of severe symptoms, and the use of treatments that are usually held back until later in the course of an infection.[543]

It has been disclosed that he has been receiving doses of zinc, Vitamin D, famotidine, melatonin, and aspirin, as well as an 8g IV dose of "Regeneron's

---

[539] Most trials continue to observe their test subjects out to about the two-year point.

[540] See https://www.wsj.com/articles/covid-19-vaccine-rollout-to-feature-app-tracking-monitoring-of-vulnerable-groups-11604582313 or https://cov.cx/a1c95

[541] 100% of all early-use studies of HCQ have shown positive effects, with the average improvement in patient outcomes being 64%. See https://c19study.com/ or https://cov.cx/a1a24

[542] See https://www.medrxiv.org/content/10.1101/2020.10.29.20222661v1 or https://cov.cx/a1c96

[543] It is not entirely clear when he first received a positive test. Some sources are suggesting some time on Wednesday 28 September, others are suggesting early on Thursday, and he made an official announcement by Twitter shortly after midnight on what had become Friday, 2 October.

polyclonal antibody cocktail"[544],[545] A couple of hours later, with some reports suggesting he was already having trouble breathing, it seems he started taking remdesivir too.[546] Then we learned on Sunday morning that he has been taking the steroid dexamethasone as well,[547] something not usually given in the early stages of an infection.

The one (or two) notable omissions in his disclosed treatments? There has been no mention of the hydroxychloroquine he had so controversially espoused some months previously, and the azithromycin that it is often combined with. But we also note that the list of medications he is being treated with may not be complete. Nowhere does it say "these are the only drugs he is being given" and there was a lot of non-transparency about when he first tested positive (possibly Wednesday rather than late Thursday night), whether he had been receiving supplemental oxygen in hospital on Friday, and his overall condition.

We note that the disclosed treatments, apart from the IV doses of the Regeneron trial product and remdesivir are all non-prescription products. While the fact Trump – presumably with his doctors' concurrence – is taking these products is not necessarily medically significant, it does show however that the claim there is nothing that can be done is open to challenge, and some of the possible things that can be done are things you can directly do yourself with a simple visit to the shelves of your local pharmacy.[548]

---

[544] The Regeron treatment is explained here – an article written a couple of days prior to Trump's infection announcement https://www.cnn.com/2020/09/29/health/regeneron-covid-19-early-antibody-treatment-results/index.html or https://cov.cx/a1c97

[545] As reported here https://www.bbc.com/news/world-us-canada-54396670 or https://cov.cx/a1c98

[546] See https://www.dailymail.co.uk/news/article-8800117/Donald-Trump-taken-Walter-Reed-hospital-COVID-treatment.html or https://cov.cx/a1c99

[547] See https://news.trust.org/item/20201004174312-useuk or https://cov.cx/a1d01 - it is unclear from the wording when he started taking the steroid but no later than some time on Saturday and possibly sooner. More details of this treatment are in this article https://www.statnews.com/2020/10/04/trump-receiving-dexamethasone-steroid-usually-given-patients-with-severe-covid19/ or https://cov.cx/a1d02

[548] To be clear, I am *not* saying "because President Trump took this drug, you should too. I am simply saying "President Trump's doctors didn't just tell him to do nothing and stay at home." The only real point here is to show that the statements from CDC/NIH/FDA/WHO/etc that there is nothing to be done during the early and mild

(continued on next page)

The bottom-line is most unfortunate. Over 2,000 more people will die today, in the US alone, and many thousands more in the rest of the world, due to inadequate treatments, and not only due to inadequate treatments, but due to possibly/probably good treatments being withheld due to lack of official approvals.

And you know the worst thing about this? Keep reading......

The Approval Delays are Unnecessary

While the FDA and CDC stubbornly insist there's nothing you can do if you get the virus, in the real world, doctors are doing things and finding, based on their front-line experiences, that some things work and don't work.

Academia and government bodies try and hide behind their claimed need for "double-blind random trials" and for sure, those are the "gold standard". But do we need the gold standard, and can we afford to wait for a gold standard, when there are already "silver standards" that are working in the real world?

Perhaps surprisingly, there is an official answer to this, and the answer might astonish you. While the official bodies insist on gold standard testing before they'll change their minds, the 21st Century Cures Act,[549] which took effect on 31 December 2016, allows and even requires the FDA to consider "real-world evidence" as well as double-blind random clinical trials.

The FDA should read their own website. This page[550] (and the links from it to other pages on their site) explain what this Act allows and obliges the FDA to now do. The FDA can now simply accept a statement like "We gave this drug to

---

stages of a Covid infection are not universal truths unquestioningly accepted and acted upon by everyone. This is not a black and white issue.

If you are in a dialog with your doctor, it is fair to ask, if told there is nothing that can be done "Why then did President Trump disclose he immediately started taking five different over-the-counter products?".

[549] See https://www.congress.gov/114/plaws/publ255/PLAW-114publ255.pdf or https://cov.cx/a1d03 for the text of the Act. Unfortunately, the simple concept of this act requires 312 pages of written content, making it difficult for normal people to digest and understand.

Yet again, we wonder how it is that the entire US Constitution – including the 27 amendments – is only 7,591 words (about 20 – 25 pages) yet a single amendment to a single act now takes 312 pages.

[550] See https://www.fda.gov/regulatory-information/selected-amendments-fdc-act/21st-century-cures-act or https://cov.cx/a1d04 and, as a further example, https://www.fda.gov/science-research/science-and-research-special-topics/real-world-evidence or https://cov.cx/a1d05

1,000 patients and all survived without getting a serious case of Covid. We didn't withhold the drug from another 1,000 patients to prove the difference in outcome, because the drug is so clearly helpful, and it would have been cruel and immoral to withhold it from anyone, but look at other statistics everywhere else to see for yourself that having 1,000 out of 1,000 survive is obviously significant and impactful and exciting".

This makes the FDA's unwillingness and slow-motion response to this fast-moving virus and evolving knowledge of practical effective treatments all the more shameful. While the Cures Act doesn't suggest the FDA should now become reckless or foolish, it allows the FDA to shift from a demand for 110% "gold standard" irrefutable proof of everything to allowing a, well, maybe 99% proof and for making decisions in areas where some grayness still exists but in which the overwhelming preponderance of evidence supports an approval, and the downsides of being possibly wrong are trivially small.

We believe that some of the treatments being proposed by responsible experts meet appropriate standards to be, if not officially approved, at the very least be given "Emergency Use Authorization" by the FDA to allow them to move out of the shadows and be more readily given to patients.

You're reading this book because you're curious, questioning, and keen to take charge of your destiny. So now we'll have a look at what some respected groups of physicians and researchers are advocating, but which officialdom has yet to respond to.

Some Unofficial Early Treatment Plans

Many doctors refuse to even talk about possible treatments with Covid patients until they are seriously unwell and need to be hospitalized. Their caution is so extreme they'll not even tell you to get some over-the-counter non-prescription supplements such as Vitamin C, Vitamin D, and zinc.

But, many other doctors will tell you about non-prescription treatments and may prescribe additional drugs, too. A survey of doctors around the world conducted September 17 – 20 showed the following responses in terms of what medications doctors would prescribe/recommend to patients with mild non-hospitalized cases of Covid.[551]

---

[551] See https://app.sermo.com/covid19-barometer or https://cov.cx/a1g08 - this is from their Study 14.

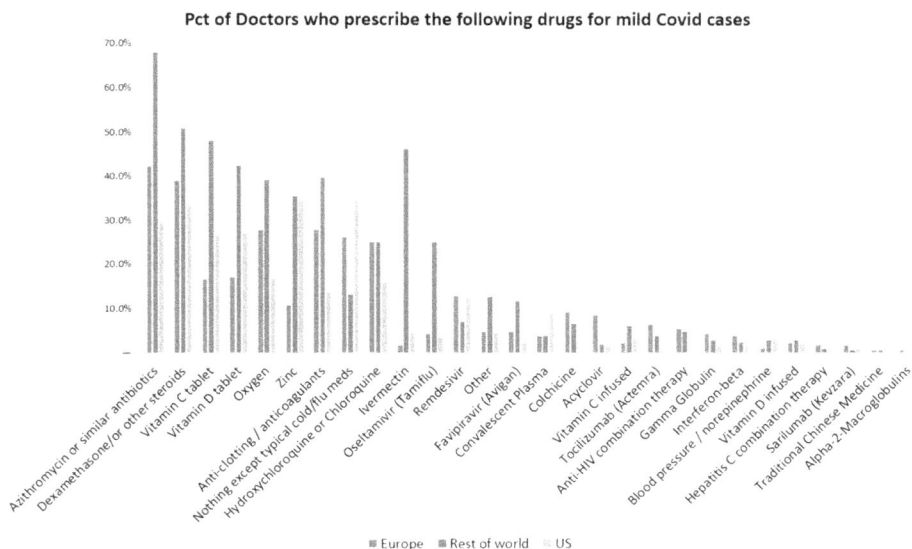

Figure 62 What doctors prescribe for mild-case Covid patients

So what do doctors actually prescribe? We see a long list in this chart, but of course not every doctor is prescribing every one of those medications to every patient. It was also interesting to note that US doctors were more likely to prescribe nothing.

We are not suggesting that choosing the best medications should be based on a popularity contest, and of course, other issues may also impact on why some doctors choose some medications in some countries, and others do something different.

But if your physician is anxious about prescribing you any of the medications we mention, you can point to this chart as interesting and hopefully reassuring evidence that other physicians, both in the US and elsewhere, are doing so currently.

We are aware of several published treatment plans that have been developed to provide a structure to what drugs to prescribe, in what quantities, and when. We know there are many others as well – many practices of multiple doctors seem to have agreed upon a consistent approach among themselves but of course, have not bothered to publish their treatment plan.

- ## *The EVMS and FLCCC Plans*

The main two early treatment plans we know of have quite a lot in common (including some of the lead people in formulating the plans).

They are the **I-MASk+ plan from the FLCCC Alliance**[552] and the **EVMS Critical Care Covid-19 Management Protocol from the EVMS Medical Group**.[553] They are well documented and explained in the links.

- ## *The McCullough Group Plan*

A third early treatment plan is advocated by a group of 23 physicians and researchers, with **Dr Peter McCullough** being the lead person advocating it.

He has suffered the virus himself, and used his program on himself, with very positive results,[554] and the group of advocates have had positive outcomes when prescribing it for their patients too.

The plan can be seen here[555] and is backgrounded and explained here.[556] There is also an interesting podcast where McCullough is interviewed.[557]

It is interesting because it suggests, if you are healthy, with no comorbidities, and under 50, you don't need to do anything if only mildly infected except take zinc supplements, and wait until/unless you become more unwell.

With the treatments being suggested for the over 50s and younger people with comorbidities being so mild and so inexpensive, I'd think it makes sense on a "better safe than sorry" basis to adopt a treatment plan, no matter what age you are.

---

[552] See https://covid19criticalcare.com/ or https://cov.cx/a1d06

[553] See https://www.evms.edu/covid-19/covid_care_for_clinicians/ or https://cov.cx/a1d07

[554] Yes, we know – simply having had the virus oneself doesn't make anyone an automatic expert on it, neither Dr McCullough nor President Trump, nor anyone else.

[555] See https://img1.wsimg.com/blobby/go/f2ee8902-0ee5-4100-996d-e73b761ae165/McCullough%20PA%20Ambulatory%20Treatment%20of%20COVID%20Up.pdf or https://cov.cx/a1d08

[556] See https://www.trialsitenews.com/this-doctor-has-covid-he-has-a-plan-for-all-of-us/ or https://cov.cx/a1d09

[557] See https://www.youtube.com/watch?v=fdbwTNNsF1E or https://cov.cx/a1d10

Sure, not nearly as many people get severe or fatal infections if they are young and healthy, but some do, and some of the survivors experience lasting lung/brain/other organ damage that impairs their quality of life (and quite likely longevity too).

There are some medical abbreviations on their plan document that need explaining – we have a table of abbreviations and their meanings in the Reference Appendix below on page 449.

- ## *The ICON Protocol*

Another early treatment plan evolved out of what has been referred to as the "Icon Study" in South Florida. This showed a significant improvement in outcomes for patients who were prescribed ivermectin.[558]

The treatment plan calls for 200 mcg/kg of ivermectin (ie 91 mcg/lb – so a 200lb person would be prescribed 18 mg) on the first and second day, with repeats on days 8 & 9 and so on (ie weekly) if the patient continues to show symptoms of Covid. In addition, doxycycline or azithromycin, atorvastatin, and various over-the-counter products are called for, and additional prescription medicines if the patient's condition becomes more serious.

Full details are here.[559]

- ## *The MGU Plan*

We are also aware of another treatment plan published by Russia's probably most prestigious university, the Moscow State University (MSU or MGU).[560]

We specifically discuss this plan here because the other two plans don't need any discussion – they are in English and reasonably well documented/explained.

The MGU plan has a primary focus on in-hospital treatment, which is beyond the scope of what we're considering. But it also features a section for people with

---

[558] See https://journal.chestnet.org/article/S0012-3692(20)34898-4/fulltext or https://cov.cx/a1g04

[559] See https://pscflorida.com/wp-content/uploads/2020/12/PSCFlorida-ICON-Protocol.pdf or https://cov.cx/a1g05

[560] See http://mc.msu.ru/m/protokol-mnoc.pdf or https://cov.cx/a1d11 - this is in Russian, but you can copy the text and paste it into a translation program such as https://translate.google.com/ or https://cov.cx/a1d12

mild to moderate symptoms who have not yet been admitted to a hospital. That section has four entries/recommendations :

1. Bromhexine - 8 mg to be taken four times a day

2. Spironolactone - 50 mg to be taken once a day

3. Rivaroxaban - 10 mg once a day OR Apixaban 2.5 mg twice a day

4. Dipyridamole - 75 mg twice a day

Bromhexine is sometimes used in cough medicines and has specific properties that seem like they might combat Covid.[561]   It has been little researched outside of Russia.

Spironolactone is a diuretic, also known as Aldactone. It is also used in acne treatments and to treat high blood pressure. There have been some suggestions that it may help with a Covid infection,[562] but it is another drug little known outside Russia.

Rivaroxaban, also known as Xarelto, is a blood thinner used to prevent blood clots. The Russian treatment is very focused on blood clot prevention. There have been articles advocating for Rivaroxaban use when patients are hospitalized and continued treatment after they have been released, but I've not found articles advocating its use in the early stages of the virus infection. That's not to argue against that part of the Russian protocol, merely to point out there are not lots of supporting studies in the west to affirm it.

Dipyridamole is another blood thinner/anti-clotting agent, and the comments above for Rivaroxaban apply similarly here, too.

It would do no harm to talk through the four drugs mentioned here with your doctor, too. We're interested in the Bromhexine, which, if you can find a cough medicine featuring it, is even available over-the-counter rather than needing a prescription.

It is also interesting to see the importance the Russians give to blood thinners/anticoagulants. But that's not to say the west ignores this completely

---

[561] This study in particular shows massive changes in outcome for patients who took Bromhexine after being admitted to hospital. https://bi.tbzmed.ac.ir/Files/Inpress/bi-23240.pdf or https://cov.cx/a1d13 There are other studies with weaker findings (particularly due to having too-small groups of people in their studies). This paper, written back in May, wonders if it might be useful in conjunction with either HCQ or quercetin. https://www.ncbi.nlm.nih.gov/pmc/articles/PMC7249615/ or https://cov.cx/a1d14

[562] See https://www.ncbi.nlm.nih.gov/pmc/articles/PMC7363620/ or https://cov.cx/a1d15 and https://www.ncbi.nlm.nih.gov/pmc/articles/PMC7191632/ or https://cov.cx/a1d16

at an early stage – see our recommendation for low amounts of aspirin, which also has an anti-clot/thinning property.

A Possible Evaluative Perspective

No matter what the official statements are from the various health agencies, there are some not-yet-officially-blessed treatments that might be showing promise and which have been endorsed and adopted, variously by some medical practitioners in jurisdictions where they are not yet officially approved, and officially in some countries that have chosen to deem them as appropriate.

As we said before, we shouldn't let desperation and disbelief drive us to inappropriate treatments, but perhaps we shouldn't also let a too-conservative approach to official approvals[563] blind us to the existence of some promising treatments where the only controversy seems to be the extent of their effectiveness rather than concerns about downside risks.

This is the approach and attitude and perspective I am adopting in this section.

The treatments that have been approved (a mere three of them, remdesivir plus two others under Emergency Use Authorizations) are focused on patients with severe symptoms, who have already needed to be admitted to hospital, and even those are far from miracle cures.

New treatment approaches and tactics using existing medications and treatment methods continue to evolve, and they are usually described in terms like "reduces mortality by 15%" or whatever – hardly transformational at all. Don't get us wrong – if we end up needing hospitalization, we'll be very appreciative of any and all such treatments, and every possible tweak of the odds in our favor. But we'd prefer larger shifts in the odds than the ones currently on offer, and most of all, we'd prefer not to get to that dire situation.

A stitch in time saves nine, and while it is reassuring to know that hospital-level treatments for severe Covid illnesses are probably improving, we'd much prefer not to need to go to a hospital in the first place. You doubtless feel the same way, as does most everyone else.

Avoiding hospitalization is also very beneficial for the healthcare system which doesn't then get overloaded. Do you remember all the panic and press coverage about a ventilator shortage in March and April (it turned out the

---

[563] There's also a question for you to ponder. Some people smugly discount the speed with which some drugs are accepted in some countries. But is the FDA's comparative slowness to approve new drugs, compared to the speed of similar bodies in other countries, proof that the FDA has higher standards? Or does it merely show the FDA to be a more slow-moving body than those in other countries?

ventilator shortage was non-existent)? The demanded solution was to urgently source more ventilators. Wouldn't it be better to focus on early and outpatient treatment options, so that patients never get to the unfortunate point of needing ventilators – so that they never even need hospitalization at all?

In other words, isn't a few dollars worth of pills, taken at home, better than three or four weeks in a hospital, in the ICU, on a ventilator, costing the high side of $100,000, and with a risk of death? Instead of, or as well as, focusing on emergency hospital facilities and urgently building more ventilators, shouldn't we be urgently seeking out existing approved medicines that can be repurposed to help Covid patients in the early stages of their infections, and keep them from becoming more serious?

Why was there so much outrage about insufficient ventilators, but no outrage about the lack of earlier stage treatments that resulted in people needing the desperate last-ditch attempt to save their lives with a ventilator (a treatment that often failed to save the patient)?

Developing early intervention measures should be an outcome that is getting every bit as much attention as the current frenzy over finding a vaccine,[564] and late-stage treatments to improve survival odds for the most severely ill patients.

This brings us to this section of the document.

Do I need to state, yet again, that I am not a doctor? In this section, I risk straying off the path of accepted conventional treatments and medicine to a greater or lesser extent. You should cautiously consider the commentary here, and act on it only after weighing the pluses and minuses of each possible option, and keep in mind that none of these things have been officially sanctioned by

---

[564] I should explain that comment. Normally, developing a vaccine is the very best of all outcomes when designing a response to a virus threat. But a vaccine is only the very best outcome if it is long-lasting, highly effective, and close to universally taken. Current vaccine candidates are showing promise in terms of their effectiveness, but we don't yet know how long they may last, and current surveys suggest at least one-third of the country will refuse to be vaccinated.

So what happens for the other third of the population? Or even for the protected people when their shot starts to wear off? And what happens if/when a new strain of the virus mutates which the vaccine doesn't protect against (as may have already happened in Denmark)?

Due to what so far appears to be an uncertain vaccine benefit, and associated with that, finite rather than enduring acquired immunity after an infection, it seems there will be a likely continuation of outbreaks and public health impacts, even after a vaccine comes along.

Maybe – hopefully – we'll uncover a better vaccine in the future. But until and if that ever happens, researchers need to be working on cures as well as vaccines.

NIH/CDC/FDA/WHO or any other US-related agency (although, to be fair, some have been officially approved in other jurisdictions).

As mentioned before, everything we ingest has side-effects. Even oxygen is harmful (in too great a quantity), as is water, too.[565] It is the same with all medicines, vitamins, minerals, and supplements in general.

There are two other sides to that statement though, which should not be ignored.

First, many things that are poisonous and harmful, even in small quantities, can be extremely beneficial and sometimes essential in much smaller quantities. Evaluating harm and benefit needs to be considered alongside the dosage levels being countenanced.

Second, many things that are poisonous and harmful have the potential to solve a greater problem. Think of chemotherapy for cancer – at the risk of gross oversimplification, basically you are poisoning yourself with many of these treatments, in the hope the cancer will die before the rest of you does. Evaluating harm and benefit needs to be considered alongside the harm of not administering the risky/dangerous treatment.

Whether you're an evolutionist or a creationist, you probably agree that our bodies have been designed to be as self-supporting, self-regulating, and self-maintaining/self-healing as possible, and if we live normal/healthy lives, with normal/healthy eating, in normal times, we shouldn't need anything more, most of the time.

But that is a lot of uses of the word "normal", which is a very vague term, and for sure, this new SARS-CoV-2 virus is not normal. It is (sort of) a new virus, and our body has little in the way of built-in defensive mechanisms to counter it, which is of course why we're all looking for the best way to help our bodies in any upcoming fights against the virus.

So with that as background, let's look at some possible steps we can take alone, or ask our doctors to help us with, that might reduce our risks variously of becoming infected, and, if infected, of having the disease become serious and possibly fatal.

We'll look at this the same way medical practitioners often categorize medicines and treatments; in four categories

- Things to take every day as a precautionary or "prophylactic" measure to reduce the chances of getting a Covid-19 infection (and/or, so that if you

---

[565] See, for example, https://indianapublicmedia.org/amomentofscience/can-oxygen-be-toxic.php or https://cov.cx/a1d17 and https://www.medicalnewstoday.com/articles/318619 or https://cov.cx/a1d18

are infected, your infection is less serious/severe than would otherwise be the case)

- Additional precautionary measures that probably aren't needed or aren't advised every day, but which make sense if you've been in a higher risk and possibly exposed situation
- What to do if you think or know you've been infected – "early treatment" and "mild illness"
- What to do if your infection becomes more serious – "late treatment" and "severe illness"

There is another stage as well, sometimes referred to as "salvage" – when a patient is critically ill and it is a case of "all hands to the pump" and using increasingly aggressive treatments. You would be hospitalized well before reaching this stage, and probably not fully able to participate in treatments at that point, so we'll not comment on that at all.

There is yet another stage or possibly even two – treatment when you get out of ICU but are still in a hospital, and further treatment once you've been discharged but before a 100% complete recovery.

This last stage is particularly important. I know people – and have read of many more – who, once discharged, discover they are far from "cured". Don't expect your recovery from Covid to be like a sore throat or most other illnesses where you quickly recover and are soon back to normal. There's a significant chance of you feeling ongoing fatigue and weakness for some time after being discharged (if hospitalized) or having "beaten the beast" if you worked your way through it at home.

Our feeling is that once you become part of the formal medical system, you're best advised to accept their expertise, although you (or another family member) could cite articles such as the EVMS guidelines[566] and ask your doctors what they think and which of the EVMS recommendations they'll either follow or ignore and why.

---

[566] I don't mean to suggest that the EVMS recommendations are the ultimate gold-standard that should be slavishly followed at all, and some aspects of their recommendations give me pause. But it is a credible set of written guidelines from a credible source, at a point where there are very few such sets of written guidelines, and as a reference point to guide a discussion with your medical team, it is as good as any. See
https://www.evms.edu/media/evms_public/departments/internal_medicine/EVMS_Critic al_Care_COVID-19_Protocol.pdf or https://cov.cx/a1d19

We'll look at possible strategies for all four of those stages, plus add some thoughts about at-home treatment and care, and the question of if you should take a vaccine if/when one becomes available.

There is an important consideration that underlies this categorization into four stages. Some remedies are not recommended and can even be harmful at some stages of a Covid infection while beneficial at other stages. This is particularly true of steroids, which are not recommended in the early stages of an infection, but may be beneficial in the later/more serious stages. This illustration from the EVMS site shows how treatment needs change over time with the Covid virus :[567]

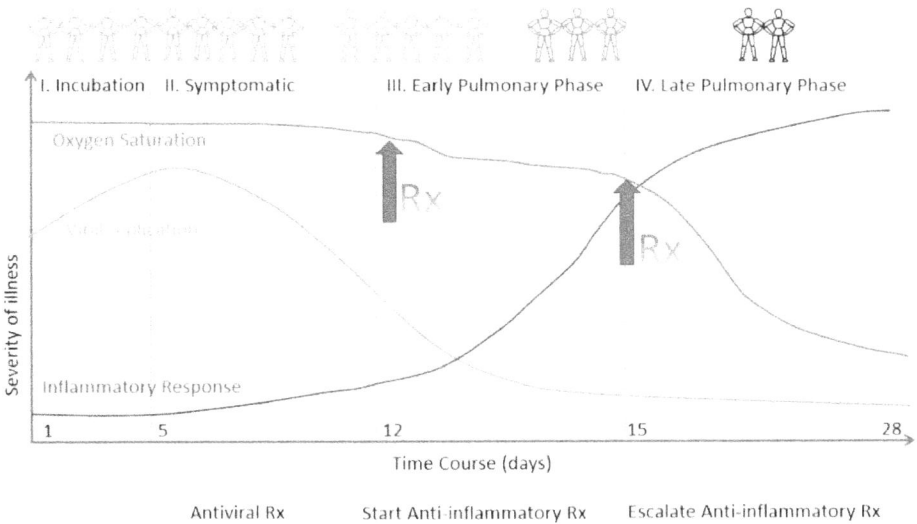

Figure 63 The changing challenges and treatment needs over time

So, please don't think that "if this can help me when I'm seriously ill, surely it will also help me when I'm not so sick". This is an example of the tricks and traps of approaching all of this without medical counsel.

As things get worse and more complex, the stakes get higher. In other words, the further along the stages, the more you should rely on medical professionals, and the less you should rely on me. That's one of two reasons why I comment

---

[567] See
https://www.evms.edu/media/evms_public/departments/internal_medicine/EVMS_Critic
al_Care_COVID-19_Protocol.pdf or https://cov.cx/a1d19

less when you get to these levels of severity. The other reason? Because I'm truly unqualified to help in such high-stakes and much more complex decisions.

One last introductory point. Please read the following sections together with the sections in the chapter below, "16. Medicines, Supplements, Vitamins, etc", starting on page 356 that provides more detailed information about each of the treatments we mention here. All the bolded items in the sections below have more details in that chapter.

1. In General, Every Day

To repeat, in case you skipped straight to this point, there are no officially[568] approved (in the US), nor even officially recommended (in the US), medicines to take to reduce your risk of infection. It is quite the opposite. The National Institutes of Health says[569]

> **Pre-Exposure Prophylaxis**
>
> The COVID-19 Treatment Guidelines Panel (the Panel) recommends against the use of any agents for SARS-CoV-2 pre-exposure prophylaxis (PrEP), except in a clinical trial (AIII).
>
> *Rationale*
>
> At present, there is no known agent that can be administered before exposure to SARS-CoV-2 (i.e., as PrEP) to prevent infection. Clinical trials are investigating several agents, including emtricitabine plus tenofovir alafenamide or tenofovir disoproxil fumarate, hydroxychloroquine, and supplements such as zinc, Vitamin C, and Vitamin D. Studies of monoclonal antibodies that target SARS-CoV-2 are in development. Please check ClinicalTrials.gov for the latest information.

So please keep in mind that everything which follows in this section is going against the NIH advice.

Having said that, we should first acknowledge part of the possible logic behind this NIH statement. It seems reasonable to at least accept the concept that a healthy body with a strong immune system is probably more resilient and better able to fight off an infection than one that is weakened and with an impaired immune system. Maybe no pre-exposure medications are needed?

---

[568] In the sense of CDC or WHO type officialdom and formal statements

[569] See https://www.covid19treatmentguidelines.nih.gov/overview/prevention-of-sars-cov-2/ or https://cov.cx/a1d20

The thing about getting a Covid-19 (or most any other) infection is there is some "minimum dose" required – an uncertain minimum number of virus particles that are needed to create a sustainable and growing infection.

The exact number of particles needed is not known and varies depending on a mixture of factors – some controllable, some almost random. In a way, it is a bit like conceiving. Only one sperm is required to fertilize one egg, and men typically ejaculate many tens of millions of sperm in a single session. So you'd think there's no problem whatsoever in a couple getting pregnant. But, astonishingly, ejaculating fewer than 40 million sperm makes fertilization difficult, and even with a high number received at a woman's most fertile time, pregnancy is not guaranteed.

That concept, while the cause of much heartbreak for some couples, is part of what is protecting us now. It is a numbers game. You have two strategies to "win" this "game". The first is to keep the number of virus particles that enter your body to an absolute minimum, and the second is to do whatever you can to help your body be able to triumph against the largest possible number of viral invaders.

What does this mean? In terms of keeping the number of virus particles entering your body to a minimum, this essentially means things like **social distancing** and **mask-wearing**. We discuss this in detail in our chapter above, "10. How to Avoid Infection – In General", starting on page 214.

As for doing whatever you can to help your body to triumph against the largest possible number of invaders, in the most general terms, this means eating and living well. You know – a **good diet**, **fresh** rather than processed food as much as possible, drinking **plenty of water** but **not too much alcohol**, **exercising**, maintaining a **reasonable body mass index**, getting **plenty of sleep**, and all that other stuff.

There's no real shortcut to getting the benefits of such things, but there are a few possible ways to ensure you're "fighting fit" and in the best medical shape, and to hopefully compensate, at least partially, for any lack of perfection in the generic concept of healthy living.

Another consideration would be to look at the list of **comorbidities** (see page 159). While you can't influence some of the risk factors that might make an infection more serious (such as age and gender) some of the comorbidities might be things you can work on improving, either through lifestyle changes or medication.

I don't know if reducing any comorbidities makes you less likely to become infected, but clearly, reducing comorbidities makes any infection you might get less threatening, and that's a very good outcome. Because these sorts of actions might take some time to implement, it is good to start working on them now.

Beyond these general concepts, here are some other specific things to consider.

1.1   Consider taking a **multi-vitamin supplement** every day.

Sure, in theory, a well-balanced diet should give you all the vitamins and minerals and everything else you need to be healthy. It is also very true that you can overdose on taking too many vitamins, minerals, and assorted other supplements. You can harm yourself, your kidneys, and your liver.

But one single "normal" level type of multi-vitamin supplement is generally considered as safe, and while probably not essential for most people in normal times, it might be prudent in these more challenging times.

However, the concept of "if one tablet is good, two are surely twice as good" absolutely does not apply. Stick to the daily single tablet dose, so as not to inadvertently overdose on some of the ingredients.

1.2   Although I just recommended you should be careful not to go too far over the recommended daily value[570] for most substances, I personally made an exception for **Vitamin D**.

Dosage recommendations vary; I decided to take an additional 50 mcg (2,000 IU) every day, which is 2 ½ times the recommended daily value and suggested here.[571]

Orally taken Vitamin D3 has a long half-life in your system – about 25 days. So if you are not already taking the vitamin via a multi-vitamin supplement, you might want to spend a couple of days with "loading doses" at 4,000 IU a day, and then move to a maintenance level of 2,000 IU a day.

1.3   I don't do this, but some people (and EVMS) recommend a **Vitamin C** boost. My multi-vitamin tablets already give me 90 mg, which is 100% of the recommended daily value.

EVMS suggests 500 mg, twice a day, and it is common to see other sources also recommending much higher "mega-doses" of Vitamin C in various situations. For no real reason other than a probably unfounded concern that there might be some correlation between my past higher level of Vitamin C taking

---

[570] The "recommended daily value" is just that – a *recommended* daily value. It is seldom/never the same as a "do not take more than this" upper limit, and possibly the recommended daily value has been arrived at with only very little underpinning medical research and scientific proof.

It is a good starting point to work from, but it is not an exact number in any way at all. It is more likely to be a minimum amount than a maximum amount.

[571] See https://newsnetwork.mayoclinic.org/discussion/mayo-clinic-q-and-a-how-much-vitamin-d-do-i-need/ or https://cov.cx/a1d21

and occasional episodes of kidney stones,[572] I'm sticking with the 90 mg for an everyday amount, but any time I feel I've been at risk, I go to the higher level dosage mentioned in the next section.

1.4 **Zinc** seems very beneficial and may be useful as a prophylactic (preventative). But don't overdose on it – be careful to see what dosage you are already getting from your multi-vitamin tablets and any other supplements you are taking.

Zinc does have definite and nasty side-effects if you take too much, so as an everyday item, stick reasonably closely to the recommended daily amount.

1.5 **Melatonin** is recommended by EVMS, with a dosage starting at 0.3 mg and possibly increasing from there as long as you experience no side-effects up to 2 mg every night, ideally in a slow-release form.

1.6 Consider getting a **BCG vaccination** (for tuberculosis). This is a possibility this may also give you some Covid resistance as well.

Note – if you are already taking, for example, Vitamin C every day, when you read about taking it in these sections, this does not mean "in addition to your everyday amount", it means "in total, you should be taking this much". The same for all other medications. Don't add the doses mentioned in each section, make sure the dose in any section is the maximum you're taking.

2. If You've Been in a Higher-Risk Situation

Again, the NIH suggests you should do nothing if you have been in a situation with an elevated risk of infection. They say[573]

> **Post-Exposure Prophylaxis**
>
> The Panel recommends against the use of any agents for SARS-CoV-2 post-exposure prophylaxis (PEP), except in a clinical trial (AIII).
>
> *Rationale*
>
> At present, there is no known agent that can be administered after exposure to SARS-CoV-2 infection (i.e., as PEP) to prevent infection. Potential options for PEP that are currently under investigation include chloroquine, hydroxychloroquine, lopinavir/ritonavir, nitazoxanide, Vitamin super B-complex,

---

[572] See https://www.kidney.org/news/newsroom/newsreleases/0150 or https://cov.cx/a1d22

[573] See https://www.covid19treatmentguidelines.nih.gov/overview/prevention-of-sars-cov-2/ or https://cov.cx/a1d20

and Vitamin D. Other post-exposure preventative strategies that are in development include the use of SARS-CoV-2 monoclonal antibodies and convalescent plasma. Please check ClinicalTrials.gov for the latest information.

If you feel it appropriate to consider taking some things as a general prophylaxis measure, you'll probably feel twice as convinced about the need for preventative measures after you've been in a risky situation.

Unless otherwise detailed, the measures we mention below should be done for a week, maybe even two weeks. It can take at least that long or longer for symptoms to appear after being exposed to the virus (which is why the standard quarantine time is 14 days).

2.1   I'll do a gargle/mouthwash upon returning home after being in a higher-risk environment. In the past, I've used either 1.5% **hydrogen peroxide** or **Povidone-Iodine** (also as a nasal spray too). I repeat before going to bed that night and do it again the next day and night, too (ie four gargles in total).

But I've now switched to **Listerine Original Formula**, which has been shown to be much more effective than either hydrogen peroxide or Povidone-Iodine. Note the study showed the gold-colored Original Formula to be much better than any of the other Listerine products.

2.2   I'll spray some **propolis** into my throat after each gargling. And possibly take a propolis capsule or two as well.

2.3   I'll take 500 mg of **quercetin**, twice a day.

2.4   This is the point where I abandon my reluctance to take larger doses of **Vitamin C**. I'll take 500 mg of Vitamin C twice a day for a week (ie 1000 mg/day) and maybe reduce it to once a day for the second week. Some sources suggest even more.

2.5   I'm also willing to now go over the RDA for **zinc**, too. One source suggests 50 – 75 mg of "elemental" zinc a day for a week. 50 mg of elemental zinc is the same as 220mg of zinc sulfate. Another source suggests not exceeding 40 mg/day.

2.6   Slow-release **melatonin**. Consider increasing your "In General, Every Day" dose up to perhaps 6mg every evening. If you'd not been taking it every day, now start taking it as per that section.

2.7   20 – 40 mg of **famotidine**, daily.

2.8   We discuss **hydroxychloroquine** in the next section. In addition to the controversy over its use as a cure, there is further controversy about its possible use as a prophylactic. It seems there may be weak evidence of some benefit of using HCQ as a prophylactic. If you have plenty of HCQ on hand, and/or know you can replace your supply if you use it now, there might be some value in using it in that form, particularly because some studies suggest it takes a while for the HCQ to build its levels in your system.

2.9   Possibly increase **Vitamin D** from 2000 to 4000 IU/day.

2.10 Although it seems likely the prime benefit of **aspirin** is in the form of reducing the risk of blood clots, it may possibly have some antiviral properties too. Because, for almost all of us, aspirin is such a benign medication, and many of us take a quarter aspirin every day "just because", I'd probably start taking a full (325 mg) aspirin every day after a high-risk experience and possible exposure to the virus.

2.11 You might want to consider taking **metformin**, in its immediate-release form, twice daily, with a 500 mg dose each time.

2.12 This might seem either excessively trivial, or excessively obvious, but one comment in particular stood out in an email forwarded to us from an HMO in California that is creating an "opinion-leader" role for itself in the fight against the virus.[574] The comment was

> Despite all measures we mentioned, the #1 factor in improvement is bed rest - complete and total.
>
> Bed. Couch. Recliner.
>
> Almost 25% suffered a relapse after recovery, and the number one factor in those cases was discontinuing bed rest.

It is true the average American tends to be sleep deprived these days, so we can understand how simply not stressing your body by lack of sleep can make it more vulnerable to infections.

Consider the possibility or reality of a Covid-19 infection as your "excuse" to treat yourself and take it truly easy for a while.

3. If You Feel You May Be Infected/Mild Illness

Of course, if you think you are infected, see about getting tested, and be careful who you're in contact with until your test results are known.

NIH becomes more equivocal when it comes to treating mild illness. They simply say[575]

Mild Illness

---

[574] Caduceus Medical Group, https://www.caduceusmedicalgroup.com/ or https://cov.cx/a1b82

[575] See https://www.covid19treatmentguidelines.nih.gov/overview/management-of-covid-19/ or https://cov.cx/a1d23

Patients may have mild illness defined by a variety of signs and symptoms (e.g., fever, cough, sore throat, malaise, headache, muscle pain) without shortness of breath, dyspnea on exertion, or abnormal imaging. Most mildly ill patients can be managed in an ambulatory setting or at home through telemedicine or remote visits.

All patients with symptomatic COVID-19 and risk factors for severe disease should be closely monitored. In some patients, the clinical course may rapidly progress.

No specific laboratory evaluations are indicated in otherwise healthy patients with mild COVID-19 disease.

There are insufficient data to recommend either for or against any antiviral or immune-based therapy in patients with COVID-19 who have mild illness.

In my world, albeit not the NIH world, if I have the disease, I'm much more motivated to do anything that promises to possibly reduce its severity. I'm not going to demand a gold-plated guarantee of effectiveness such as NIH seems to require; as long as I'm convinced a treatment doesn't have any downsides, I'll consider it and possibly adopt it.

3.1   I will take two doses of **ivermectin** (aka Stromectol).

3.2   If not already taking it, I'll take 500 mg of **Vitamin C** twice a day, maybe increase to 1000 mg twice a day, depending on my symptoms.

3.3   If you have a way of measuring your cardiac **Qt interval** (see medical equipment, below) then you might wish to consider **hydroxychloroquine**, in conjunction with **zinc**, and *perhaps* adding **azithromycin** as well. Your QTc should be less than 470 msec.[576]

In terms of controversy and risk, taking zinc is probably the safest of these three medicines, with a possible dosage of zinc (from all sources) of around 220 mg a day (in the form of zinc sulfate), taken once a day for five days.

Then comes the HCQ. One source suggests 200 mg twice a day for five days, with an extra 200 mg for the first dose, so 400 mg once then nine doses of 200 mg.

NIH reports a dose (but doesn't endorse it) in one study of 800mg on day one then 400 mg a day for six further days. This is very similar to the other source.

---

[576] This is a great flow-chart for evaluating Qt risk
https://www.massgeneral.org/assets/MGH/pdf/news/coronavirus/QTC-monitoring-guidance.pdf or https://cov.cx/a1d24

NIH reports a common dosage for AZ is 500 mg on the first day, then four doses of 250 mg, one each on days 2 – 5.

Both HCQ and AZ are prescription medicines. If you can't find a doctor to prescribe these, you'd have to order them from an off-shore pharmacy (see the Resources chapter, below).

3.4   Continue daily **aspirin**, anything from a quarter dose (about 80 mg) to a "full" dose (325 mg). I'd take a full dose myself.

3.5   Consider increasing your **melatonin** dose some more. EVMS suggests up to 12 mg, I've seen other literature saying there is no such thing as "too much" melatonin and suggesting what seem like ridiculously large amounts. I hesitate to link to this or say how much!

3.6   Increase your **famotidine** dose to 40 mg/day.

3.7   Continue your **quercetin** (2 x 500 mg).

3.8 If you have a fever or are troubled by aches and pains, take acetaminophen as per its normal dosage directions and be careful to ensure that in total you take no more than 3,000 mg of acetaminophen, from all sources, a day.

3.9   Continue taking **metformin**, in its immediate-release form, twice daily, with a 500 mg dose each time.

3.10 Please   note   -   a   **corticosteroid**   like   dexamethasone   or methylprednisolone seems best for later in an illness – ask if hospitalized, but *probably not before*.

4. Considerations if Hospitalized

This should go without saying, but just to be clear, when you are admitted, be sure to tell the hospital staff about every medicine and supplement you have been taking. Don't keep things a secret.

Don't automatically discontinue everything – if someone says "stop taking that", ask why. "What harm does this cause?" is an appropriate question to ask. The answer is almost certainly "It probably doesn't cause any harm, but it does no good" or some similar variation "It has not been approved for use" or "there is no proof it helps" – statements that are almost reflexive in nature and which seldom mean "I am aware of all the studies including the ones suggesting some possible benefit, and after careful analysis, have clearly determined that for sure there is no benefit to be derived".[577]

---

[577] Be careful of people who do say they are familiar with all the studies. That is more likely to actually mean "I am aware of the studies I am aware of, but I am not aware of
(continued on next page)

While "there is no proof it helps" might be considered a reasonable parameter for some healthcare professionals to recommend discontinuing treatments <u>in cases where they have other choices that are proven to work</u>, that is not the case with Covid.   Remember we are now in a situation where you have a life-threatening illness, against which there is nothing that has been proven to work 100% and for sure quickly cure you.

A fair question to ask in reply is "Other than possibly supplementary oxygen in the future, what will you prescribe, right now, that will be more beneficial than the treatments I have been self-administering?". If the answer is "Nothing", then surely the logic and sense support continuing any course of treatment that has no risks attached to it and which might possibly – even if only to a very unlikely degree – help you in your struggle to get better.

You should ask the doctor(s) if they are familiar with the EVMS treatment guide, and the MATH+ treatment protocol advocated by the Front Line Covid-19 Critical Care Alliance,[578] and the ICAM treatment developed by AdventHealth in Ocala, FL.[579]

These are treatment plans that have been developed by "real" doctors who care for Covid-infected patients every day. They might not be scientifically "proved" to the n-th degree, but these experienced doctors who are actually working with patients and battling the disease have found positive outcomes when they use such treatment plans.

---

the studies I am not aware of" – that seems like an obvious statement, but it is surprising/dismaying how many people fall into that trap.

I can't tell you how often I've heard people say "<u>All</u> the studies show HCQ provides no benefit and may actually be harmful". But the person who makes that statement absolutely never has carefully evaluated, themselves, all the HCQ studies (205 as of mid-December and shown on this site https://c19study.com/ or https://cov.cx/a1a24) – not only that, but whatever source they're relying on probably has not done a complete and careful review, either.

Closely linked are the people who say things like (as was the case in a well-watched YouTube video I don't want to glorify with a link to) "There have been over 1,000 HCQ studies and not a single one has shown any benefit". It beggars belief that the person making that statement has actually found 1,000 different studies, let alone carefully evaluated each one, and consistently found that every positive study, even the refereed ones, are invalid, and every negative study, even the ones that are not refereed, are valid.

[578] See https://covid19criticalcare.com/math-hospital-treatment/ or https://cov.cx/a1d25

[579] See https://www.ocala.com/story/business/2020/09/22/ocala-developed-covid-19-therapy-local-study/5865410002/ or https://cov.cx/a1d26

You want your doctors to at least be familiar with these plans, and if they choose not to adopt them, to be able to articulate and explain why they have decided to ignore them and <u>tell you what treatments they will use instead and why they are better</u>.

If you're now in hospital, doing nothing and hoping for the best is no longer an option.

At-home Treatment if Infected

We've read several accounts from people who suffered from the virus but didn't go to a hospital.

There have been some good suggestions in some of these accounts about items to have and to stock up on beforehand.

- An electrolyte type drink such as Gatorade or Pedialyte.
- Cough medicine to reduce the coughing you might experience.
- Something to reduce your fever. Acetaminophen is a good choice.
- Possibly an anti-nausea drug if you are vomiting a lot.
- Possibly a humidifier if you have dry air which might make some symptoms worse.
- Consider sometimes sleeping on your stomach, which can help your breathing.

But don't stay at home when things get to the point when you should go to a hospital for advanced care. When is that? See back to our section "When Should You Go to Hospital?" in the chapter "6. How to Know if You Have the Virus".

Post-Illness Recovery

One of the distinctive things about this virus is that many people continue to feel less than 100% recovered, even though they've been officially pronounced as "cured". We discuss this in the earlier chapter, "7. How Long Does an Infection Last", and report that 12% of sufferers report lingering malaise 30 or more days after symptoms first appeared. An Irish study puts the number much higher.

Sadly, this is one of the relatively unexplored elements of the virus, and also gets into the realm of Chronic Fatigue Syndrome, which is not a well-understood phenomenon.

We hope there will be more focus on this element of the infection; of course, researchers have focused first on how to reduce mortality and the severity of infections; but with a growing number of people who are now past the worst of their infection but still suffering reduced quality of life, it is time to look at this issue in more detail.

We found a web page that offers eight possible treatments to help people get through the chronic fatigue remains of a Covid infection.[580] The page offers up links to support its various recommendations, although the linked articles vary in persuasiveness such that there's nothing we feel able to unambiguously endorse. But once you are no longer taking meds for the virus infection itself, and if you still feel fatigued, say a week after you are officially "cured", you definitely should consider approaching your doctor, article in hand, and discussing the pluses and minuses of each of the eight possible treatments recommended.

Should You Take a Vaccine

The promise of a vaccine is on the cusp of becoming a reality. In the earlier worst-case scenario, there were fears that any vaccine might be as low as 50% effective, and might only last for three months.[581] But now, the most promising vaccine candidates in mid-December vastly exceed such modest expectations and seem to offer very high efficacy rates and may offer an extended duration of protection.

We discuss issues relating to vaccine development in detail in the section "Vaccination" in our chapter "3. When Will the Virus Finally Go Away?", above, starting on page 102.

For higher-risk people, however, even a 50% reduction in risk would be valuable, and the need for possible quarterly booster shots acceptable. But if you have only a moderate degree of risk, should you get the vaccine if/when one is finally released?

The simple answer is "yes, of course you should". But the question behind the question is "Should you rely upon the vaccine as giving you total protection against the virus?".

A large part of the answer to that question is influenced not only by your personal degree of risk, but by the potential downside if the vaccine doesn't work for you, or if a new virus strain comes along that obsoletes the earlier vaccine. The good news is there are an evolving range of treatments and cures that might allow for most or even all people who become infected with the virus to simply

---

[580] See https://www.thailandmedical.news/news/covid-19-rehab-supplements-that-could-help-with-chronic-fatigue-syndrome-myalgic-encephalomyelitis-manifesting-in-recovered-covid-19-patients or https://cov.cx/a1d27

[581] See https://www.cnbc.com/2020/08/07/coronavirus-vaccine-dr-fauci-says-chances-of-it-being-highly-effective-is-not-great.html or https://cov.cx/a1d28

"take one pill a day for a week" and have the virus go away as quickly and easily as is the case at present when taking antibiotics to cure a sore throat.

But, as of today, no such miracle cure exists, but as the range of treatments possibly extends and becomes more universally accepted, it is possible the risk element might therefore reduce, making it less obviously essential to be vaccinated.

I am not an anti-vaxxer. I abhor the illogic of people who rail against vaccines. The public health benefits of vaccines have been irrefutably proven and should be obvious to all. I do acknowledge there is an extremely small number of people who develop side-effects and complications from a vaccine, but it is a very simple equation cost/benefit equation to evaluate. If a vaccine benefits 1,000 times more people than it harms, doesn't it make sense to vaccinate? Why should the 1,000 people who can benefit from a vaccine be withheld it because of the one person who was harmed – a person who may potentially be harmed more, in any event, by the virus the vaccine was designed to treat?

But when it comes to a Covid-19 vaccine, there may be credible cause for caution based on what seem to be extraordinarily rushed and compressed testing and validation protocols.[582] A normal vaccine takes years to wend its way through the three phases of trials and evaluation before eventually receiving approval, but a Covid-19 vaccine will spend perhaps only six months going through the same process.[583]

---

[582] I was astonished to see this WSJ article reporting on how people who are vaccinated will be given a smartphone app to track if they develop any serious side effects. The article says

"Government health officials and drugmakers plan to roll out extra tools to detect whether Covid-19 vaccines cause any serious side effects once the shots are cleared for widespread use, aiming to fill gaps in existing safeguards given the expected speed and scope of the rollout"

The article goes on to say that instead of the usual six months of monitoring test subjects for side-effects, the FDA is allowing only a two-month period. Maybe we should wait another four months then before choosing if we're vaccinated or not?

This seems to be an open admission that a vaccine will be approved and released without the normal degree of rigorous testing. Personally, I'd prefer to wait for a well-tested vaccine rather than be given one of unknown risk and a smartphone app I can use to report any serious side-effects subsequently! See https://www.wsj.com/articles/covid-19-vaccine-rollout-to-feature-app-tracking-monitoring-of-vulnerable-groups-11604582313 or https://cov.cx/a1d29

[583] This article has an interesting timeline in it – several months for phase 1 trials, several months to two years for phase 2, and 1 – 4 years for a phase 3 trial. There's

(continued on next page)

Furthermore, we all have to acknowledge that the proposed Covid vaccines are not vaccines in the traditional sense of the last 200+ years. A traditional vaccine involves introducing inactivated or related virus particles into the person, thereby training/teaching the body's immune system to recognize a new virus and to work out how to attack it. That "lesson" on a "safe" type of virus is then remembered and can be used to subsequently defend against the real virus threat.

These new mRNA vaccines use a different approach. The approach might work brilliantly and safely. But for twenty years, all attempts at developing safe mRNA vaccines to use against other coronaviruses have failed. Maybe there truly has been a breakthrough and these new vaccines are safe and effective. But are just two or three months of testing, on some small number (less than 100,000) subjects sufficient to guarantee this? I really don't know, but the level of disaster to humanity as a whole if there is a late-onset problem, after hundreds of millions of people have taken the vaccine, defies the imagination and sounds like a James Bond movie villain's plan to depopulate the earth. I have no specific concerns about specific issues, and absolutely don't know enough to be able to have such concerns. But the history of mankind has been filled with hubris and collapse – when people believe they've conquered a problem, only to discover that they completely have not, because they failed to understand the reality of the problem or the limits of their solution.

This was true in the classic case of the "unsinkable" Titanic, and it has been true in biological sciences with various actions in the past, particularly introducing a new species into an ecosystem to combat an existing threat (or just because they seemed like "nice cuddly pets"), only to have the new species become an even greater threat. Examples abound, in my home country of New

---

even a post-approval fourth phase of trialing in many cases, too. So, taking the middle points, and ignoring all the time prior to phase 1 (there is likely a phase 0 trial with human subjects, previous trials with animals, and prior to that, in vitro evaluations in the laboratory with cultured mediums), and all the paperwork preparation time and FDA response times, that is over 3 ½ years on average, and possibly longer than 6 ½ years on the normal timetable. See https://www.fda.gov/patients/drug-development-process/step-3-clinical-research or https://cov.cx/a1d30

What is being sacrificed on this expedited timetable? If the answer is "nothing", then why aren't all drugs tested and evaluated at the same speed? Clearly, something is being marginalized or lost in this expedited trial scenario.

As this second article says, one of the purposes of a phase 3 trial is to evaluate the efficacy and safety of the new drug in the medium and long term. "Medium and long term" is a phrase that demands to be measured in years, not weeks. See https://symbiosisonlinepublishing.com/pharmacy-pharmaceuticalsciences/pharmacy-pharmaceuticalsciences65.php or https://cov.cx/a1d31

Zealand our native kiwis and other birds are now struggling to survive against the threat of imported animals like weasels and stoats, and cuddly rabbits and "deer for hunting" are ravaging the landscapes, while in Australia, the cane toad problem continues to take over the entire country with no apparent solution.

So I don't believe we can be certain, now, that we fully understand every dimension of these new mRNA vaccines, and the consequences of something going wrong could be quite unlike any other disaster we've ever brought upon ourselves.

It is possible the "normal" process (and for normal drugs and vaccines) is unduly leisurely and perhaps also overly cautious. But how far can we compress the timeline and how much assurance of safety can we compromise on before the risks change from "1,000 people benefit for every one person harmed" and become some much less favorable number due to some emergent and previously unanticipated issue?[584]

While this is an essential and necessary question to ask and answer, it is far from certain we will have an accurate answer at the time a vaccine is initially introduced. Yes, for sure, there will have been a Phase 3 trial in which some (hopefully tens of) thousands of people are given the vaccine, and that will provide a reasonable base point of safety data in terms of any side-effects.

But there are two other aspects to that trial to consider. The first is that typically trial volunteers, especially in the early phases, tend to skew more to the healthy side of the spectrum. If you have the same medical profile as the trial volunteers, then the trial data may validly correspond to what you can expect, yourself. But if your medical profile doesn't match that of the people who were participating in the trials, there is more uncertainty about what to expect.

The second concern is the greater one. An accelerated two or three-month trial, unavoidably, can only observe what happens during that period. It can't guarantee the future, and what might happen in four or five months or some years later. Side-effects and unexpected issues might very well not appear immediately, and might only reveal themselves at some future time, and in some unexpected way.

Examples of delayed effects – "late-onset reactions" that could potentially appear in the future include auto-immune disease, infertility, and cancer.

Certainly, it is not likely that some mysterious and negative "X factor" will appear after four months or four years, but it is not impossible. Two vivid

---

[584] What would that number be? Is it a simple majority – if slightly more than half the people who are vaccinated suffer no harm, is that enough? But it isn't just a simple counting of numbers. There are degrees of harm – both in terms of reactions to a vaccine, and in terms of reactions if/when infected by the virus.

examples will indicate how that can sometimes happen. Neither are vaccines, but they might still be helpful examples.

The first is DDT. It was hailed as a wonder pesticide and worked brilliantly well at killing mosquitos and other insects. It was developed in 1874 and brought into widespread use during the early 1940s (ie World War 2), and it took a further 30 years until it was withdrawn in 1972, due to unexpected impacts on other creatures, in particular, the thinning of shells on bird eggs that endangered a vast number of species.[585]

The second is Thalidomide. This drug was discovered in 1953 and first marketed in 1957. It wasn't even a prescription medicine in West Germany, the country that first offered it for sale. Anyone could buy it in their local pharmacy.

It was used to treat anxiety, insomnia, coughs and colds, headaches, and morning sickness, and was deemed to be safe for pregnant women (as of course any drug for morning sickness necessarily must be!). It wasn't until 1961 that its use was associated with a rise in birth defects, and the drug was withdrawn from the market at that time.[586]

Okay, both those examples are many decades old. We are cleverer now – hopefully. But the thing is that at the time, just like back with the Titanic, we thought we were sufficiently clever then, and the problem both then and now is that we don't know what we don't know. We also note that both these cases took years to discover.

An extended trialing program with hundreds of thousands of volunteer subjects with widely varying backgrounds, lifestyles, health, and everything else, and running for a year or longer, provides more time and opportunity for unexpected issues to arise. I've no idea what those unexpected issues might be. Maybe there won't be any at all. But maybe there will be.

It is happily true there have been no spectacular tragedies with vaccines that have been developed and released to date. The CDC has only a very short list of problems with past vaccines that were approved.[587] However, keep in mind that vaccine technology has become a well-developed science over the last 200+ years, but these new "vaccines" are not vaccines in the historical and understood sense of the word. They are entirely new technology, which should demand a closer and more extended study, rather than be rushed through a compressed trial.

---

[585] See http://npic.orst.edu/factsheets/ddtgen.pdf or https://cov.cx/a1d32

[586] See https://en.wikipedia.org/wiki/Thalidomide or https://cov.cx/a1d33

[587] See https://www.cdc.gov/vaccinesafety/concerns/concerns-history.html or https://cov.cx/a1d34

Another point to consider – is the excellent safety record of traditional vaccines because they are inherently safe to start with, or is it a testament to the value of a long evaluation process and extended Phase Three trial? It is generally quoted that about 40% of drugs that make it to a Phase Three trial end up being rejected at this final step in the process.[588]

Phase three testing is not a mere rubber stamp. It is a valid part of the process and causes two out of every five candidate drugs to be rejected. It would be interesting to know whether the 40% that are rejected manifest their problems within the first month or two, or if issues don't appear until after a year or two of extended rigorous testing. There are clear benefits in a full Phase Three trial.

Now let's consider the implication of the worst-case scenario - a vaccine that is 50% effective.[589] If you take a vaccine that is 95%+ effective (as the two mRNA-based vaccines from Moderna and Pfizer and the non-mRNA vaccine from AstraZeneca claim to be), you probably don't give the disease you've been vaccinated against a second thought. You view that risk as having been reduced down to a level that is no longer significant.

But what about a much less effective vaccine, especially one that is barely 50% effective? Will you happily abandon your mask, stop social distancing, and feel entirely relaxed at joining large crowds of loud people in restaurants, bars, night clubs, churches, and sporting events?

For many of us, the answer might be (and probably should be) "No". Reducing our risk by 50% is the same as just adding a coin-toss into the equation, isn't it. "Heads you have the same risk of getting the virus as before, tails you avoid it".

Furthermore, if you're in the unlucky 50%, you *might* get the virus as severely as if you weren't vaccinated at all. [590] So if you're a high-risk person, you might

---

[588] See for example https://academic.oup.com/biostatistics/article/20/2/273/4817524 or https://cov.cx/a1d35

[589] I believe the definition of "effective" being used is "did not get an infection serious enough to require a visit to a doctor". And note also that the 50% level is the minimum effectiveness the FDA is requiring as a condition of approving the vaccine, but it is possible that ultimately approved vaccines may be much more effective than this.

[590] There is a possibility that a vaccine might also provide "some" benefit by causing infections to be weaker than they'd otherwise be, and so while not zeroing out infection rates or hospital admissions, the partially effective vaccine might be more impactful in terms of ultimate mortality/survival rates.

So there could be an entire spectrum of outcomes after being vaccinated. Some people will never get any type of measurable infection, some will get a weaker infection than

(continued on next page)

choose to get the vaccine and also continue with all your current safety procedures. The vaccine is helpful, but not life-changing, if that description fits you.

There's also the uncertainty about how long the vaccine lasts. I don't know, but guess this period of effectiveness is not a binary situation. The vaccine doesn't provide full 100% protection for a certain period of time, and then the next day, its protection level has dropped overnight to 0%. Instead, its protection probably stays at close to whatever its maximum is for a certain period, then at the expiry of that first period, the protection level starts fading away, either in a straight line or in an opposite type of geometric curve – it loses half its effectiveness in a certain time, then in the next same period of time, it loses half of its remaining effectiveness, and so on.

Whether it is a linear or geometric reduction doesn't matter for us right now. What I'm curious about is at what point between "working as well as it ever can" (which, keep in mind, might mean that it is 50% effective) and "no longer works at all" the authorities declare the vaccine needs to be renewed. In other words, if we're told a vaccine that is (say) 90% effective on the day it is administered remains effective for 90 days before you need a booster shot, what is the situation on the 89th day? How effective is it then? Still 90%? Or is 50% the cut-off? Maybe only 25%? Or what?

A related question is does the vaccine's period of effectiveness vary from person to person? Maybe you only have a 60 or 30 day period. Or maybe you have a 180 or 270 day period. Unless you want regular expensive blood tests to check your antibody levels, you have no way of knowing.

One more thing about vaccine effectiveness. If you're in a "high-risk" group due to age or comorbidities, keep in mind that the current very limited trial data may not give any indication of how effective the virus is for your risk category. Don't automatically assume that it will work as well for you as it does for people in lower-risk categories.

There's also the potential for sudden vaccine obsolescence if a new virus strain mutates. This may have already happened in Denmark.[591] If it happens once, it will probably continue to happen in the future.

Another thing that is not yet known is whether a vaccinated person might still get a mild dose of the virus – not severe enough to be inconvenient or life-

---

before, and some will still be impacted much the same as if they'd never been vaccinated.

The current measurement and criteria is very inadequate.

[591] See https://www.theguardian.com/environment/2020/nov/04/denmark-announces-cull-of-15-million-mink-over-covid-mutation-fears or https://cov.cx/a1d36

threatening to the vaccinated person, but an infection that could be passed on to other people. The CEO of Pfizer conceded, in early December, that they don't know if their vaccine will stop people from getting mild doses of the virus and passing it on to other people or not.[592] That's a huge unknown issue that surely should be better understood.

I also feel that with so many vaccines in development at present, and using different approaches to defending against the virus, it might be wise to hold back and see if "better" vaccines appear in the next several months, rather than rushing to take the first vaccine that comes available.

Lots of unknowns.

I find it hard to be too enthusiastic about a vaccine based on a totally new medical process that has been rushed through its testing and trials. It is better than nothing, but it is far from the magic cure-all solution to this scourge that many people are desperately hoping it will be.

I'm going to be selfish, and I'm not going to rush to be among the first to be vaccinated. I'll hold back and allow the people who do get vaccinated to become a very public further validation of the vaccine before holding out my arm for a shot.[593]

So I guess what I'm saying is you should get vaccinated to give me the reassurance I seek to subsequently be vaccinated too!

And hopefully, you don't live in Australia. Australia already is a bit different from most other democratic free countries – voting in elections is mandatory, and the authorities will track you down and fine you if you don't vote (albeit only A$20 for first-time offenders).

It was suggested Australia might make the Covid vaccine mandatory.[594] The suggestion was quickly withdrawn again. But there is a certain sense and logic to making a Covid vaccination mandatory, and (perhaps paradoxically) the more likely it is that people will not wish to be vaccinated, the more beneficial mandatory vaccination becomes as a public health measure.

But three months later, the concept resurfaced in Australia in mid-November, when Qantas, their national airline, announced it would require proof of

---

[592] See https://thehill.com/news-by-subject/healthcare/528619-pfizer-chairman-were-not-sure-if-someone-can-transmit-virus-after or https://cov.cx/a1f95

[593] There's actually a formal name for this. It is called a Phase 4 trial. See https://www.news-medical.net/health/What-is-a-Phase-4-Clinical-Trial.aspx or https://cov.cx/a1d37

[594] See https://www.msn.com/en-us/news/world/coronavirus-vaccine-should-be-mandatory-in-australia-pm/ar-BB187BNS or https://cov.cx/a1d38

vaccination before allowing people onto their international flights.[595] This was a slightly empty announcement when made, not only because no vaccines are yet available, but also because Qantas has canceled all its international flights until probably the second quarter of 2021. My sense is that this is Qantas "encouraging the other airlines in public" to join it in this move, and indeed, their CEO indicated that other carriers are favorably responding to the idea. Probably they said to Qantas "You announce that you'll do it, then we can all wait and see how the public responds".

It all comes back to the herd immunity challenge – the need for 60% or possibly more of the population to become immune so that an infectious person doesn't find other at-risk people to infect. The logic of vaccination, in that respect, is similar to the logic for wearing a mask. When you decide to get vaccinated, you're not only protecting yourself, you're also helping to project everyone else around you too.

And that is how the concept of compulsory vaccination comes about – the people around you may demand your participation in the vaccine program, not for your sake, but for theirs.

- *In Summary*

I've taken a roundabout look at the pluses and minuses of the current likely vaccines we might be offered. The most important point to me is they are based on new medical techniques and are being rushed to market with less testing and trialing than is normally given to well known traditional vaccine development programs. I'm not an anti-vaxxer, and I agree with and support just about all currently offered vaccines, before Covid, so my caution about the Covid vaccine does not spring from an underlying suspicion of vaccines per se.

Surprisingly, we have a high tolerance for unknown risk with these new vaccines, but a low tolerance for almost zero risk with treatment medicines that have been in use for decades and are known to be safe (but not necessarily yet known to be fully effective in treating the Covid virus). This is a strange and unsettling disconnect.

Should you be vaccinated? If you are at high risk – both in terms of a high risk of having a severe or possibly fatal case of the virus if infected, and in terms of likelihood of being exposed and infected, then the vaccine becomes more appealing.

But if you can minimize your risk, and if the chances are that an infection may not necessarily be life-threatening, and if you have access to the potential treatments discussed in the next chapter, then maybe delay a vaccine as long as

---

[595] See https://www.bbc.com/news/world-australia-55048438 or https://cov.cx/a1d39

you can, allowing others to continue to be a "Phase Four" trial of their safety. At the same time, you're giving time for other vaccines, using other methodologies, to appear. There's absolutely no reason whatsoever to believe that the very first vaccine to request Emergency Use Authorization is also the very best vaccine, quite possibly, a vaccine that completes testing in the future might be more appropriate and appealing.

As long as you are sure time is on your side, and assuming you don't need to "give in" and be vaccinated as a condition of your work, or because you want to travel internationally, it might make sense not to be among the first wave of people to be vaccinated.

16. Medicines, Supplements, Vitamins, etc

T his section details the various products we mention in earlier sections, provides some details about each and explains why some people are advocating their use in Covid treatment plans.

One important point, in case you're speed reading through this. **Just because a product is listed does not mean we're actually endorsing or recommending it**. Several of the products appear on the basis of "do *not* take this". Others appear because they have been suggested elsewhere so we mention them to give you information on them, but their mention is more neutral rather than positive.

Some of the products we mention require a prescription and some do not. You might think that you can freely take any over-the-counter (OTC) medications without a second thought because, if there were risks with them, they'd be limited to prescription use only. You might think that even more strongly when it comes to vitamins and other "healthy supplements" because how could such "good" things ever be bad? Those are appealing thoughts, but somewhat of an oversimplification, particularly if you're going to be taking three or four or more different medications, vitamins and supplements simultaneously.

Even choosing OTC medicines, vitamins and supplements is something that is best done in consultation with a doctor or pharmacist – there may be interactions between some of the medications and others, or possibly interactions between the OTC and any prescription medicines.

The prescription medicines are often not specifically intended to be used to treat Covid-19 – how could they be, with the virus only becoming an issue in about March of 2020?

But that doesn't mean that drugs primarily used for other purposes can not lawfully be prescribed for Covid-19 treatments, too. Perhaps I should start this chapter with an explanation on that point.

Off-Label Use

There has been a lot of activity trying to find existing drugs that have already been proven to be safe, and which now show positive impacts on virus patients.

To get a new drug approved requires two things to be established – obviously that the drug is helpful, and secondly that it is safe. If there is an existing drug that has already been shown to be safe, that is a huge saving in time and money and resource, and allows the focus on the existing drug to be primarily whether or not it helps people with Covid.

Every prescription drug has been FDA approved and is required to have a "label" (usually quite a large-sized sheet of paper rather than a small label) that describes the drug, its *approved* uses, dosage information, and assorted other information too. But, there's an interesting issue – while the FDA controls what medicines can and can not be prescribed in general; it does not control the medical profession and so can not and does not approve, control, or restrict the purposes for which the medicine can be used.[596]

That would seem a bit counter-intuitive and to create a major loophole in the otherwise vast and intense regulatory framework. Yes, indeed it does. Drugs have to go through a validation process to demonstrate their efficacy at *something*, and have to have a label describing their approved use(s). But doctors are then free to prescribe the drug for *anything they wish*, with their only restrictions being common sense and professional competency, ethics, liability worries, and what insurance companies will pay for.

While these are indeed major constraints, it is interesting to note that fully one in every five prescriptions written in the US these days is thought to be for off-label purposes.[597] Most of us also prefer the concept of being able to decide in conjunction, one-on-one, with our personal physician, about what is best for us, rather than relying on a bureaucracy that is trying to make "one size fits all"

[596] See https://www.drugwatch.com/health/off-label-drug-use/ or https://cov.cx/a1d40 for a thoughtful discussion of the topic

[597] See https://www.webmd.com/a-to-z-guides/features/off-label-drug-use-what-you-need-to-know#1 or https://cov.cx/a1d41

regulations, and which is unavoidably months, probably years behind the latest research and potential uses of every drug out there. So whether this is a deliberate policy or an accidental loophole, most of us will be pleased it is out there.

We suspect doctors might sometimes choose to shelter behind not-completely-correct statements of the form "this drug isn't approved for that purpose". Maybe the drug is not approved for a specific purpose, but just because it is not formally approved does not mean it is illegal for the doctor to prescribe it for other purposes if he chooses to do so.

If your doctor tries to kill the discussion with a statement like that, say "Yes, I understand that, but I also understand there are no restrictions on you using your discretion and best professional judgment to prescribe it on an off-label basis for this purpose". That signals to him that you can't be bluffed by vague half-truths.

One more point about off-label use. It costs a lot of money for a drug company to go through a formal process to add a new "indication" – a new disease for which its drug is "indicated" as a suitable treatment. If there is a large *and profitable* market opportunity, the drug manufacturer will probably choose to go through the process, because it is a sensible business decision, particularly because drug manufacturers are not allowed to specifically promote their drugs for off-label uses.

But if it is a small market opportunity, or not profitable, it makes no business sense to go through the process, even though the evidence and support for adding a new treatment indication to the drug's label may be very obvious and incontrovertible. Particularly for older drugs with expired patents, it is quite likely there is no commercial sense in applying for a new indication because that means any other company can then manufacture the same drug for the same indication too. With a much narrower profit margin and the ability of competitors to benefit from a new use approval, the costs of the application may be too high compared to the benefits from the approval.

The point we are making here is simply to say that just because a drug use is off-label does not mean it is necessarily any more risky or any less beneficial than the drug's on-label use.[598] The approved uses for a drug are as much an expression of "which uses can we make money from" as they are an expression of "what are the most beneficial purposes for this drug".

---

[598] This is a good explainer about off-label use, written from a Canadian perspective but generally applicable to the US too
https://www.cadth.ca/sites/default/files/pdf/off_label_use_of_drugs_pro_e.pdf or
https://cov.cx/a1d42 and this is a more technical article that tells you a great deal more
https://www.ncbi.nlm.nih.gov/pmc/articles/PMC3538391/ or https://cov.cx/a1d43

So by all means approach your physician and after discussing your situation say "Will you please prescribe me a course of (drug name) as an off-label treatment for this". It is, after all, your body, and as long as you are making a well-informed decision, surely you should have at least an equal say in how your illnesses are treated.

There's one other "card to play" when asking your doctor for prescription meds. "If President Trump got all the various medications he did, immediately he first came down with symptoms, why can't I get the same things he did?" That's a fair question to ask, isn't it, although we don't recommend the same apparent treatment regime and timing as President Trump received, we do recommend that you don't wait until "too late" to start taking anti-virals and other drugs to help fight the virus and its effects.

The Volatility of This Information

It is important to appreciate that the truth, as we think we understand it, continues to change and evolve when it comes to Covid treatments. Even in the short several months I've been writing this book, there have been changes – a drug that was thought to be harmful to use (ibuprofen) has now been exonerated of blame and deemed safe to use. Other things that had only weak support (Vitamin D) are becoming more strongly recommended, and entirely new treatments such as ivermectin are becoming prominent, too.

We will keep this section reasonably updated in the Kindle eBook, and believe there is a way you can get updated versions of the eBook at no cost as part of how Kindle eBooks "work". We'll make several updated revisions available before publishing a completely new edition at some future point.

We also note there is an abundance of articles on the internet on every one of the items we list in this section. Some are positive and some are negative. Some are more convincing and reliable than others.[599] I've only cited two or three articles to support each of the products I'm calling to your attention here. After having done a dispassionate search of the good and bad for any product, I've then

---

[599] We recommend you re-read the footnote way back near the beginning, in our first chapter, about internet "recommendation management" companies that can magically cause negative articles to disappear and flood the internet with positive articles. It can sometimes be very difficult to separate the serums from the snake oils.

We also repeat the awkward statement that just because a person is a credentialed doctor does not make them an unassailable authority and automatically "ex officio" an expert on and correct about every element of medical science. There are some truly strange doctors out there. If you'd like a relevant direct example, there is this https://www.npr.org/2020/10/01/914433778/web-of-wellness-doctors-promote-injections-of-unproven-coronavirus-treatment or https://cov.cx/a1d44

deliberately featured primarily what I feel to be credible articles sufficient as to at least encourage you to then do further research yourself.

If you find anything unconvincing – whether it is something I say,[600] something a healthcare professional says, or something you encounter in any other context, do your own additional research.

The FDA is trying its best to shut down websites that make direct claims of efficacy for various substances that have not been proven, to FDA standards, to actually work to reduce the impact of a Covid infection. It is interesting and helpful to read their page of information and to see some of the warning letters they have sent to offenders, to understand what is and is not acceptable to say about such products and to ensure that you're not allowing your enthusiasm to run away with you to the point that implied claims on websites and elsewhere are interpreted more positively by you than they should be.[601]

Make Your Own Decisions

Do your own due diligence – do Google searches for the various items here using search phrases like "(drug name) Covid" and see what newer information appears.[602] Be careful to make sure you are indeed reading new information and studies – sometimes articles appear long after a study they are quoting has been published – try and see the original study paper so you can understand how up to date each study is. And, just like most other topics, the original headlines tend to linger on long after the tiny retraction/correction is subsequently issued.

---

[600] Within reason, and time allowing, I try to reply to emails in the spirit in which they are written. If you send me a thoughtful email and reasoned argument that does not align with my own, I'll try to respond in kind. Your emails and opinions help me as I seek to continue to evolve and enhance this document, for all our future benefits.

[601] See https://www.fda.gov/consumers/health-fraud-scams/fraudulent-coronavirus-disease-2019-covid-19-products or https://cov.cx/a1d45 At the time of writing (8 October) there are 118 warning letters listed. Four weeks later, the total had swelled to 127 warning letters.
But please understand that the absence of an FDA warning letter does not mean that any product is approved, or safe, or accurately described. It might just mean the FDA hasn't received a complaint about the product yet.

[602] I recommend you use exactly that simple search string. By just mentioning the name of the drug/treatment and the word Covid, you cast the widest net for both positive and negative articles, rather than influencing the results with a question seeking specific types of articles. But, of course, search every which way that seems to give you the best information.

Bad information has a life all of its own, and at times, it seems to thrive more than the good.

Be sure to look at the side-effects associated with every one of these products and make sure they don't apply to you and the interactions with other things you might be taking (see our section "Drug Interactions" in the chapter, "14. Include Your Doctor in Your Decision-Making", above).

When we say things like "can't hurt" or "no downside" we are not guaranteeing that everyone can take the product in question, free of any possible risk. We are saying that risks are unlikely and uncommon, but **you always need to check your own situation against the products being described**.

You'll also need to set your own parameters for what will persuade you to add a new product to the ones you may already take or plan to take.

For example, if you read five refereed papers that all show a certain drug is of no benefit whatsoever, and then find a sixth paper, not refereed, that points to some significant benefit, what do you do? Allow the five negative findings to outweigh the one positive?

That's a trick question. The five refereed papers are not essentially negative. They are neutral. They are saying "in this set of test conditions, with these particular people, and with the following definitions of what constitutes beneficial outcomes, we have failed to observe the beneficial outcome we require to deem it a success". That is not necessarily a negative outcome, *other than within the narrow test scenario it exists within*.

But don't overgeneralize, and remember the saying "absence of proof is not the same as proof of absence".[603]

It is a bit like fishing – you might go fishing for an hour and catch nothing. That doesn't mean there are no fish there, it just means you didn't catch any. But if you go fishing and you do catch a fish, then you know there was at least one fish there and might be more.

---

[603] It is possible to construct high-quality trials that actually will go most of the way towards providing a proof of absence, but there are so many ways that researchers can unwittingly create flawed tests, or do a flawed analysis of the results, that there often remains some ambivalence as to whether a negative outcome is more generally applicable as a "proof of absence" or narrowly a mere "absence of proof" in the scenario that was tested.

This is also not to say that any test with apparently positive results is automatically right, whereas tests with apparently negative results are automatically wrong. It truly is all very complicated, with sincere experts sometimes arguing totally opposite sides of an issue, all convinced of the rightness of their opinion and the wrongness of the other opinion.

In this hypothetical example, I'd take note of the five negative studies, but if I could see some relevance and correspondence in the one positive study, then I'd find that more meaningful and influential.

A classic example of this is hydroxychloroquine. Some reasonably convincing studies show no benefit from HCQ use. But they need to be considered in the context of what they were testing. Were they testing HCQ in the early stages of the disease, or as a last-ditch hope for people on ventilators? What was the dose of HCQ being administered? Was it used alone, or in conjunction with other medications? What was the success/failure test? How long were the test subjects evaluated for?

Other reasonably convincing studies show HCQ providing significant benefits. See if you can determine what the difference between the scenarios for positive and negative use are, and then, if your case falls within the positive outcome scenarios, you should feel encouraged.

The other thing to consider is safety and negative outcomes associated with the use of these products. If there are risks associated with using a particular drug, you'd obviously be more reluctant to use it "just in case" and more demanding of a high degree of certainty that the possible benefits more than outweighed the possible negative consequences.

Similar "swings and roundabouts" apply to issues of cost and availability.

An obvious example of these considerations would be aspirin or Vitamin C. Negative consequences of taking either of these products? For most of us, about as close to none as possible. Possible positive consequences? Uncertain, unproven, but possibly there might be some benefit and lessening of severity if you have contracted the virus. Cost? Very low. Availability? Very readily available.

If that's a decision-making approach that appeals to you, you'd probably decide to take some aspirin and Vitamin C accordingly. "Can't hurt, doesn't cost, might help" being the bottom-line conclusion you might reach.

Good luck!

The List

You'll see frequent references to EVMS, FLCCC, and ASHP as support sources. Rather than link every time, here is the information about them :

ASHP : The American Society of Health-System Pharmacists' Assessment of Evidence for Covid-19-Related Treatments.[604] Note that this is regularly

---

[604] See https://www.ashp.org/-/media/assets/pharmacy-practice/resource-centers/Coronavirus/docs/ASHP-COVID-19-Evidence-Table.ashx or https://cov.cx/a1d46

updated. What you see might not be what I saw, so if the version of their document you see contradicts what I said was in their document, clearly there has been new information added. They do show when items are updated, but they only show it as updated for a short while before removing the indicator.

EVMS : The Eastern Virginia Medical School's pages on Covid Care for Clinicians. We recommend the lengthier complete protocol, but the two-pager gives you a good summary of the longer 30-page document.[605]

FLCCC : The Frontline Covid-19 Critical Care Alliance – a group of physicians and teaching professors who have formulated both a preventative (prophylactic)/early treatment program they call I-MASK+ and a program for hospitalized patients they call MATH+. A leading figure in this group, Dr Paul Marek, is also a prominent member of the EVMS group, so there is some overlap in opinions and approaches.[606]

NIH : The National Institute of Health's Covid-19 Treatment Guidelines.[607]

The following list is in alphabetical order. At the top of each product is a quick summary on two lines, the first line showing which scenarios the particular product is recommended for, and the second line showing if the product can be freely purchased, or if a prescription is required.

If a product can be freely purchased, we usually include an Amazon link, although there is probably not a lot of need for that when it comes to some of the most commonplace things such as aspirin.

If a prescription is needed and you can't find a doctor who will agree to prescribe the product, you can see our discussion in the appendix "Appendix - Resources", below on page 444.

---

[605] Main page https://www.evms.edu/covid-19/covid_care_for_clinicians/ or https://cov.cx/a1d47
Summary two pages
https://www.evms.edu/media/evms_public/departments/internal_medicine/Marik-Covid-Protocol-Summary.pdf or https://cov.cx/a1d48
Detailed protocol
https://www.evms.edu/media/evms_public/departments/internal_medicine/EVMS_Critical_Care_COVID-19_Protocol.pdf or https://cov.cx/a1d49

[606] See https://covid19criticalcare.com/ or https://cov.cx/a1d06

[607] Main page https://www.covid19treatmentguidelines.nih.gov/ or https://cov.cx/a1d51
PDF including all sections of their guidelines
https://files.covid19treatmentguidelines.nih.gov/guidelines/covid19treatmentguidelines.pdf or https://cov.cx/a1d52

- *Alcohol*

Use only in moderation

Alcohol depresses the immune system.

It is best to be moderate with your alcohol intake, and if you feel you're at risk or infected, you should stop drinking alcohol entirely until you are recovered.

- *Aspirin*

Every Day	After Exposure	Mild Infection

No Prescription Needed	Prescription Required

Perhaps the original "wonder-drug", you might be as surprised as I was to see aspirin on the EVMS list of recommended treatments for mild Covid infections.

EVMS doesn't explain the reason for its inclusion, but we surmise it probably is because of its blood-thinning and anti-clotting properties.[608]

Aspirin is also on the very similar to EVMS FLCCC I-MASK+ protocol. They suggest 80-100mg of aspirin daily as a prophylaxis and 325 mg as an early-stage treatment, while making the note "unless contraindicated".

The McCullough plan also calls out aspirin, primarily as a blood thinner/anticoagulant, and also countenances perhaps adding other drugs too.

There are also suggestions that aspirin may have some antiviral properties which might give a degree of protection against acquiring a Covid infection in the first place.[609]

Aspirin is one of those "probably won't harm and possibly might help" type treatments (as are essentially all the others mentioned). It is extremely low cost and non-impactful in other ways for most people, and many people are already

---

[608] See https://medicalxpress.com/news/2020-05-blood-thinners-treatment-covid-science.html or https://cov.cx/a1d53 although the article cautiously does not go as far as to recommend aspirin usage

[609] See this article from the International Aspirin Foundation – although perhaps not the most obviously impartial of sources! https://www.aspirin-foundation.com/forum/aspirin-and-covid-19/ or https://cov.cx/a1d54

taking a quarter dose (ie about 80 mg) of aspirin every day because of other possibly beneficial properties.

President Trump's treatment, after he was tested positive, included aspirin.

- *Azithromycin*

Every Day	After Exposure	Mild Infection

No Prescription Needed	Prescription Required

Azithromycin (AZ) has primarily been proposed as a possible Covid treatment in conjunction with hydroxychloroquine, rather than as a standalone treatment. AZ is an antibiotic, and as such would seem to have no impact on a virus whatsoever, although there are suggestions that it may have some antiviral properties too.[610]

There is an article in response to the linked article above that argues against using AZ,[611] but it does so due to concern that its over-prescription is encouraging the growth of antibiotic-resistant bacteria. [612] This anti-AZ article does not challenge the original article's claims about AZ having antiviral properties.

But if we found ourselves definitely with Covid-19, and if we had sufficient comorbidities as to make it a risky infection for us, we'd probably work on the basis of "a bird in the hand is worth two in the bush" and ask for azithromycin treatment now to solve the immediate disease, rather than hold off on it because

---

[610] See https://www.ncbi.nlm.nih.gov/pmc/articles/PMC7290142/ or https://cov.cx/a1d55

[611] See https://www.ncbi.nlm.nih.gov/pmc/articles/PMC7438973/ or https://cov.cx/a1d56

[612] We certainly understand and are similarly concerned about the growing and very worrying problem of drug-resistant bacteria and the underlying massive over-prescription of antibiotics.

Sometimes it seems doctors prescribe antibiotics more as a placebo than out of any real expectation it will do any good, and because patients demand it and it is easier to prescribe it than to spend extended time attempting to educate a patient. There may even be, in the minds of some doctors, concerns about getting a bad rating on one of the growing number of websites that allow patients to rate their doctors.

of concern about reducing our treatment options for some hypothetical future infection that we might not even live to experience!

The main reason for prescribing AZ in conjunction with HCQ is controlling inflammation and bacterial lung infections as a secondary/side-effect of the Covid infection. In this respect, it might also be valuable as a standalone treatment for severe Covid cases.[613]

Azithromycin is perhaps not as controversial as HCQ, but both have the same possible side-effect of slowing down your heart's Qt interval. **Taking AZ and HCQ together therefore poses more of a possible risk than taking either alone**.

Get your doctor to explain this to you and determine if it is something to be concerned about (ie have your doctor test your Qt interval, and ideally then monitor it during your treatment plan).[614]

The AZ dosage has been suggested at 500 mg once on the first day then 250 mg for each of the next four days. This is lower than a typical AZ dosing plan when used alone as an antibiotic.

It is mentioned by NIH, although largely in a negative manner in conjunction with HCQ use.

The McCullough plan suggests either using AZ or doxycycline. Doxycycline does not have the risk of heart Qt interval prolongation, and so might be a better choice if this is a possible concern/issue.

- *BCG Vaccination*

Every Day (One Time)	After Exposure	Mild Infection

No Prescription Needed	Prescription Required

---

[613] See https://www.thelancet.com/journals/lancet/article/PIIS0140-6736(20)31863-8/fulltext or https://cov.cx/a1d57

[614] If it is not practical for ongoing monitoring in your doctor's office, consider getting the AliveCor KardiaMobile 6L so you can monitor your Qt interval at home, possibly in conjunction with sending your results over the internet to your physician or any other interpreting service to double-check what is happening to your Qt interval.

See our chapter on Medical Equipment and Supplies You Should Have for more information on this device.

This is one of our more speculative recommendations, and we justify it on the basis that it might be a useful and beneficial thing to have anyway.

The BCG, or to give its full name, the Bacillus Calmette–Guérin vaccine was first used in 1921 and is primarily a vaccine against tuberculosis. It is on WHO's list of Essential Medicines and is given to about 100 million children, globally, every year.

What has this to do with Covid, you might ask? Well, there seems to be a possible correlation between a country's level of BCG vaccination and its level of Covid activity. There has long been a major puzzle as to why some countries have very high levels of Covid activity while other seemingly identical and even adjacent countries have very much lower levels. It seems unlikely to be climate or geography based, and not even race or lifestyle based.

Some sort of other national difference appears to exist, and one possibility that is being suggested is that countries that have been widely vaccinating children against TB with the BCG vaccine appear to have lower Covid case rates than countries that have not had this policy. Studies seem to confirm this correlation at a national level,[615] and other studies of specific case by case individuals also point to a major reduction in Covid activity in people who have had the BCG vaccine.[616]

While relatively uncommon in the US, TB is still present.[617] Tuberculosis rates are dropping slowly, worldwide, but it is still prevalent in some countries such as India, China, Indonesia, the Philippines, Pakistan, Nigeria, Bangladesh, and South Africa. Worldwide it is one of the top ten causes of death, with 1.5 million people dying in 2018. And because tuberculosis is becoming increasingly drug-resistant, being vaccinated is prudent.[618]

---

[615] See https://www.ncbi.nlm.nih.gov/pmc/articles/PMC7395502/ or https://cov.cx/a1d58 and https://www.ncbi.nlm.nih.gov/pmc/articles/PMC7432030/ or https://cov.cx/a1d59 and https://www.medicalnewstoday.com/articles/mandatory-bcg-vaccination-may-slow-spread-of-covid-19 or https://cov.cx/a1d60

[616] See https://www.ncbi.nlm.nih.gov/pmc/articles/PMC7360951/ or https://cov.cx/a1d61

[617] See https://www.cdc.gov/tb/publications/factsheets/statistics/tbtrends.htm or https://cov.cx/a1d62

[618] See https://www.who.int/news-room/fact-sheets/detail/tuberculosis or https://cov.cx/a1d63

So, on the basis that a BCG vaccination has other benefits and no downside,[619] why not get one and hope for some Covid resistance, too. The vaccine is available in the US, but the CDC is unenthusiastic about its general use.[620] The bottom-line? A BCG vaccination can't hurt and might help.

- *Budesonide*

> **Not (Yet) Recommended**

Budesonide is a corticosteroid. There have been suggestions that when taken in an inhaler it may help minimize the severity of a Covid infection.

The advocacy seems to come almost exclusively from a controversial doctor in Texas, Dr Richard Bartlett. As best we can tell, he is basing his enthusiasm for budesonide on an analysis of two patients he treated with the inhaled drug.[621] It should go without saying that a two-patient study of this type has no valid significance whatsoever. We don't know if the patients wouldn't have recovered by themselves without taking the budesonide, we don't know if there was a placebo effect, we don't really know much at all.

The weakness of his advocacy has been pointed to in several responses.[622] We find ourselves more persuaded by the dissenters than by Dr Bartlett.[623]

While there may be a difference between taking steroids in tablet form and in a nebulizer that delivers the dose directly into the lungs, and perhaps this difference is beneficial both in terms of directly attacking the virus and not impacting so much on the body's immune system, we feel this is a case where the downside may be greater than the upside. Our concern is the budesonide may

---

[619] See https://www.bbc.com/news/health-54465733 or https://cov.cx/a1d64

[620] See https://www.cdc.gov/tb/publications/factsheets/prevention/bcg.htm or https://cov.cx/a1d65

[621] See http://covidsilverbullet.com/wp-content/uploads/2020/07/Bartlett_COVID_Case_Study.pdf or https://cov.cx/a1d66

[622] See https://www.factcheck.org/2020/08/asthma-medicine-not-proven-as-covid-19-cure/ or https://cov.cx/a1d67 and https://fortune.com/2020/07/24/budesonide-coronavirus-covid-richard-bartlett/ https://cov.cx/a1d68 or (and many others)

[623] It is very untrue to suggest "David has never met a quack treatment he doesn't embrace"! I'm as skeptical as anyone, but I'm also open to wherever persuasive studies lead me.

depress the overall immune system and reduce its ability to fight off the virus infection, which would of course be quite the opposite outcome to that hoped for.

So for that reason, we do not recommend budesonide, at least not based on this one only positive report. There are clinical trials that are due to start reporting in November/December, and maybe they will confirm Dr Bartlett's findings. But until then, this is one possible treatment we'll be avoiding.

- *Corticosteroids*

> Not Appropriate for Home Use

Corticosteroids such as dexamethasone, prednisone, methylprednisolone, and hydrocortisone should **NOT** be used for preventative or early illness use, but they do seem to have clear benefit for patients admitted to hospital when the disease gets to a point where such drugs can help rather than hinder the body's fight against the virus.

Corticosteroids can reduce the body's immune system activity. This is a bad thing when your body is first fighting the virus – it needs all the help it can get. But, later, after having lost the first few "battles", your immune system can "panic" and go into dysfunctional "overdrive" – at this point you want to "calm it down", and corticosteroids can help at this point. But when is that point? That's not a determination you should make, unaided.

NIH comments on corticosteroid use here.[624]

President Trump started taking dexamethasone on, we believe, Saturday 3 October while hospitalized. This is surprisingly early in an infection to take a steroid. Either he had an unusually rapid progression of the virus, or he may have had the virus for longer than the stories of the first positive test being on Thursday (or even Wednesday) suggest.

The McCullough plan prefers prednisone, and the reason for the preference is discussed in this podcast with Dr McCullough.[625]

---

[624] See partway down this page
https://www.covid19treatmentguidelines.nih.gov/tables/table-3a/ or
https://cov.cx/a1d69 and the dedicated section
https://www.covid19treatmentguidelines.nih.gov/immune-based-
therapy/immunomodulators/corticosteroids/ or https://cov.cx/a1d70

[625] See https://www.youtube.com/watch?v=fdbwTNNsF1E or https://cov.cx/a1d71 –
from memory, it is mentioned 1/3 to 1/2 of the way through.

- *Famotidine*

Every Day	After Exposure	Mild Infection

No Prescription Needed	https://amzn.to/2PzjKKV or https://cov.cx/a1f47

Famotidine is best known as a heartburn relief product sold as Pepcid. In addition to its properties in that respect, it has been shown to do two other good things that help combat a Covid infection.[626]

The first is it can inhibit viral replication, so the virus doesn't grow as quickly, giving your body time to build up an effective defense against a weaker attacker.

The second bonus feature is it stimulates the immune cells, helping them to effectively combat the virus.

According to this article,[627] hospitalized patients who took famotidine were 45% less likely to die and 48% less likely to need a ventilator. In other words, your chances of avoiding the most severe of the virus effects, and most of all, your chances of surviving, almost double if you're taking famotidine.

President Trump's treatment, after he tested positive for Covid-19, included famotidine.

- *Favipiravir*

Every Day	After Exposure	Mild Infection

No Prescription Needed	Prescription Required

---

[626] See the detailed discussion and links here https://covid19criticalcare.com/math-hospital-treatment/scientific-review-of-covid-19-and-math-plus/#1596446829797-a8266904-e8a9 or https://cov.cx/a1d72

[627] See https://hartfordhealthcare.org/about-us/news-press/news-detail?articleId=28305&publicid=497 or https://cov.cx/a1d73

Favipiravir (also known by the brand Avigan) is a relatively new drug and was first marketed as an antiviral drug to help combat influenza.[628] It has been shown to inhibit 53 different types of 'flu viruses. It has also been shown to have a positive impact on assorted other virus diseases too,[629] although trials for use against Ebola have demonstrated only weak effectiveness in that specific role.

It was used by the Chinese in their Wuhan outbreak early in 2020, and since then has been used, with varying degrees of official approval, in countries such as varied as Italy, Japan, Russia, Ukraine, Uzbekistan, Moldova, Kazakhstan, Saudi Arabia, UAE, Turkey, Bangladesh, Egypt, and India. Both Canada and the US have trials currently underway.[630]

Studies suggest it is most beneficial when given to people with mild to moderate rather than severe cases of the virus.[631] It seems that benefits are positive but not overwhelming, although who among us would not refuse any benefit and improvement in our experience and survival odds?[632]

One of its benefits is it can be given orally rather than intravenously, making it better suited for outpatient use. It is commonly given in a dose of 1800 mg

---

[628] Please keep in mind that although the symptoms of influenza and Covid-19 are similar, the viruses causing each are totally different. So it doesn't automatically follow that an anti-viral agent that works against the various influenza viruses will also work against the SARS-CoV-2 virus that causes Covid-19.

[629] See https://www.ncbi.nlm.nih.gov/pmc/articles/PMC7467067/ or https://cov.cx/a1d74

[630] See https://www.contagionlive.com/news/fda-clears-favipiravir-covid19-facility-outbreak-prevention-study or https://cov.cx/a1d75

[631] See https://www.ncbi.nlm.nih.gov/pmc/articles/PMC7467067/ or https://cov.cx/a1d76 and https://www.trialsitenews.com/the-dhaka-trial-clear-cut-evidence-favipiravir-effective-against-covid-19-with-compelling-results/ or https://cov.cx/a1d77 and https://www.sciencedirect.com/science/article/pii/S1876034120305931 or https://cov.cx/a1d78 and https://www.trialsitenews.com/can-favipiravir-compete-against-remdesivir-in-north-america-targeting-covid-19/ or https://cov.cx/a1d79

[632] See https://www.trialsitenews.com/avigan-favipiravir-meets-endpoints-in-phase-3-japanese-clinical-trial-sponsor-will-register-as-a-therapy-for-covid-19/ or https://cov.cx/a1d80

twice on the first day, and then 800 mg twice a day for 13 more days.[633] In India, the cost of this complete course of treatment is US$100.[634] The drug patent expired in 2019 and a growing number of companies are now making it in generic form, and we expect its cost will drop as a result.

Overall, it seems the evidence to support the efficacy of favipiravir is currently mild rather than compelling, but at the same time, it is encouraging rather than discouraging. It is featured in one of the treatment options in the McCullough plan, but we are not certain if the drug is available in the US.

We note a suggestion that you should be careful if using it in conjunction with acetaminophen, if you are a pregnant woman, and to be aware that it too may lead to Qt interval prolongation (mentioned in the ASHP document).

- *Homeopathic Remedies*

Every Day	After Exposure	Mild Infection

No Prescription Needed	

This entry, and the subsequent entry on Traditional Chinese Medicine and Folk Medicine are added primarily for completeness and to ensure you don't overlook them. But they are not added as recommendations per se.

Homeopathy is a bizarre concept. It starts off from a curious claim – the same things that cause illnesses in large doses can cure them in small doses – and then it builds on that concept by making the small doses really really small. Vanishingly small.

Indeed, not just vanishing, but vanished – the dilution of products is so extreme that often you'll end up with a homeopathic remedy that has been so diluted that there isn't a single molecule of the medicinal substance remaining in each pill.

So how can a pill containing nothing except filler and dried pure water (that's essentially a nonsense concept, by the way – dried pure water leaves nothing behind!) work at all? Homeopathic advocates claim that the process of vigorous

---

[633] See https://www.ncbi.nlm.nih.gov/pmc/articles/PMC7467067/ or https://cov.cx/a1d81 Note that the entire 14-day course is not needed if the patient has fully recovered prior to then.

[634] See https://www.trialsitenews.com/favipiravir-sales-skyrocket-in-india-targeting-mild-covid-19-cases/ or https://cov.cx/a1d82

agitation before each stage of dilution – a process they call "succussion" somehow mysteriously causes the water to "remember" the presence of the active ingredient that is now being diluted away to nothingness.[635]

Some studies have suggested some effectiveness from some homeopathic remedies for some ailments. I've sometimes felt that using Oscillococcinum has helped me get over colds more quickly. But maybe there is a placebo effect, and I've never actually analyzed any study to see how rigorous its procedure is and how statistically significant its findings are.

If you like exploring alternative medicines, you'll find a lot of people who believe in homeopathic remedies, so you're in good company. I am not endorsing it at all, but I'm similarly not going to criticize it just because I don't understand it, either. Do your own due diligence and perhaps consider any such remedies to be in addition to other treatments you might be taking.

This seems like a reasonably fair and comprehensive explanation of homeopathy, although obviously from the perspective of supporters of the field.[636] Here's an interesting report on the success of homeopathy in a very small trial in Italy.[637] And this website has some Covid/homeopathy resources.[638] Here's a surprising additional source of information about homeopathic remedies for regular 'flu – Kaiser Permanente.[639]

I recommend you to cautiously proceed with an open mind.

[635] Cynics have wondered that if water remembers such things, when does it forget? Maybe never? Does all water on the planet "remember" everything that has been dissolved in it? And so on. Homeopathy really is a bizarre concept.

[636] See https://arizonahomeopathic.org/homeopathy-and-covid-19/ or https://cov.cx/a1d83

[637] See https://homeopathic.com/italian-mds-study-results-on-homeopathic-treatment-of-50-covid-19-patients-none-of-whom-needed-hospitalization/ or https://cov.cx/a1d84

[638] See https://www.homeopathyusa.org/ or https://cov.cx/a1d85

[639] See https://wa.kaiserpermanente.org/kbase/topic.jhtml?docId=hn-2236006 or https://cov.cx/a1d86

- *Hydrogen Peroxide Gargle*

Every Day	After Exposure	Mild Infection

No Prescription Needed	https://amzn.to/34zUBXG or https://cov.cx/a1f48

This is an interesting concept that seems to be underpinned by simple common sense. The basic concept is that the virus is breathed in, and needs to descend from its original point of entry (mouth or throat) and get into one's lungs. So if you can "head it off at the pass" – ie before it goes down your throat – you may have beaten the infection. The concept is described in a series of articles linked below.[640]

Note we also feature Povidone-Iodine mouthwash/gargling, below, which uses the same concept, just a different chemical to kill the virus particles, and Listerine, which seems to be most beneficial of all.

Hydrogen peroxide is readily available and inexpensive. You should dilute it (if necessary) with regular tap water down to about a 1.0% to a 1.5% solution. So if you get a 3% solution, simply mix it 50:50 with water. There's no need to get the proportions exact, a reasonable approximation, measuring by sight in a glass with parallel sides, is good enough.

There are stronger concentrations also available, but there's no advantage to getting these. You still need to dilute them, and the exact proportions become slightly more important.

The advocating website (Loico.com) suggests 60 seconds of gargling each time, which can be either a continuous 60 seconds, or two 30 second gargles, or any other combination. They also say "up to four times a day" and stress the evening gargle.[641]

Of course, spit the gargling liquid out after gargling. Try not to swallow any.

---

[640] See https://loico.com/international-researchers-pick-up-loicos-idea-of-throat-disinfection-to-counter-covid-19/ or https://cov.cx/a1d87 and https://loico.com/update-on-preventive-throat-disinfection-antisepsis-to-counter-covid-19/ or https://cov.cx/a1d88 and https://loico.com/update-on-covid-19-and-oral-antisepsis/ or https://cov.cx/a1d89

[641] See https://loico.com/the-logic-of-surviving-the-coronavirus-pandemic/ or https://cov.cx/a1d90

- ## *Hydroxychloroquine (HCQ)*

Every Day	After Exposure	Mild Infection

No Prescription Needed	Prescription Required

One of the most unfortunate aspects of the entire virus experience has been how hydroxychloroquine has been viewed. We should all be asking why HCQ is not being prescribed for Covid-19 after 74% of studies deem it effective and safe.[642]

The facts are simple and straightforward. Hydroxychloroquine is a safe drug with an 80-year exemplary record and which might now save tens of thousands more lives – those of Covid-19 sufferers. Why is it not being prescribed to everyone as soon as they are diagnosed with the virus?[643] Instead, physicians tell their patients there is nothing to be done except rest and drink plenty of fluids.

Of 94 studies (in September) into HCQ's use against Covid-19, an astonishing 74% have shown positive results, either when used alone or together with zinc and possibly also azithromycin. These studies are from hospitals and universities all around the world, including several in the US such as the Henry Ford Health System (MI) and the Icahn School of Medicine (NY). Many have been published in refereed journals.

Particularly when taken at an early stage, *the evidence is overwhelmingly in favor of HCQ use.* The studies show that, on average, it prevents 64% of all infections from progressing into the virus's serious and potentially fatal stages.

HCQ is a very commonly prescribed drug in the US, is in wide use worldwide, and is so important it is on WHO's shortlist of essential (and very safe) medicines. Its patents have expired, so a course of treatment for Covid-19 costs maybe a dollar or two.

Because it is a widely used drug, its possible side-effects (primarily a potential change to one aspect of your heartbeat rhythm – an elongation of the QT interval)

---

[642] See https://c19study.com/ or https://cov.cx/a1a24 (I see the count is rising - on 6 October, up to 128 studies, on 4 November, 161 studies, and on 17 December, 205 studies, 139 of them being peer-reviewed)

[643] This article cogently makes exactly that point : https://www.newsweek.com/key-defeating-covid-19-already-exists-we-need-start-using-it-opinion-1519535 or https://cov.cx/a1d91

are well known and judged sufficiently minor to allow for its longstanding use and for extended periods to prevent malaria and to treat arthritis and lupus.

Although the vast preponderance of trials shows HCQ as benefiting patients, what about the few that don't? A common feature of the negative trials is they are not testing HCQ the way the positive studies indicate.

The trials with negative results have typically not tested HCQ with zinc, and have only been administered to hospitalized patients in the later stages of the disease – but even then, the positive studies outweigh the negative by a factor of two to one.

In some cases, the negative outcomes are based on erroneous interpretations. In two high-profile cases, refereed articles that first hailed as persuasive proof of HCQ being of no value were subsequently retracted due to outright fraudulent data.[644]

In August, 42 American, British and Brazilian professors, statisticians, mathematicians, and doctors wrote an open letter about misinterpreted data in the negative cases, with the lead author saying, "This misinterpretation in statistical tests is well known and explained in most undergraduate books in the field."[645]

The possible failure of HCQ alone in late and severe case scenarios does not invalidate its use, with zinc, as soon as possible after the virus has been detected. Indeed, in every case where HCQ was administered early – all 26 of the early studies thus far – the results were positive.

But a group of naysayers are choosing to selectively focus on the 24 negative trials (mainly later stage), while ignoring the 70 positive trials, and have spread the word that HCQ does not work, and is too dangerous to even trial anymore. Both points are wrong.

HCQ is not dangerous. A peer-reviewed study published on 20 August confirmed there have been no deaths reported as a result of HCQ use and went further to show that HCQ treatment substantially reduced cardiac mortality and decreased thrombosis, arrhythmia, and cholesterol in treated patients.[646]

---

[644] See https://www.thelancet.com/journals/lancet/article/PIIS0140-6736(20)31180-6/fulltext or https://cov.cx/a1d92 and https://www.sciencemag.org/news/2020/06/two-elite-medical-journals-retract-coronavirus-papers-over-data-integrity-questions or https://cov.cx/a1g09

[645] See https://veja.abril.com.br/saude/especialistas-contestam-estudos-que-nao-viram-beneficios-na-cloroquina/amp/ or https://cov.cx/a1d93

[646] See https://www.sciencedirect.com/science/article/pii/S2052297520300998 or https://cov.cx/a1d94

Rather than being potentially harmful to the circulatory system, HCQ was actually beneficial.

Covid-19 is fatal, and now is the third most common cause of death in the US. Lupus and rheumatoid arthritis are nasty afflictions, but not fatal. If HCQ is safe for lupus and arthritis sufferers, why is it not safe for Covid-19 sufferers?

Shouldn't researchers be chasing down the positive elements of the 70 affirming studies, while using the 24 negative studies to clarify when not to dispense it?

This is a literal life and death matter. Numbers have gone up and down; in mid-December the US is averaging almost 2,500 deaths daily from Covid-19. It is expected that 69,715 more people will die in December and 76,562 in January – that's almost 2,500 a day in January.[647] The rest of us are also suffering due to social distancing, mask-wearing, our jobs either lost or at risk, and the entire economy very fragile. The cost of the outbreak, so far, is anyone's guess – over $5 trillion, maybe $10 trillion, and rising.

While everyone hopes a vaccine will be developed, it may not ever be the complete solution. While the new vaccines now being given Emergency Use Authorizations show high rates of effectiveness, those are for "average people" not for elderly people, and we know much less about how effective the vaccines will be for those types of people. It could work for as few as half the people who take it, might last no more than three months, and might be rendered useless by a new virus mutation. Sure, we need a vaccine; until then – and in cases where the vaccine fails and a person still comes down with the virus, HCQ (and other promising treatments) is available today.

As often happens these days on the internet, HCQ-hate has become an echo chamber where a few early negative studies keep getting cited, while the more recent positive studies are never looked at.

It seems HCQ may be most beneficial when used together with zinc, and when you take the two drugs (or three if you add AZ) as quickly as possible after coming down with the virus. Its efficacy seems to drop drastically with each extra day of delay.[648]

---

[647] The IHME projection dated 19 November, see the current projection at https://covid19.healthdata.org/united-states-of-america?view=total-deaths&tab=trend or https://cov.cx/a1d95

[648] See https://hcqtrial.com/ or https://cov.cx/a1d96

It has been suggested that if you have a Qt interval greater than 500 msec, you should not take HCQ.[649] If you do take HCQ, and especially if you add AZ to your treatment plan, you should monitor your Qt interval and discontinue treatment if it extends too long. Ideally you need your doctor involved in this supervision.

HQC is mentioned by NIH (who recommends against its use). It is featured in the McCullough treatment plan, together with azithromycin or doxycycline and zinc.

Lastly, it is worth mentioning that according to a September survey of doctors around the world, front-line doctors are quietly prescribing HCQ for their patients. 15% of US doctors admitted to prescribing it, and 25% of doctors in the rest of the world are also prescribing it.[650]

- *Ivermectin*

Every Day	After Exposure	Mild Infection

No Prescription Needed *	https://amzn.to/30Fwzta or https://cov.cx/a1f49
No Prescription Needed	Prescription Required

Ivermectin (sometimes sold under the brand Stromectol) is a derivative of a related product, avermectin, that was discovered in Japan in the 1970s. Its two finders won half the Nobel Prize for Physiology/Medicine in 2015 as delayed recognition of the importance of their discovery. It has been described as a wonder-drug, due to being beneficial in many different applications.[651]

Evidence in support of ivermectin as an antiviral drug has been steadily growing.[652] In late October it received a resounding endorsement by a group of

---

[649] See https://www.dicardiology.com/article/fda-reports-deaths-and-injuries-use-antimalarial-hydroxychloroquine-covid-19-patients or https://cov.cx/a1d97

[650] See https://app.sermo.com/covid19-barometer or https://cov.cx/a1g08 - this is from their Study 14.

[651] See https://www.ncbi.nlm.nih.gov/pmc/articles/PMC3043740/ or https://cov.cx/a1d98

[652] See https://c19study.com/i or https://cov.cx/a1d99

physicians, the Front Line Covid-19 Critical Care Alliance (FLCCC),[653] making it the key ingredient of their new I-MASK+ early/at-home care plan.[654]

Whereas most other studies have focused on using ivermectin as a treatment, the FLCCC I-MASK+ protocol adds two other possible uses. One is as a prophylaxis for high-risk individuals (that would be determined by your age, other comorbidities, and the degree of exposure to potential infection you have to experience), in which case they suggest taking a weekly dose of 0.15 – 0.20 mg/kg of body weight. The second case is for anyone who has had a definite exposure to the virus, and in that case, they suggest two doses, three days apart, each of 0.2 mg/kg. As an early-stage treatment, the protocol suggests 0.2 mg/kg a day for two days.

It seems that ivermectin has little or no side-effects, and may significantly reduce the number of people who, after exposure to the virus, become infected (if given at the onset of symptoms), and may also reduce the time people spend in a hospital if given later in an illness.

Here's an interesting observational study that looks at death rates in Peru before and after a wide distribution of ivermectin for patient treatment.[655] The reduction in deaths is substantial, and while there may well be other factors and considerations, it is certainly another suggestion/hint that ivermectin might make a major difference to Covid case outcomes.

ASHP is guardedly positive about ivermectin use and EVMS notably much more positive.[656] It is also one of the recommended treatments in the McCullough plan.

---

[653] See https://covid19criticalcare.com/ or https://cov.cx/a1d06

[654] See https://covid19criticalcare.com/i-mask-prophylaxis-treatment-protocol/ or https://cov.cx/a1d50

[655] See https://www.trialsitenews.com/real-world-evidence-the-case-of-peru/ or https://cov.cx/a1e02 and https://www.researchgate.net/publication/344469305_Real-World_Evidence_The_Case_of_Peru_Causality_between_Ivermectin_and_COVID-19_Infection_Fatality_Rate or https://cov.cx/a1e03

[656] See EVMS and ASHP and https://www.sciencedirect.com/science/article/pii/S0166354220302011?via%3Dihub or https://cov.cx/a1e04 and https://www1.racgp.org.au/newsgp/clinical/insufficient-evidence-to-currently-support-ivermec or https://cov.cx/a1e05

The recommended dose is 70-90 mcg (micrograms) per pound of body weight, generally at the 90 mcg end for Covid-19 infections.[657] If expressed in terms of mcg per kilogram of body weight, this converts to 150 – 200 mcg/kg.

On the other hand, a recently reported positive study in Argentina showed more positive results, based on a three times higher dose - 600 mcg/kg.[658]

Some studies suggest taking two equal doses (each of 150-200 mcg/kg), one or two days apart, others suggest a single dose and waiting two weeks before a second dose.

Take ivermectin with a glass of water on an empty stomach and an hour or two before a meal. It is a prescription drug, although you can get the drug for animals over-the-counter or from a vet or Amazon (link above) (just be sure it is pure ivermectin, without any other chemicals added).

NIH recommends against using ivermectin, but apparently not due to any safety concerns but rather due to a lack of convincing evidence in favor of its use.[659]

We also note that their negative statement was last updated on 27 August. As of the time of writing this section, that is over two months out of date, and much of the new evidence in support of ivermectin has come out since then.

It is regrettable that NIH isn't more up to date with the discoveries and developments in Covid-19 treatments. Rather than being helpful, they are being actively unhelpful with such a long lead time and slow response to promising developments such as ivermectin may possibly be.

---

[657] So, if you weigh 150 lbs, your dose would be 150 x 70 mcg = 10.5 mg at the low end or 150 x 90 mcg = 13.5 mg at the higher end. See also https://www.trialsitenews.com/zagazig-university-randomized-controlled-ivermectin-study-results-confirms-pi-hypothesis-drug-effective-against-covid-19/ or https://cov.cx/a1e06

[658] See https://www.trialsitenews.com/argentina-study-supports-ivermectin-for-covid-19/ or https://cov.cx/a1e07

[659] See https://www.covid19treatmentguidelines.nih.gov/antiviral-therapy/ivermectin/ or https://cov.cx/a1e08

- *Listerine*

Every Day	After Exposure	Mild Infection

No Prescription Needed	https://amzn.to/3kVav5X or https://cov.cx/a1f50

We discuss mouthwash/gargle products under the hydrogen peroxide and Povidone-Iodine entries. Both seem to have some efficacy.

But a new study[660] shows the very best performing product of all is Listerine Original Mouthwash – the golden-colored product. It performs much better than any of the other Listerine products and much better than hydrogen peroxide or Povidone-Iodine too.

So that is now our go-to product for mouthwash/gargling.

- *Melatonin*

Every Day	After Exposure	Mild Infection

No Prescription Needed	https://amzn.to/2I4VwrJ or https://cov.cx/a1f51

Melatonin is another of the perhaps unexpected entries on this list. It became prominent (at least to me) a couple of decades ago, as a wonder-drug with many magical properties claimed. One of those was as a possible way of reducing jet-lag and accelerating one's adjustment to a new time zone.[661]

In the Covid context, it is recommended by EVMS as a possible treatment for Covid-19. This is a good article that explains some of the ways melatonin might help Covid-sufferers but gives no specific case examples of how it has helped.[662] However, feeling comfortable with any type of treatment is always boosted if one understands exactly how the treatment might work and benefit you, so it is an

---

[660] See https://onlinelibrary.wiley.com/doi/10.1002/jmv.26514 or https://cov.cx/a1e09

[661] Here's an article I wrote way back in 2002 on the topic. https://old.thetravelinsider.info/2002/0517.htm or https://cov.cx/a1e10

[662] See https://www.tandfonline.com/doi/full/10.1080/08830185.2020.1756284 or https://cov.cx/a1e11

interesting article, even if not conclusive proof of melatonin actually doing anything at all.

Melatonin is also advocated in the FLCCC I-MASK+ protocol. It recommends 6 mg daily as a prophylaxis and 10 mg as an early-stage treatment. They also point out that melatonin causes drowsiness, so suggest taking it at bedtime.

Here's an open-minded look at some of the arguments for and against melatonin use.[663] And this article identifies some possible positive outcomes while noting there are almost no side-effects or problems with very high dosage levels.[664]

I find melatonin gives me "lucid dreams"; I used to use it as a way to reduce jet-lag and more quickly adjust to new time zones, and after great success using it in that context, starting taking it every night "just because" and for a better quality of sleep. But once I identified the "lucid dream" correlation, I stopped taking it every day, and these days seldom use it when traveling across multiple time zones, either. However, if I've acquired or am at risk of a Covid infection, I'll accept the lucid dreaming as a fair trade-off.

In the past, I've taken between at least 0.3 and up to 2 or 3 mg of melatonin each evening. The suggested doses for Covid-19 treatment are substantially higher, with a suggestion you start low and work yourself up to whatever level you are comfortable with.

President Trump's treatment, after he was tested positive, included melatonin.

- *Metformin*

Every Day	After Exposure	Mild Infection

No Prescription Needed	Prescription Required

Metformin (common brands being Glucophage, Riomet, and Glumetza) is primarily used for people with Type 2 diabetes and modifies how the liver

---

[663] See https://www.discovermagazine.com/health/the-latest-supplement-touted-as-a-covid-19-treatment-melatonin or https://cov.cx/a1e12

[664] See https://www.sciencedirect.com/science/article/abs/pii/S0024320520303313 or https://cov.cx/a1e13

produces glucose.[665] It is the most popular glucose reducing drug worldwide, and has held that position for at least two decades and is on the WHO list of Essential Medicines.

Researchers have noted that having diabetes makes a Covid infection more impactful (ie, it is a comorbidity), but have also noted a strong difference in patient outcomes between those who have been taking metformin and those who have not been taking it.[666]

It also seems to be most strongly effective in women rather than men.

Although metformin use seems to be reasonably convincingly shown to benefit diabetics, it has not been tested on "normal" non-diabetic patients. Will it also provide some protection and benefit to people more broadly? That has not yet been confirmed, but it seems like it may be active in other areas (such as having some anti-inflammatory properties) giving it some credible ways of benefiting people with Covid-19.[667]

Metformin is another very low-cost drug in common use and has been prescribed since the 1920s. It has few side-effects and is generally safe in use, although it is not recommended for people with reduced function of the kidneys or liver, congestive heart failure, other severe acute illnesses, or dehydration.

It therefore seems possible to conclude that metformin may indeed provide some protection against the SARS-CoV-2 virus, particularly in the early stages of a Covid infection. It seems to fall in that happy category of "can't hurt, might help, has little or no downside, and is very inexpensive."

However, do check possible interactions between metformin and any other drugs you might be taking, and also please note it is not recommended to drink

---

[665] See https://www.diabetes.co.uk/diabetes-medication/biguanides.html or https://cov.cx/a1e14

[666] See https://www.medicinenet.com/diabetes_drug_metformin_may_reduce_covid_19_death-news.htm or https://cov.cx/a1e15 and https://www.medrxiv.org/content/10.1101/2020.07.29.20164020v1 or https://cov.cx/a1e16 which reports a 70% reduction in mortality. This article lists other research findings https://www.diabetes.co.uk/news/2020/jul/more-evidence-suggest-metformin-could-help-treat-covid-19.html or https://cov.cx/a1e17

[667] Table 1 of this document summarizes potential ways metformin might positively impact on Covid-19 https://www.ncbi.nlm.nih.gov/pmc/articles/PMC7395819/ or https://cov.cx/a1e18 and this report goes into more detail on some of the possible benefits https://www.ncbi.nlm.nih.gov/pmc/articles/PMC7190487/ or https://cov.cx/a1e19

alcohol while taking metformin. Ibuprofen, naproxen, and other similar anti-inflammatories may also be a problem.

It is recommended to take metformin with meals.

A new study is believed to now be underway, evaluating metformin's value both as a preventative measure and as a treatment. Results are not expected until September 2021.[668]

- *Multi-Vitamin Supplement*

Every Day	After Exposure	Mild Infection

No Prescription Needed	https://amzn.to/33BGiTd or https://cov.cx/a1f52

I have no specific reference to support this recommendation, and in my normal life before the virus appearing never took vitamin supplements.

But there are so many "low science" recommendations to take extra of this or that vitamin/mineral/supplement that it seems on the basis of "can't hurt, might help, and costs next to nothing" it may be a prudent thing to do, "just in case". On the other hand, some studies show that taking too much multi-vitamin supplement might actually be harmful[669] and others suggest the benefits might be "all in the mind" (but we should never underestimate the benefits of the placebo effect).[670]

You'll see (or should see), on any container of these types of products, information on the active ingredients and usually a statement of how much of the ingredient is included and what percentage it is of the "Daily Value" (DV) or "Recommended Dietary Amount" (RDA). Some ingredients might not show any percentage, because they are not items included in the DV/RDA schedules.

There is another helpful parameter that is seldom disclosed, but good to know. This is the Tolerable Upper Intake Level (UL) which represents the maximum amount of each vitamin or mineral you can safely take each day

---

[668] See https://clinicaltrials.gov/ct2/show/NCT04510194 or https://cov.cx/a1e20

[669] See https://www.bbc.com/future/article/20161208-why-vitamin-supplements-could-kill-you or https://cov.cx/a1e21

[670] See https://www.studyfinds.org/health-benefits-multivitamins-in-mind/ or https://cov.cx/a1e22

without risk of an overdose or serious side-effects. The margin between the RDA/DV number and the UL number can vary widely, as can the consequences of exceeding the UL value.

I now take a Costco Kirkland Signature brand "Daily Multi" tablet every day. Many others are similar. Choose one that doesn't have aggressively high doses of anything within it – up to 100% of the recommended daily value is fine, but because you probably get some of each substance through normal eating and drinking, don't go way over that with the supplement.

Here's an example of a multi-vitamin that in my opinion has too much of several of the products.

Supplement Facts

Amount Per Serving	Serving Size 1 Capsule	%DV*
Vitamin A (as natural beta carotene)	750 mcg RAE (2,500 IU)	83%
Vitamin C (as calcium ascorbate/ascorbyl palmitate)	120 mg	133%
Vitamin D3 (as cholecalciferol)	75 mcg (3,000 IU)	375%
Vitamin E (as natural Crystalline Vitamin E)	60 mg (90 IU)	400%
Vitamin B1 (as thiamin hydrochloride)	10 mg	833%
Vitamin B2 (as riboflavin)	10 mg	769%
Niacin (as niacinamide/chromium nicotinate)	20 mg	125%
Pantothenic Acid (as calcium pantothenate)	20 mg	400%
Vitamin B6 (as pyridoxine hydrochloride)	10 mg	588%
Vitamin B12 (as methylcobalamin - protected Coenzyme B12)	250 mcg	10,417%
Folate Complex (as L-methylfolate/folic acid)	533 mcg DFE (200 mcg folic acid)	133%
Biotin	500 mcg	1,667%
Calcium (as calcium carbonate/ascorbate)	100 mg	8%
Magnesium (as magnesium oxide)	50 mg	12%
Zinc (as zinc oxide)	15 mg	136%
Selenium (as sodium selenite)	200 mcg	364%
Copper (as copper oxide)	2 mg (2,000 mcg)	222%
Manganese (as manganese sulfate)	2 mg (2,000 mcg)	87%
Chromium (as chromium nicotinate)	200 mcg	571%
Molybdenum (as molybdenum glycinate)	75 mcg	167%
Boron (as potassium borate)	200 mcg	†
Vanadium (as vanadyl sulfate)	50 mcg	†
Lutein	1 mg (1,000 mcg)	†
Lycopene	1 mg (1,000 mcg)	†
Zeaxanthin Complex	500 mcg	†
Branched Chain Amino Acids (Leucine, Valine)	5 mg	†
Silicon (as silicon dioxide)	3 mg	†

* Percent Daily Value (%DV) based on a 2,000 calorie diet. † Daily Value not established

Other Ingredients: Gelatin capsule, Proprietary Protective Methyl B12 Matrix.

Figure 64 Typical labeling on a multi-vitamin package

- *Povidone-Iodine*

Every Day	After Exposure	Mild Infection

No Prescription Needed	https://amzn.to/36ADxDL or https://cov.cx/a1f53

The rationale for this is the same as for the hydrogen peroxide gargle mentioned above.

In addition to the Loico articles advocating some type of virucidal gargle, there is another article that specifically calls out gargling and rinsing (both oral and nasal) with Povidone-Iodine.[671]

We recommend you read the comments above about hydrogen peroxide for further information and discussion and the reason for this and also consider Listerine, which seems likely to be a superior alternative.

- *Propolis*

Every Day	After Exposure	Mild Infection

No Prescription Needed	https://amzn.to/33CU0Fs or https://cov.cx/a1f54

Evidence in support of propolis as a Covid-19 treatment is plentiful but weak rather than strong.[672] It also seems that part of the reason for this weakness might be due to the paucity of formal testing, and I draw comfort from the reference to viricidal action in the citations referenced immediately above.

---

[671] See https://www.medrxiv.org/content/10.1101/2020.05.25.20110239v1 or https://cov.cx/a1e23

[672] See https://www.webmd.com/vitamins/ai/ingredientmono-390/propolis or https://cov.cx/a1e24 and https://www.healthline.com/health/propolis-an-ancient-healer or https://cov.cx/a1e25 and https://www.ncbi.nlm.nih.gov/pmc/articles/PMC7415165/ or https://cov.cx/a1e26 and https://www.sciencedirect.com/science/article/pii/S0753332220308155 or https://cov.cx/a1e27 and https://onlinelibrary.wiley.com/doi/10.1111/dth.13780 or https://cov.cx/a1e28

Propolis is a product formed by bees and is used as a coating to build their hives. We are starting to become increasingly aware of the various benefits of honey and other bee-related products, particularly New Zealand's manuka honey.

"Royal Jelly" is another honey derivative albeit maybe with a stronger profile than it deserves.[673] Bee venom is another bee product that is claimed to have assorted benefits (please note we're not recommending either of these for anti-Covid purposes).

Perhaps propolis is another bee/honey derivative with exciting benefits just waiting to be better appreciated? Perhaps it is, and of course, perhaps it isn't. I'd certainly not bet my life on it having any special powers, but as part of a multi-layered system of defenses, it might help and surely doesn't hurt. It is reminiscent of the fold-remedy of taking some warm honey and lemon water for a cold – maybe the presence of propolis is part of the reason for that time-hallowed suggestion?

It seems the worst-case scenario is just that propolis does not do anything, which encourages one to try some "just in case". Other than in very rare cases of food/honey type allergies, there's no reason to suspect any harm coming from propolis, and when I was a child, I used to love to go to the apiary just a mile from where I lived in New Zealand and get some fresh raw honey, still in the comb, and eat the honey and honeycomb on bread or toast. Goodness only knows how much propolis I'd eagerly have as part of an ordinary lunch, back in those long-past halcyon times.

Propolis isn't unduly expensive and is easy to take as a spray or capsule. I use the BeeKeeper's Naturals throat spray and the Healthcare Australia capsules, both available through the link to Amazon, above.

- *Quercetin*

Every Day	After Exposure	Mild Infection

No Prescription Needed	https://amzn.to/3fwvwAC or https://cov.cx/a1f55

Quercetin is another natural product that may be hiding its anti-Covid light under a bushel, a lot like propolis. Indeed, that's not the only similarity between

---

[673] See https://www.webmd.com/vitamins/ai/ingredientmono-503/royal-jelly or https://cov.cx/a1e29

them; quercetin is found in propolis and is one of the active ingredients that may make propolis valuable. Quercetin also appears in many other products, including (but not limited to) red onions, berries, red wine, green tea, buckwheat, and apples.

Interestingly, quercetin was originally known as Vitamin P and was discovered by the same Nobel Prize winner who discovered Vitamin C (Albert Szent-Györgyi).[674]

So why not just take propolis by itself, and get your quercetin that way? By taking quercetin as well, you can boost the amount of quercetin without needing to take an enormous amount of propolis, and by still taking the propolis, you continue to get benefits from the several other active agents within propolis that may also be beneficial in fighting Covid.

Quercetin use is supported by the EVMS protocol. They note there have been rare reports of hypothyroidism being associated with prolonged high dose use of quercetin.

The FLCCC I-MASK+ protocol recommends 250 mg of quercetin daily as a prophylaxis and 250 mg twice daily as an early-stage treatment.

Some supporting articles in favor of quercetin can be found in the footnoted links.[675] A less enthusiastic article can be seen here.[676]

I use the Amazing Formulas 500 mg brand. There are plenty of others, all at the Amazon link.

- *Traditional Chinese Medicine & Folk Medicine in General*

Every Day	After Exposure	Mild Infection

No Prescription Needed	(Doctor visit recommended)

---

[674] See https://www.frontiersin.org/articles/10.3389/fimmu.2020.01451/full or https://cov.cx/a1e30

[675] See EVMS, and https://www.medpagetoday.com/infectiousdisease/covid19/87373 or https://cov.cx/a1e31 and https://www.ncbi.nlm.nih.gov/pmc/articles/PMC7392107/ or https://cov.cx/a1e32 and https://www.mountsinai.org/health-library/supplement/quercetin or https://cov.cx/a1e33

[676] See https://www.ncbi.nlm.nih.gov/pmc/articles/PMC7392107/ or https://cov.cx/a1e34

I add this entry mainly to open your eyes to the enormous amount of non-western medical treatments that are out there. I am not recommending any specific traditional Chinese medicines (TCM) in this section, but I do encourage you to not overlook the potential of TCM and all other sorts of folk remedies and country medicines.

It is easy to turn away from the concept of making medicines by boiling up mixtures of various plants and leaves and animal parts and other natural substances, but just because it doesn't seem "scientific" does not mean it is not valid.

Many of our most impactful medicines today have come directly from natural products. Penicillin, birth control pills, and aspirin are all directly derived from natural products in a manner that was originally much the same as how traditional Chinese medicine still works today – but minus the participation of the multi-billion dollar pharmaceutical companies. Much of the speculative research into new medicines involves identifying active chemicals in plants, their potential use in medicine, and then coming up with ways to commercially manufacture them.

Perhaps a key difference with TCM is that instead of getting a little jar of flavorless pills, you get a brown bag of strange looking stuff that you have to steep in boiling water and then drink, and which often has the most awful of tastes. And, instead of getting a product that has had millions of dollars spent on scientific studies to prove its value and its safety to a skeptical FDA, you get a product that requires you to trust the person who mixed it up from assorted raw materials, and based on many thousands of years of tradition rather than "hard science".

It is common to find that even western type "old wives' tales" and "country medicines" are not nonsense at all, but are based on real active ingredients in the products being offered up. As an example, this is an interesting article about licorice;[677] it is surprising to see all the active and beneficial substances contained within it. Many natural plants are full of active ingredients of varying properties and strengths, and there's a huge amount we could learn from further analysis and adapting some of these ingredients into more active forms.

Over a billion Chinese people have been relying on TCM for over 6,000 years. That's a fairly good market test!

One of the uncomfortable elements of TCM is there is no real quality control. You have to rely on the expertise and honesty of the practitioner, both in terms of their diagnosis of your ailment, and then secondly, you don't know if the

---

[677] See https://www.ncbi.nlm.nih.gov/pmc/articles/PMC4629407/ or https://cov.cx/a1e35

substances they are giving you are fresh or stale, strong or weak, compared to some sort of reference standard.

It is this lack of quality control that gives concern to many of us. But if you can find a TCM doctor who you know can be trusted, you might be well advised to consider and heed their advice, especially if it is inexpensive (as is usually the case) and doesn't preclude your ability to take western medicines as well.

In this context, my preference is to visit a TCM doctor in-person and to have him/her "examine" me directly[678] and then mix up a potion of assorted active ingredients, rather than buying something online.

Having said that, if you are curious, this is an interesting article about TCM and Covid in general,[679] and this set of six pages has "recipes" for specific possible cures._[680]   It might be something to show and discuss with any practitioner you visit. Here's a skeptical response to that article[681] and a second response only slightly less negative.[682] We're not sure we'd go as far as a quoted "expert" who says there is no good evidence to support using TCMs, and therefore its use is not just unjustified but dangerous.

This article, while urging caution, also notes that some TCM remedies have been officially approved by the Chinese government.[683] That is not the same as being approved by the FDA, and we suspect the Chinese government is more predisposed to look positively on TCM than the FDA does.

It would only be dangerous if TCM was used instead of best-practice western medicines too. And noting there are no officially approved western medicines out there and commonly available at present, there is no danger of that

---

[678] The reason for the quotes around the word "examine" is because the examinations that have been conducted, at least for me, have been very superficial seeming, comprising little more than checking pulse rate, looking at my tongue, and that seemed to be about all.

[679] See https://massivesci.com/notes/traditional-chinese-medicine-covid19-treatment-trials/ or https://cov.cx/a1e36

[680] See https://covid-19.chinadaily.com.cn/a/202003/17/WS5e702f52a31012821727fa19.html or https://cov.cx/a1e37

[681] See https://www.nature.com/articles/d41586-020-01284-x or https://cov.cx/a1e38

[682] See https://www.bbc.com/news/world-asia-53094603 or https://cov.cx/a1e39

[683] See https://www.thelancet.com/journals/lancet/article/PIIS0140-6736(20)31143-0/fulltext or https://cov.cx/a1e40

happening and perhaps, therefore, more reason to consider TCM based approaches as well as (but not instead of) the other ones mentioned here and elsewhere.

We think this article is a fair overview of some other folk medicines[684] and here's another article about herbal recipes for Covid-19 in general.[685]

- *Vitamin C*

Every Day	After Exposure	Mild Infection

No Prescription Needed	https://amzn.to/2XuJGfq or https://cov.cx/a1f56

Another medical product that seems to crop up as suitable for many different types of ailments is Vitamin C, and it is being advocated as a Covid treatment, too.

Vitamin C has always been a bit controversial, with some of its supporters attributing near-miraculous powers to it, most famously the Nobel Prize-winning chemist, Linus Pauling.[686] As for Pauling's claims that Vitamin C extends one's life-span, it is perhaps relevant to note that he lived to the ripe old age of 93, ultimately dying of prostate cancer. Most of us would view 93 years as a win.

Vitamin C is recommended in the EVMS treatment schedule and discussed in the ASHP document. Note that the EVMS treatment schedule refers both to oral Vitamin C and in later stages, IV administered Vitamin C. As this article points out,[687] intravenous Vitamin C concentrations can go to very much higher concentrations than oral levels.

---

[684] See https://www.athenahealth.com/knowledge-hub/clinical-trends/natural-remedies-and-the-fight-to-treat-COVID-19 or https://cov.cx/a1e41

[685] See https://www.healthline.com/health-news/herbal-remedies-covid-19-what-to-know or https://cov.cx/a1e42

[686] This article is a bit overly critical, perhaps, but very readable https://www.vox.com/2015/1/15/7547741/vitamin-c-myth-pauling or https://cov.cx/a1e43

[687] See https://lpi.oregonstate.edu/COVID19/IV-VitaminC-virus or https://cov.cx/a1e44

Vitamin C is featured in the FLCCC I-MASK+ protocol. They recommend 1000 mg of Vitamin C twice daily as a prophylaxis and 2,000 mg two or three times daily as an early-stage treatment.

This article sees two benefits of Vitamin C use – a moderate dose in the early stages of the disease to address early problems of virus growth, and a high dose in the late stages to minimize cytokine storms.[688]

The multi-vitamin I take has 90 mg – 100% of the daily value for Vitamin C, and I'm considering that enough as a prophylactic measure. I take more when coming down with a cold, and in such cases, I take another 500 mg – 1,000 mg of additional Vitamin C each day.

If you can, get a "slow-release" or "time-release" product. I use a Boots product that I buy when in the UK – 500 mg of "sustained release" Vitamin C; but I've not seen it for sale in the US. Amazon has slow-release products available at the link, above.

There are no clear dosing recommendations, and similarly, no clear maximum doses or cautions when taking high doses. This website[689] suggests a maximum daily dose of 2,000 mg and lists possible side-effects of mega-doses as being

- Diarrhea
- Nausea
- Vomiting
- Heartburn
- Abdominal cramps
- Headache
- Insomnia

If you are taking large doses of Vitamin C before being admitted to a hospital or before a blood test, you should mention this because Vitamin C can affect the accuracy of point of care glucometers.

High doses of Vitamin C can also interact with some other drugs such as Tylenol (acetaminophen), NSAIDs, and some others too.[690]

NIH says there is insufficient data to justify a recommendation for Vitamin C use.

---

[688] See https://www.sciencedirect.com/science/article/pii/S0899900720302318 or https://cov.cx/a1e45

[689] See https://www.mayoclinic.org/healthy-lifestyle/nutrition-and-healthy-eating/expert-answers/vitamin-c/faq-20058030 or https://cov.cx/a1e46

[690] See https://www.stlukes-stl.com/health-content/medicine/33/000994.htm or https://cov.cx/a1e47

- *Vitamin D*

Every Day	After Exposure	Mild Infection

No Prescription Needed	https://amzn.to/30WwrpB or https://cov.cx/a1f57

The evidence in support of Vitamin D helping with Covid-19 was originally weak.[691] But after that early study, there have been a growing number of further studies,[692] and the evidence in favor of taking Vitamin D now seems strong and persuasive.[693]

Even the much-praised and respected Dr Fauci takes a Vitamin D supplement every day (and speaks positively of Vitamin C too).[694]

Here is a good general explainer about Vitamin D.[695]

NIH says there is insufficient data to support a recommendation for Vitamin D use. However, their statement was last updated July 17, and there seems to be growing support for Vitamin D use in the 3½ months since then. As we've said elsewhere, it is a very great disappointment that NIH isn't more up to date with developments in Covid-19 treatments.

---

[691] See https://jamanetwork.com/journals/jamanetworkopen/fullarticle/2770157 or https://cov.cx/a1e48

[692] This study in particular is very optimistic – a 25-fold reduction in the rate of ICU admissions apparently due to Vitamin D. See https://medium.com/microbial-instincts/the-first-clinical-trial-to-support-vitamin-d-therapy-for-covid-19-906a9d907468 or https://cov.cx/a1e49 . We also find this study supportive of Vitamin D - https://www.ctvnews.ca/mobile/health/more-than-80-per-cent-of-hospitalized-covid-19-patients-had-vitamin-d-deficiency-study-1.5162396 or https://cov.cx/a1e50

[693] See https://c19study.com/d or https://cov.cx/a1e51

[694] See https://www.cnbc.com/2020/09/14/supplements-white-house-advisor-fauci-takes-every-day-to-help-keep-his-immune-system-healthy.html or https://cov.cx/a1e52

[695] See https://www.yalemedicine.org/stories/vitamin-d-myths-debunked/ or https://cov.cx/a1e53

NIH suggests a maximum daily dosage of 4,000 IU.[696] I take 50 mcg (2,000 IU) of Vitamin D each day (in addition to the 10 mcg/400 IU in my daily multi-vitamin supplement). I take a Kirkland Signature D3 2,000 IU soft gel, but there are plenty of similar products on Amazon.

President Trump's treatment, after he was tested positive, included Vitamin D. The FLCCC I-MASK+ protocol recommends 1000-3000 IU of Vitamin D daily as a prophylaxis and 4,000 IU/day as an early-stage treatment.

- *Zinc*

Every Day	After Exposure	Mild Infection

No Prescription Needed	https://amzn.to/36FUiNU or https://cov.cx/a1f58

Zinc is widely understood to be beneficial to immune-cell development and has also been associated with both reducing the risk of respiratory infections and reducing the length of such things. Its use as a preventative/treatment for the common cold is widely known.

Approximately 30% of the US adult population are said to be deficient in their zinc levels, so taking a moderate dose is a good thing if that 30% includes you, and might be a good thing anyway. This article[697] tracks a correlation between zinc levels and outcomes for Covid patients – the more zinc they had, the better their experience was, with a 2.3 times lower risk of death among people with higher zinc levels in their blood than people with lower levels. Other studies have had generally similar findings.[698]

EVMS recommends zinc, although I wonder if their recommendation for 50-75 mg a day as a precautionary dose might not be a bit too far on the high side.

---

[696] See https://www.stlukes-stl.com/health-content/medicine/33/000340.htm or https://cov.cx/a1e54

[697] See https://medicalxpress.com/news/2020-09-zinc-blood-death-patients-covid-.html or https://cov.cx/a1e55

[698] See https://medium.com/microbial-instincts/more-studies-shed-light-on-the-value-of-zinc-in-covid-19-a4595271270d or https://cov.cx/a1e56

However, to reduce that concern, this page says that doses of up to 180 mg a day for up to two weeks have been taken with no problems.[699]

Zinc is one of the elements of the FLCCC I-MASK+ protocol. They say you should take 100 mg of zinc daily as a prophylaxis and 200 mg a day as an early-stage treatment.

The McCullough plan recommends 220 mg of zinc sulfate as a treatment for all patients.

The level of supplement you should take of course depends on how much zinc is in your diet already. Six oysters alone can give you 51 mg of zinc. A 5 oz chuck steak has 15 mg. A single chicken leg has 5 mg.[700]

NIH[701] recommends against going over the recommended dietary allowance for zinc when used as a preventative measure and says there is insufficient evidence to support using zinc to treat Covid-19.

Something to beware of is that zinc supplements may inadvertently also contain significant levels of cadmium. Elevated levels of cadmium are harmful and can lead to kidney failure. It is easy for a zinc supplement to omit mention of any cadmium impurities – they can be dismissed as generic impurities or "other inactive substances" on any analysis.

According to this source,[702] zinc gluconate products are least likely to have unwanted cadmium. Other zinc sources can have up to 37 times more cadmium in them than the lowest sources.

A stated concern with higher levels of zinc is that it causes depressed copper levels;[703] hopefully your daily multi-vitamin provides additional and sufficient copper to counter that.

President Trump's treatment, after he was tested positive, included zinc.

---

[699] See https://lpi.oregonstate.edu/mic/minerals/zinc or https://cov.cx/a1e57

[700] This page lists high-in-zinc foods https://www.myfooddata.com/articles/high-zinc-foods.php or https://cov.cx/a1e58

[701] See https://ods.od.nih.gov/factsheets/Zinc-Consumer/ or https://cov.cx/a1e59

[702] See https://www.webmd.com/vitamins/ai/ingredientmono-982/zinc or https://cov.cx/a1e60

[703] See https://ods.od.nih.gov/factsheets/Zinc-HealthProfessional/ or https://cov.cx/a1e61

Possible Future Treatments

As we said before, the truth is changing, and there are new developments regularly occurring. Keep an eye on our website for updates and maybe sign up for the free emailed updates,[704] and we believe there's a way we can update the Kindle version of this book for free through Amazon. If that is so, we'll do several free updates of the book until we get to a point where it fairly deserves to be rewritten and sold again as a new edition.

Some of the possible new treatments that I'm keeping an eye on include metformin[705] (update – I've now moved it into the main list), baricitinib,[706] colchicine, [707] Polyoxidonium,[708] and the possibility of ivermectin to be used as a 1 – 3 month injectable prophylactic.[709]

This site tracks the progress of (currently) 281 different treatments being studied and 42 different vaccines being developed.[710] New studies are coming

---

[704] See https://thecovidsurvivalguide.com or https://cov.cx/covid

[705] See https://www.trialsitenews.com/university-of-minnesota-medical-school-investigators-to-lead-study-investigating-efficacy-of-metformin-targeting-covid-19/ or https://cov.cx/a1e62

[706] Cited in the ICON treatment plan and here : https://www.theguardian.com/science/2020/dec/11/coronavirus-uk-scientists-identify-drugs-that-may-help-severe-cases or https://cov.cx/a1g07

[707] Colchicine is a low-cost anti-inflammatory drug currently used to treat gout and rheumatic disease. See https://www.ncbi.nlm.nih.gov/pmc/articles/PMC7367785/ or https://cov.cx/a1e63 and https://www.medrxiv.org/content/10.1101/2020.08.06.20169573v2 or https://cov.cx/a1e64 . It is also featured in the later stage treatments in the McCullough plan.

[708] See https://www.msn.com/en-us/news/world/russia-s-richest-man-seeks-global-market-for-local-covid-19-drug/ar-BB1bkTSK or https://cov.cx/a1e65

[709] See https://www.medrxiv.org/content/10.1101/2020.10.29.20222661v1 or https://cov.cx/a1e66 for positive results in India (300 micrograms/kg rounded down in two doses, three days apart, then a single top-up dose monthly subsequently) and a study showing 73% effectiveness https://www.medrxiv.org/content/10.1101/2020.10.29.20222661v1 or https://cov.cx/a1e67 and also https://www.trialsitenews.com/france-based-medincell-initiates-ivermectin-clinical-trial-targeting-covid-19-with-prophylactic-strategy/ or https://cov.cx/a1e68

[710] See https://racetoacure.stanford.edu/ or https://cov.cx/a1e69

out regularly, and sometimes contradict earlier studies, for example, a new promising study on tocilizumab[711] seems to rebut earlier more neutral or negative studies.

Early November saw reports of a possibly promising nasal spray – just a squirt a day might be all that is needed to keep the virus from infecting you.[712] But, as of that time, there had not yet been any human studies at all, and the one study in ferrets, while completely positive, was with very few ferrets. There's a long way to go through human testing and gaining FDA approvals before this could ever appear on a local pharmacy's shelves, but it is a hope for the future.

Another possible drug has also been mentioned by President Trump, oleander. This is a plant derivative that is very deadly if taken in appreciable quantity, which critics were fast to note. But in appropriate small quantities, it might have some beneficial qualities. Studies are ongoing.[713]

Who only knows what other promising products might be uncovered. Possibly even, according to this article, honeysuckle.[714]

Talking about products such as honeysuckle, here's a scientific formal study/trial of a folk medicine in the Philippines.[715] It is encouraging to see some of these folk medicines being formally studied.

The website trialsitenews.com is a good source of what is happening.

---

[711] See https://www.theguardian.com/world/2020/nov/19/rheumatoid-arthritis-drug-tocilizumab-appears-to-help-covid-patients-in-icu or https://cov.cx/a1e70

[712] See https://www.nytimes.com/2020/11/05/health/coronavirus-ferrets-vaccine-spray.html or https://cov.cx/a1e71 and https://www.trialsitenews.com/columbia-university-led-study-identifies-powerful-nasal-spray-to-combat-covid-19-as-prophylaxis/ or https://cov.cx/a1e72

[713] See https://www.biorxiv.org/content/10.1101/2020.07.15.203489v1.full.pdf or https://cov.cx/a1e73

[714] See https://www.nature.com/articles/s41421-020-00197-3 or https://cov.cx/a1e74

[715] See https://www.trialsitenews.com/philippines-trial-sites-enrolling-patients-for-regulatory-approved-investigation-into-use-of-folk-medicine-for-covid-19-adjunctive-therapy/ or https://cov.cx/a1e75

17. Medical Equipment & Supplies You Should Have

T he chances are you already have a thermometer at home, and a "first aid kit" that has some plasters and bandages in it, although probably not very much else.

Happily, you won't need to invest heavily into rare and specialized medical equipment, nor will you need to add much more in the way of bandages to your first aid kit. But a few items would be beneficial.

Because supplies have been unreliable and often scarce, and deliveries have sometimes been slow, we urge you to get – now – anything and everything you think you might want/need in the future. Although supplies of many items are better now (November) than they were in spring, they are still not back to "normal" levels, and we fear that with the major increases in cases at present and who knows how bad they'll get over the upcoming winter, supplies and delivery services may become problematic again.

The FDA Approval Role

You will sometimes see references to FDA approval, and perhaps a statement that a product has been "FDA cleared" or "FDA approved".

The FDA is a very large bureaucracy employing about 15,000 people and with an annual budget of around $3.2 billion. It has a role in regulating a variety of generally health-related things – some foods (others are regulated by the USDA), drugs, cosmetics, tobacco, radiation-emitting items (including microwave ovens), and medical devices.[716]

It not only approves items, but it also may restrict their distribution and who can buy/own/use them.

The exact nature of its oversight and whether some type of FDA "approval" is needed varies widely, based on what to an outsider can sometimes seem like subtle distinctions between similar items.

Specific information about its role for the various products it has some oversight over can be seen here.[717]

This article helps understand what the varying concept of FDA approval means.[718] In brief, some products can be automatically approved merely by the manufacturer sending in a statement describing the product and explaining why a specific review is not needed.

When it comes to medical equipment, the FDA has three categories of products – Class I (least restrictive), Class II, and Class III. Nearly half of all medical "products" (a term that can extend to rolls of bandage and tongue depressors) are categorized as Class I, and 95% of those products are exempt from any regulatory process.

Class II items are viewed as posing a medium risk. These range from wheelchairs to the Apple Watch ECG app. Some are not regulated, but most require a premarket notification (a 510(k) submission) that explains what the product is and why it is exempt from further scrutiny). Almost half of all products fall into this second category.

The remaining approximately 10% of products are Class III items – high risk (if they fail) items that are life-sustaining or which, in some other way, could have bad consequences if they fail. Those all need to have formal Premarket Approval (PMA).

All medical devices must be FDA registered. But being registered is not the same as FDA approved or endorsed or evaluated. Registration simply means the company is in the FDA database, and its products have been advised to the FDA.

---

[716] See https://www.fda.gov/about-fda/fda-basics/what-does-fda-regulate or https://cov.cx/a1e76

[717] See https://www.fda.gov/news-events/approvals-fda-regulated-products or https://cov.cx/a1e77

[718] See https://www.fda.gov/consumers/consumer-updates/it-really-fda-approved or https://cov.cx/a1e78

Class III devices generally need to be FDA approved. Class II items may be less stringently FDA cleared and most/all Class I items are FDA cleared - you'll read below of items that are FDA cleared.

FDA cleared simply means that the device has been described as being similar to an existing accepted device that at some previous stage was formally Premarket Approved.

This article explains the process a bit further.[719]

Health Monitoring Equipment

You want to be able to measure your "vital signs" and also your environment. These are the items you'll want to have.

- *Thermometer(s)*

Thermometers are inexpensive, often costing less than $10. See https://amzn.to/3a6DhMy or https://cov.cx/a1f31

As we already said, the chances are you already have a thermometer. But do you have one for every person in your home? Do you have any spares?

We suggest that each person in your residence has their own thermometer. That makes it harder for cross-contamination of infection.

We also suggest you have one or two spare thermometers. Why? Obviously, in case you break one, but that is not the main reason. If you use two (or better three) thermometers, you get a better sense of the real temperature being measured. Your first thermometer might be reading a bit high, your second might be reading a bit low, and the two together will average out to a more accurate reading. Hopefully (and often) multiple thermometers will show almost the same reading, and in that case, you are confident about the accuracy of your reading.

I have a regular "mercury" type "under-the-tongue" **thermometer** as well as newer digital thermometers. These days no thermometers have actual mercury in them, but the concept of an "analog" instrument seems to be potentially more accurate and you never have to worry about a dead battery. Because, for most of us, thermometers are rarely used, if you have a battery-powered unit, there's always a chance that the next time you need your thermometer, the battery has died.

If you are choosing to get an old-fashioned analog thermometer, make sure it is a "medical" thermometer rather than a scientific one. Scientific thermometers

---

[719] See https://www.aspenlaser.com/the-difference-between-fda-registered-fda-approved-and-fda-cleared/ or https://cov.cx/a1e79

cover a wide range but are not as accurate as a medical one, which covers only a narrow range from somewhere in the low 90s up to the low 100s (°F – the same as mid/high 30s for °C).

Do you also want an IR thermometer so you can measure the temperature of everyone who visits you? We have no specific opinion to offer on that,[720] but if you think it isn't too socially gauche to insist on temperature checks before allowing visitors in, good for you![721]

The same as for an oral thermometer, choose one specifically designed for the purpose, not a broad range IR thermometer that will read anywhere from very cold to extremely hot. Carefully understand the claimed accuracy of the device when comparing such devices, and read the reviews, trying to find credible reviews rather than meaningless praise.

Expect to pay over $30 for one of these.

This item[722] claims to be FDA cleared and claims a test/retest reliability of +/- 0.5°F (+/- 0.3°C). That's not quite the same as saying the number it shows is within half a degree of the actual temperature, but it is better than nothing.

We'd do some testing with such a unit on ourselves before relying on it. This is hypothetical because we've not bought one, but if we did, we'd test several different scenarios that on the face of them seem like they might lead to false results.

We'd do some vigorous exercise and then immediately test our skin temperature and our under-the-tongue temperature with a regular thermometer. We'd come inside from a hot day and do a test. We'd come inside after being in the rain, or after being outside on a cold day, and test. That would give us some feeling for how the numbers align to reality. Our guess is that skin temperature could vary based on these sorts of factors – as well as things such as wearing a

---

[720] Well, we would observe that only 2/3 of all people with a Covid infection develop a fever, and that most people are at their most infectious before they develop symptoms. So a temperature test works in only one way rather than two. A high temperature might mean the person has the virus (or some other issue causing their temperature to rise), but a low temperature does not guarantee they are free of the virus.

But, on the basis of risk *reduction* rather than risk elimination, it is a strategy to consider.

[721] This article on 7 October says 30% of Americans will check the temperature of their guests before allowing them in for Thanksgiving parties this year.
https://www.studyfinds.org/hosting-pandemic-americans-temperature-checks/ or
https://cov.cx/a1e80 . We wonder if these people will also check their own family's temperatures at the same time!

[722] See https://amzn.to/33ErT93 or https://cov.cx/a1e81

hat and taking it off immediately before the temperature check or having recently wiped/washed one's face with a wet wipe, although there is an artery in the forehead (the temporal artery) that gives a quick refresh of "normal temperature" blood, as long as you're pointing the thermometer in the right place.

Ear ("tympanic") thermometers are more accurate, but they are becoming appreciably more intrusive.

Oh – in case you're obsessive about getting the most accurate temperature possible, it seems the recommended procedure for the most accurate temperature reading involves a rectal thermometer. Good luck asking your guests to submit to that before allowing them into your house!

A related issue is at what temperature reading would you turn people away? We'd have a low tolerance for any elevated temperatures. Anything over perhaps 99.5°F (38.5°C) – a "low-grade fever" would be enough for us to ask the person to not come inside.

This may well result in some people being turned away (and offended!), and possibly without having an infection, either (infrared thermometers can have appreciable rates of false-positive readings, depending on the brand and how the reading is taken). But if you're going to get one of these devices, what is the point of having it, using it, and then ignoring the results?

- *An Apple Watch?*

One doesn't immediately associate an Apple Watch with equipment needed for Covid-19 healthcare. But that's why you're reading this, right? To learn the things you don't know!

The Apple Watch Series 4 introduced an interesting new health feature. Watches prior to that time could detect pulse rate, but the Series 4 Watch was the first to be able to do a simple type of ECG reading. This feature extended unaltered to the Series 5 Watch, and the latest Series 6 Watch too.

In addition, the Series 6 Watch has added another feature – an oximeter, a device that can determine the oxygen content of your blood.

Both ECG and oximeter features are useful, and there are of course plenty of standalone units that provide either an ECG or oximeter feature (and discussed below).

You definitely should not buy a Watch just to get these two capabilities.[723] But if you have a Watch, can you sensibly use and rely on/trust the data you are getting from its ECG or oximeter functions?

An ECG device detects the electrical impulses that control your heart muscles. ECG units can have any number of sensors ranging up to a maximum of 12 (well, there's no reason why there couldn't be a device with more than 12, but it really wouldn't provide any more useful data; even a 12 lead ECG machine is starting to get into the realm of diminishing returns for most purposes).

The different sensors are placed on different parts of your body – some places get clearer readings of some of the electrical signals than other places.

An expert can then analyze the timings and shapes of these signals to determine various things to do with your heart.

The Apple Watch is essentially a "two-lead" ECG, and it has its own "built-in" expert which will analyze your ECG pattern to determine if there is a risk of atrial fibrillation, a type of irregular rhythm, or not.

The Watch is surprisingly good at this, even with only one pair of "leads" (a contact on the back of the watch and a contact on the side of the watch). It has been FDA cleared[724] and has been tested to have a 99.6% accuracy at detecting a normal sinus rhythm and a 98.3% accuracy at detecting an Afib (atrial fibrillation) pattern.[725]

In our case, however, you are probably most interested in being able to monitor your Qt interval. This is because several of the medications that you might use to minimize your risk of Covid, or to treat an infection if you become infected, can potentially lengthen the Qt interval.[726]

The Watch does not have a built-in Qt interval measuring function.

---

[723] An Apple Watch 6 starts at $399. A separate ECG device and pulse oximeter, together, can cost as little as $120 and may be more accurate than the $399 Watch (particularly the oximeter).

[724] This is a much less rigorous status than FDA approval and denotes more of a passive acceptance by the FDA of a manufacturer's statement of functionality.

[725] See https://www.wareable.com/apple/how-to-take-ecg-reading-on-apple-watch-6817 or https://cov.cx/a1e82

[726] This is a good explainer of the Qt interval and also the "corrected" Qtc interval. https://www.nursingcenter.com/journalarticle?Article_ID=1123271&Journal_ID=417221&Issue_ID=1123211 or https://cov.cx/a1e83

But there are articles online showing you have you can determine your Qt interval from your ECG chart.[727] You could try doing this and see how easy you find it to measure, and you could get an idea for your accuracy of measuring by doing several measurements, trying to see what the numbers would be if you measure one way or another way in terms of where you choose to define the start and stop of the interval.[728]

I've done it and it isn't all that difficult – it ended up easier than I expected, and while my result was probably +/- 40 msec, that seemed to be accurate enough and reassured me I have a normal Qt interval (around 400 msec). This is a helpful site that gives you more information on where to start and stop your measuring.[729] There are also apps that can help you with your measuring and calculating.[730]

Alternatively, if you're not comfortable and confident in your measuring, you can send an electronic copy of your ECG to a doctor. If you want a "better" report to start with, from more sensors, we detail specific ECG devices below.

The other function, new on the Series 6 Watch that was released on 18 September 2020, is a built-in pulse oximeter. This monitors your blood oxygen concentration, and it is an important measurement of how well you're doing during a Covid infection. It is particularly important because you might not always sense exactly how your body is managing with oxygen, and small changes in oxygen level make a big difference to your health,[731] so you not only want to be able to measure your blood oxygen level, but to do so accurately.

---

[727] This page has a relatively straightforward method
https://medium.com/@aerobatic/how-to-read-your-qt-interval-5dffb04717dc or
https://cov.cx/a1e84 . This page goes into more technical detail
https://www.ahajournals.org/doi/pdf/10.1161/CIRCULATIONAHA.120.048253 or
https://cov.cx/a1e85 and says that "adequate" Qt measurements were achieved in 85% of tests, increasing to 94% when the watch was placed on other parts of the body for the reading. Some expertise is required to make these readings in terms of judging where the start and end of the Qt interval can be found on the chart.

[728] The interval can vary from beat to beat, you should try measuring one specific beat's interval in several different ways.

[729] See https://litfl.com/qt-interval-ecg-library/ or https://cov.cx/a1e86

[730] See https://apps.apple.com/us/app/ep-calipers/id982313078 or https://cov.cx/a1e87 and https://apps.apple.com/us/app/qtc-calculator/id1354439139 or https://cov.cx/a1e88

[731] In approximate terms, 97% - 99% = normal, 96% = okay, 95% = less than normal, 94% = get ready to go to hospital. So the range between the low end of good and "dial 911" is only about 3%.

So how accurate is the pulse oximeter built into the Watch 6? This article doesn't give an exact answer but suggests it would necessarily be less accurate than a dedicated device.[732] Apple itself says "not intended for medical use", which is unlike the much prouder claims about its ECG function. Actual reviews are generally negative about the accuracy of its oximeter.[733]

Our interpretation is that possibly you might either not worry about your Qt interval or accept your ability to interpret the ECG chart prepared by the Watch. But you probably will want to have a separate standalone pulse oximeter (happily, not very expensive), because accurately understanding your blood oxygen level is an important part of tracking your health and how your body is fighting a Covid infection.

- ## *ECG Reader*

If you want to monitor your heart condition and don't already have an Apple Watch Series 4, 5, or 6, there are standalone devices you can buy. Our research suggests that AliveCor products are probably the best, and they have two products of interest.

Their **KardiaMobile Personal EKG**[734] seems better than the functionality in the Apple Watch. It not only can detect Afib, but it can also detect Brachycardia and Tachycardia. Amazon says it lists for $100 and they are currently selling it for $90. https://amzn.to/30KB7hU or https://cov.cx/a1f32 It works together with a Bluetooth phone to display and report its findings, and is a two-lead device that provides a single line of data in the report.

If you want a more detailed report, you can get their **KardiaMobile 6L** unit that creates a six-line display of six different perspectives of your heart signals (although you use it with both hands and placing the unit on your knee or ankle)

---

[732] See https://spectrum.ieee.org/view-from-the-valley/biomedical/devices/should-you-trust-apples-new-blood-oxygen-sensor or https://cov.cx/a1e89

[733] This review compared the Apple Watch to an FDA approved pulse oximeter and found results varied from 0 points all the way to seven points, with the Watch showing a lower reading. In other words, you might become very alarmed from your Watch reading for no good reason. https://www.washingtonpost.com/technology/2020/09/23/apple-watch-oximeter/ or https://cov.cx/a1e90 Low readings have been reported in other reviews such as this one, too. https://www.inc.com/jeff-haden/the-new-apple-watch-6-may-have-a-problem-oddly-enough-thats-okay.html or https://cov.cx/a1e91

[734] An ECG (electrocardiogram) is exactly the same as an EKG, which is simply an abbreviation of the German spelling of the word (elektrokardiogramm).

– six signals but three points of contact. Both the two units have a similar small little unit that reads your heart signals :

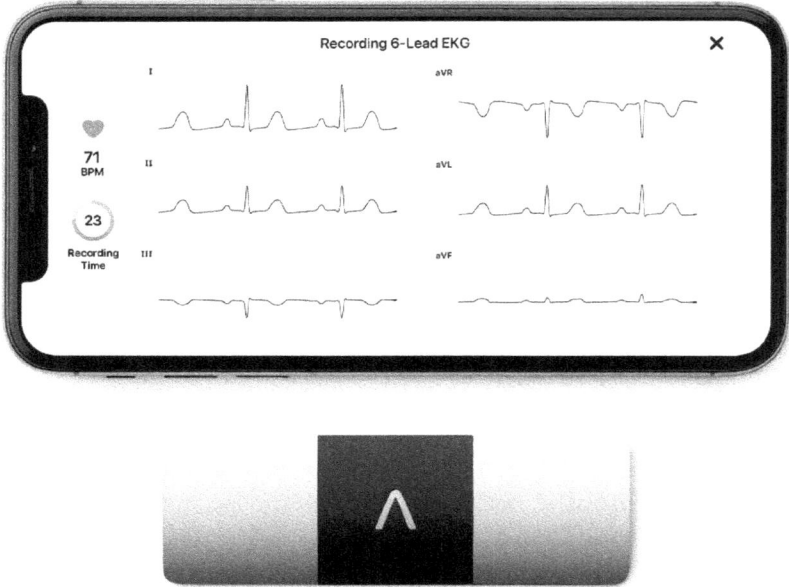

Figure 65 An example of an AliveCor KardiaMobile 6L device and its readings

Amazon has this unit for \$149.   https://amzn.to/39Yk6nU   or https://cov.cx/a1f33

If I was taking HCQ and AZ, I'd get one of these upgraded units so I could have my heart's Qt interval monitored.[735] It is possible to do this yourself direct from the EKG graph, or you can have a physician arrange to do it and interpret it for you (simply email them the electronic results of your tests).

It is probably a good idea to get some readings while you are still healthy and "normal" so you have a baseline set of data to compare to and understand if your Qt interval is normal to start with.

---

[735] See https://www.acc.org/latest-in-cardiology/articles/2020/03/27/14/00/ventricular-arrhythmia-risk-due-to-hydroxychloroquine-azithromycin-treatment-for-covid-19 or https://cov.cx/a1e92

- *Pulse Oximeter*

A **pulse oximeter** is almost essential for tracking how your body is handling a Covid infection. Happily, they are also inexpensive (around $20) and easy to use, so you've no reason not to get one. This is an example of a typical unit (they all look very similar).

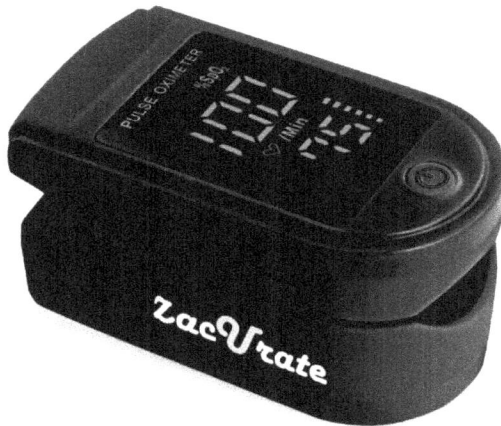

Figure 66 A typical pulse oximeter

As you can see, with the unit in the picture above, the display shows (at the top) your blood oxygen rate (sometimes referred to as the SpO_2 percentage), and below that your pulse rate and (the six-bar scale) how clearly your pulse rate is detected. There's also an on-switch (it switches off automatically when you've stopped using it).

In a regrettable example of idiotic officiousness, the most accurate pulse oximeters with FDA certification are sold only to healthcare professionals, because the FDA says they are "prescription medical devices".

The FDA, in its "infinite wisdom", thinks it would be dangerous to allow you to buy an *accurate* oximeter, but safe to allow you to buy an inaccurate one. Seriously. Does this make sense to you?

To sell directly to us, an oximeter manufacturer has to label their device as "not for medical use". I'm not quite sure what alternate use one would have for a pulse oximeter.[736]

An interesting 2018 study compared eight non-medical pulse oximeters with a formal medical pulse oximeter and found that the non-medical units tended to be close to the medical unit, showing up to five points difference in the key range between about 90% and 98%. This chart summarizes their findings :[737]

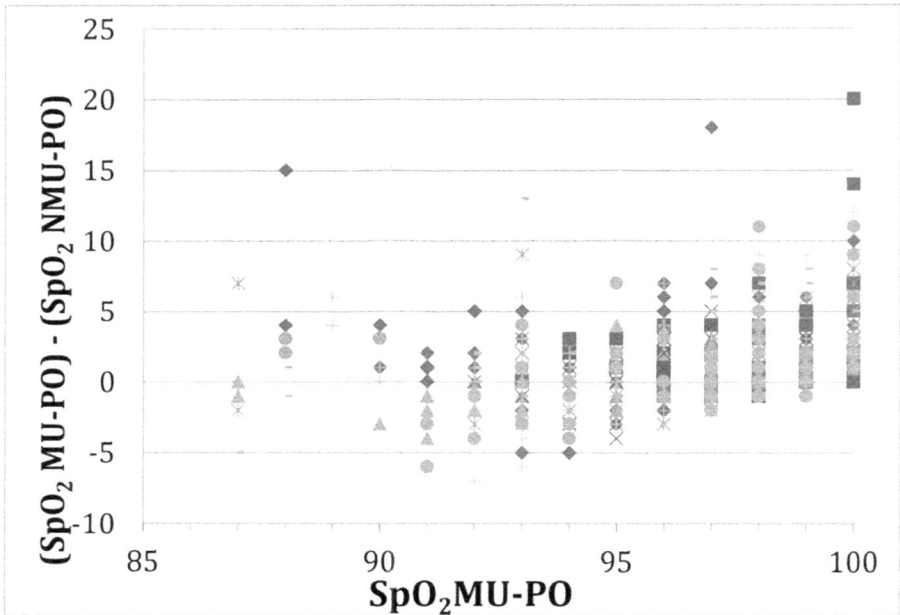

MU-PO = medical use pulse oximeters; NMU-PO = nonmedical use pulse oximeters; SpO2 = oxygen saturation.

Figure 67 Accuracy of non-medical pulse oximeters

---

[736] Actually, there are other non-medical uses. For example, in sports and aviation for evaluating blood oxygen levels as a fatigue and endurance factor in sports and to check on oxygen sufficiency when flying at higher altitudes.

But whatever the use, wouldn't people, no matter what purpose, always want the most accurate oximeter possible – especially when the difference between "good" and "bad" levels is so close?

[737] See Supplemental Figure 1 in
https://www.ncbi.nlm.nih.gov/pmc/articles/PMC6231944/ or https://cov.cx/a1e93

I've looked at four current units, and all claim accuracy to be either +/- 2% or +/- 2 units. That is a greater accuracy claim than tests showed on the devices tested in 2018, so it is hard to know if the accuracy claim is itself accurate.

If correct, with readings in the high 90s, that means the value displayed might be exact, might be two points too high, or two points too low. As mentioned above when talking about the oximeter function in an Apple Watch, because the difference between safe and dangerous oxygen levels is so small (94% and below and you're usually advised to seek hospital care with Covid; and most people tend to have 97% - 99% as normal) there's only a very few percentage points between normal and alarming.

You should definitely get one of these units, and "calibrate" it by using it on yourself in normal times to see what your normal range is. Don't worry if it reads lower than you might think, if you feel healthy with no trouble breathing, it might just be the meter under-reading.

If you visit your doctor, why not bring your pulse oximeter with you and compare its reading to the reading of an official medical grade unit in your doctor's office. That would be helpful to know as well.

The key thing is to watch whatever that number is, and if it starts dropping below your normal level, then you should start to consider seeking medical advice.

Amazon has plenty to choose from. I can't recommend any one over any other one, because all the ones I've checked quote the same accuracy. Make sure the unit shows how clear your pulse signal is, that is probably the only extra feature to look for. https://amzn.to/3a4orWU or https://cov.cx/a1f34

Make sure you have spare batteries (most units seem to use a pair of AAA batteries and include a set with the unit).

Here are some tips for getting as accurate a reading as possible.

- Use your index or middle finger; avoid the toes or ear lobe
- Only accept values associated with a strong pulse signal
- Observe readings for 30-60 seconds to identify the most common value
- Remove any nail polish from the finger on which measurements are made
- Warm your cold extremities before measurement
- Avoid bright lights, especially fluorescent lights – use it in the shade
- Don't place too much pressure on the probe

- *Hygrometer*

We shift now from testing you to testing your environment.

It is beneficial to maintain humidity in your environment – at work and at home – in a range of about 50% - 60%. Getting a hygrometer – a meter that measures humidity – is an essential first step, so you know what the humidity is.

They're inexpensive, and of course they only measure the humidity at the place they are located, so we'd recommend getting several and placing them around your home or work. Most seem to come with a thermometer as well. They're not necessarily very accurate, but accuracy isn't essential, you just want a general idea of if the humidity is a bit low, a bit high, or about right.

If you get two or three or four at once, put them all in the same location for a day or two and see if they all read the same as the humidity varies in that area. That will help you to know if they at least agree with each other, or if one is consistently too high or too low. It doesn't tell you if they are all reading correctly, it just tells you if they all read the same.[738]

Amazon of course has plenty to choose from. https://amzn.to/34CrLWG or https://cov.cx/a1f35

Once you know the air humidity, you can then decide if you need to boost it (with a humidifier) or reduce it (with a de-humidifier).

- *Air Quality Meter*

Is there a way to measure the air around you and see on some sort of gauge if the air is safe or not? Yes and no. There is nothing that will be real-time continuously sampling virus levels in the air, but there are some other devices that might give you hints as to your general air quality.

---

[738] This points to the distinction between precision and accuracy. This is a distinction you probably never need to know, but if you are interested, by all means, now that you're here in the footnote anyway, keep reading.

They are both measures of the quality of a measurement, but they measure different aspects. Precision measures how repeatable a measurement is. For example, if you have four hygrometers, and they all consistently show the same value, they are probably very precise. Accuracy measures how close to the exact correct value an instrument shows.

So say the true humidity is 50%. You have one hygrometer that sometimes shows 49%, sometimes 50%, and sometimes 51%. You have a second hygrometer that always shows either 45% or 46%. The first hygrometer is more accurate, even though it varies more. The second hygrometer is more precise, even though its reading is further away from the actual value.

Which is better? If you can calibrate the precise unit so you know how to adjust from its precise reading to the true value, it is better than an accurate unit. But, to now come back to the real world of low price hygrometers, it doesn't really make much difference for your purposes (but would be much more relevant with pulse oximeters…..).

PurpleAir makes air sensors that detect the amount of particulate matter in the air they are sampling, including particles approximating the size of the virus when in droplet or aerosol form.[739] These can be indoors or outdoors, and to guess at virus levels, you want primarily the indoor sensors, but it is helpful to have an outdoor sensor too because that shows the level of background air pollution.

If you know both indoor and outdoor readings, you then know how much better or worse than the "fresh" air outside your indoor environment is. Just knowing the indoor level of particulate matter is meaningless – it might be very low, but if outdoors is even lower, it is elevated compared to "normal" (ie outside). Or it might be very high, but if outdoors is even higher, it is better than "normal".

Your objective would be to get the PM2.5 reading as low as possible on your indoor sensors, and certainly lower than whatever the outdoor reading is.

PurpleAir also publishes a great map showing internet-connected sensors around the country which can be interesting to see for understanding smoke and smog type pollution, but of no value for understanding virus particle levels.[740] But if you didn't want to buy two sensors, maybe there are some existing nearby outdoor sensors that you can see on the map and which will give you sufficiently helpful information to be able to interpret your indoor reading.

There are other companies with similar sensors, too, of course, and this article gives an interesting introduction to a new measuring system that combines several different sensor elements.[741]

There are also what I'd term "batch sampling devices" that suck in a quantity of air and then test that sample for the virus, using slow PCR testing that might take a day for a result to be returned. That's a long way short of real-time information, and would not be helpful in situations such as a retail store (knowing that someone out of all of yesterday's customers was infected isn't very useful) but in a closed office environment with only ten or so "high value"

---

[739] See https://www2.purpleair.com/collections/air-quality-sensors or https://cov.cx/a1e94

[740] See http://www.purpleair.com/map?mylocation or https://cov.cx/a1e95

[741] See https://spectrum.ieee.org/tech-talk/telecom/wireless/indoor-airquality-monitoring-can-allow-anxious-office-workers-to-breathe-easier or https://cov.cx/a1e96

employees, then the information can be more helpful, although still slow and cumbersome and, oh yes, expensive, too.[742]

You'd use an air purifier, if necessary, to hopefully "clean-up" your indoor air if it shows a high particulate matter count. Indeed, you'd probably choose to do this regardless of whether a high indoor count was due to something inside your home or "just" because the outdoor air also suffers a high particulate matter count.

Medical Care Gear

Now that you've got various monitoring equipment, you'll now want some items that can make changes to your environment in response to the data received from the monitoring equipment.

Carrying on from a discussion of air quality immediately above, it seems logical to first look at air purification strategies.

- *Air Purifier and/or Furnace Filters*

If you're going to be sharing an environment, either at work or home, with other people who may be "doing their own thing" and incurring their own set of risks for contracting the disease, the last thing you want to do is to increase your own exposure risk by having risky contact with roommates and others you can't easily avoid.

Apart from distancing measures, one practical risk reducer is to have air purifiers processing the air in your parts of the shared environment (and by all means in shared spaces and even in their personal areas, too. The sooner you can have air purifiers grab any exhaled viral particles and trap them in a filter, the better). You want the purifier to get to these particles before you breathe them in.

If you have a central air system, the risk is it may suck up infected air from people sharing the same system, and then blow the infected air out in the area where you are. It reduces the effectiveness of social distancing within your home.

---

[742] See https://spectrum.ieee.org/the-human-os/sensors/chemical-sensors/devices-monitor-coronavirus-in-the-air or https://cov.cx/a1e97

A partial solution to this (other than turning off your central air and using only local area and ideally radiant rather than fan heating units[743]) is to replace your system's filters with new MERV 13 filters and replace them regularly. Amazon has MERV 13 filters in most common sizes. https://amzn.to/2GGxPoR or https://cov.cx/a1f36

Check with the furnace manufacturer to see if you may need to adjust the fan speed setting to compensate for the greater "blockage" factor that MERV 13 filters sometimes have compared to other regular filters. Sometimes you can change a set of jumper leads inside the control box to vary the fan speed.[744]

An air purifier for your room or work area is also a great idea. I now have a couple, because, a bit like humidifiers, they are typically rated for only relatively small areas. Needless to say, Amazon have many to choose from. https://amzn.to/3lpRt7O or https://cov.cx/a1f37

Some purifiers will also quote a CADR number – a Clean Air Delivery Rate. This is a number of cubic feet per minute, and is the product of multiplying the airflow rate through the unit by its efficiency at removing particles.[745] There are different CADR numbers calculated for the removal of dust, pollen, and environmental tobacco smoke. You want to use the tobacco smoke rating – if it is provided – to understand how well a unit can deliver virus-free air.

Our understanding is these ratings are self-assessed by each manufacturer, so use them with a degree of skepticism. But there is an independent verification authority too, which some manufacturers choose to pay to be verified and listed

---

[743] If you can't control the air in the entire residence (or office) the other approach is to minimize the sharing of the air. In that case, radiant air heaters with no fans provide a way to heat an area with the least amount of air movement.

[744] This can be more important than you might guess. If the fan speed lowers too much, that means that cool air is taking away enough of the heat being generated and the furnace gets too hot and fails.

In summer, it means the hot air isn't taking away enough of the cold from the cooling coil, which then freezes and becomes less efficient, and potentially risks the coolant not evaporating, and very bad (ie expensive) things happening to the compressor.

[745] Well, in the US, usually CADR ratings are based on cubic feet per minute (cfm). But be careful. Sometimes, and in Canada, for example, CADR ratings are more commonly expressed in terms of cubic meters per hour. To convert from cubic meters/hr to cubic feet/minute, multiply the cu m/hr number by 0.59 and you'll get cu ft/min. For example, 100 cu m/hr = 59 cu ft/min.

by – AHAM Verifide. Their helpful website collects CADR ratings for a number of air purifiers.[746]

The number of air changes an hour you want will vary depending on the number of risks present – ie, the number of other people you are sharing the space with. The more air changes an hour the better and there's no exact formula for how to balance the number of potentially infected people in a room with the rate of air changes for the room.

The main thing in larger spaces is to be able to have a steady flow of purified air blowing around your personal space so the air you are breathing is low risk.

Also, and for the same reason as humidifiers, you may need to run them most/all of the time, because your home or work probably "leaks" air in and out through gaps in doors and windows and siding, and also because if you have other people sharing your air, they may be steadily exhaling virus particles. It is a nonstop job to keep the air pure, especially if one of the problems is impure outside air (although this is not likely to be impure in the sense of laden with virus particles unless you're in an unusual place).

Most air purifiers have replaceable HEPA filters. But one of mine – a **Honeywell** unit – has a washable filter made out of a special material that continues to work well, even after multiple washes (they say "lifetime", although they do need to be occasionally cleaned). Several other Honeywell units also use the same type of filter technology.

We really like the fact that Honeywell's items are usually listed in the CARB list of approved air purifiers and also are rated by the AHAM Verifide program. Maybe there are cheaper Chinese units available (although the Honeywell units seem fairly priced) but at least we know the Honeywell units are safe and can truly evaluate how effective they are. They are available on Amazon, of course - see https://amzn.to/30VeBTD or https://cov.cx/a1f38

Normal HEPA filter based units seem to need their filters replaced every three months or so – be careful you get a unit that uses readily available filters and understand the cost of the replaceable filters – you don't want to get trapped in a "cheap printer/expensive ink" type situation! For that reason, I like the concept of the very-long-lasting washable filter.

We recommend you check the California Air Resources Board (CARB) list of approved air purifiers. It doesn't guarantee that units are effective, but it does affirm they meet basic safety standards and that they don't emit

---

[746] See https://www.ahamdir.com/room-air-cleaners/ or https://cov.cx/a1e98

harmful ozone or have other negative effects.[747] Not all the profusion of Chinese branded/generic air purifiers are on this list, so not being on the list is not necessarily a negative downcheck, but being on the list is definitely a positive upcheck.

See also the CARB's list of potentially hazardous air purifiers.[748] This list is probably much more incomplete than their list of approved products, but still should be checked (whether you are in California or not).

- *Fans*

If you don't have air purifiers, maybe you can at least use one or two fans to get the air in your personal spaces steadily being replaced with new fresh and likely cleaner/safer air from outside.

Ideally have at least two fans – one placed in a window that sucks air from outside and blows it into your area, and a second fan placed in another window that sucks air from inside and blows it outside. (Keep the two fans as far apart as possible so you aren't just recycling the same air in and out.)

There is no value to you in having a fan that just blows air around a room. You want every fan to either be blowing fresh safe air into your room, or exhausting less safe air out of the room.

If you only have one fan, we'd tend to give the highest priority to a fan that blows fresh safe air into your room. If you only have an exhaust fan, you need to understand where the replacement air is coming from. Air must always come in from somewhere to replace the air that goes out – there's every possibility that an exhaust fan might end up sucking replacement air in from shared other parts of your environment – replacement air that is more likely to have virus particles in them than the air in your personally controlled environment.

That would be very much an "own goal".

Fans can be very inexpensive, although some are inexplicably quite costly. Of course, Amazon has plenty to choose from. https://amzn.to/3oIoqEv or https://cov.cx/a1f39 There are even some already designed to fit into window spaces, such as this one : https://amzn.to/3d8wovC or https://cov.cx/a1f40 We like how it can move air in either direction.

---

[747] See https://ww2.arb.ca.gov/our-work/programs/air-cleaners-ozone-products/california-certified-air-cleaning-devices or https://cov.cx/a1e99

[748] See https://ww2.arb.ca.gov/our-work/programs/air-cleaners-ozone-products/potentially-hazardous-ozone-generators-sold-air or https://cov.cx/a1f01

- *Humidifier and/or Dehumidifier*

In the winter, the heating in our homes tends to dry the air out. In summer, rather than doing the opposite, a/c units in their cooling mode also remove moisture from the air. So most people are more likely to need to boost their indoor humidity with a **humidifier**, rather than to dial it back with a dehumidifier.

Even in normal times, many of us would benefit from a humidifier. It is common, when running heating or cooling a lot, that our homes might have humidities in the twenties or thirties percent range – half the ideal level.

When evaluating humidifiers, choose one with a very large capacity, so you won't need to be constantly refilling it. We suggest one gallon (4 liters) as a minimum size, and we prefer ones that you can "top fill" by simply bringing a jug of water to the unit and pouring it in, rather than one where you have to remove the water container, take it to a tap, fill it, take it back to the unit, re-insert it, and then restart the unit.

Some have the equivalent of a heater's thermostat – they'll shut off when a given humidity level is reached. That's a great extra feature to have.

Most humidifiers are rated for smallish areas rather than whole-home coverage, so you might need to get several.

There are several different ways that a humidifier works. The most common are either ultra-sonic, impeller (can be or become noisy), or wick (evaporative) based units. Some units simply heat and boil water to create the water vapor – these have the highest energy cost.

It is important to maintain a humidifier, changing the water every two or three days (assuming the tank hasn't emptied by itself), and occasionally cleaning the unit, perhaps with hydrogen peroxide or vinegar or even tea tree oil.

Amazon of course has plenty to choose from. https://amzn.to/30KZ3lj or https://cov.cx/a1f41

A less common requirement is a **dehumidifier**, which is basically an a/c unit without the heating/cooling function.

When choosing a dehumidifier you ideally want one that you can program the target humidity into so it doesn't overachieve – dehumidifiers generally seem to be more powerful than humidifiers in terms of the area they can serve and the impact they can have.

You also should think about how you want to handle the water it is collecting – your choice is either a collection tank that you'll need to regularly empty or a hose that can be run to a drain somewhere. The latter is less hassle but might require some thought as to where you locate the unit. If getting one with a collection tank, a bigger tank will be less bothersome than a smaller tank, of course.

Amazon has plenty of models. https://amzn.to/2I4tLQc or https://cov.cx/a1f42

- ## *Oxygen Concentrator*

An oxygen concentrator is hopefully not something that most of us will need in the foreseeable future. It primarily starts to be beneficial if your blood oxygen level goes way low, and normally, in such a case, you'd simply go to a hospital and be cared for there.

But if case numbers continue to increase as they are again in early November, there's a possibility that hospitals might start to fill up as they did earlier in 2020, making access to health care less assured and, if available, more chaotic.[749] In any case, you might want to do all you can to keep out of a hospital.

One of the most likely reasons you might need to be admitted to a hospital is if you need supplementary oxygen. If that is all (and it rarely is), an oxygen concentrator can be a great way to boost your oxygen intake, and you can continue to monitor your blood oxygen level with a pulse oximeter (as described above) to ensure that the concentrator is compensating for your reduced lung function.

But, please don't do this on your own. If you're at a point where your blood oxygen level is falling to seriously low numbers, you need professional medical intervention. The problem is not so much the need for extra oxygen, but fixing your lungs before they get worse.

However, if your doctor agrees that you could stay at home and use your own supplemental oxygen, and hopefully also prescribes you some medicines to take to address the problem in your lungs, then subject to your self-monitoring your blood oxygen level and no other symptoms providing extra cause for concern, it might be nice to at least have the option to do this if you wish; and if prudent, it is likely that overstaffed local hospitals will be extremely appreciative, too.

The cheapest approach to providing supplemental oxygen is to have one or many bottles of oxygen. We don't argue against that, but we note that for a while earlier this year there were stories of medical oxygen getting in short supply. Who only knows if this might become even more a problem in the future.

---

[749] This article in mid-November reports over 1,000 hospitals already with severe staff shortages, and expects the number of struggling-to-keep-up hospitals will increase - https://www.npr.org/sections/health-shots/2020/11/20/937152062/1-000-u-s-hospitals-are-short-on-staff-and-more-expect-to-be-soon or https://cov.cx/a1f02

Being self-sufficient by nature, I like the concept of having my own oxygen concentrator.[750] That reduces my reliance on external things to merely needing electricity to run it (and yes, I do have a standby generator!). An oxygen concentrator "never runs out", because it simply, as the name implies, concentrates the amount of oxygen that is already in the air (there is about 21% oxygen in the air).

Oxygen concentrators were common and as little as $350 on Amazon earlier this year. Now it is harder to find them and they're generally more expensive. https://amzn.to/3kdPlA2 or https://cov.cx/a1f43 Some concentrators can only be sold to people with a prescription authorizing the purchase of one – the FDA again at work "protecting us" (from ourselves).

Some models are "portable" – they can run on batteries as well as mains power. That might be a useful feature to look for – both from the portability point of view and also from the "just in case of a power cut" perspective.

Because of the critical nature of a concentrator – that is, if you are at the point of needing one, and if you are a long way from a hospital, this is not an item that you'd want to buy the cheapest model and hope it doesn't fail. At the very least, have a small emergency backup bottle of oxygen too, so if your concentrator fails, you can rely on your oxygen bottle while getting to a hospital.

Bulk and Area Cleaning/Disinfecting

This was a topic of great focus in the early stages of the virus outbreak, back when health experts claimed the primary route for infection was by us touching an infected surface, then putting our contaminated hand in our mouth or nose, or rubbing our eye with it.

While there is a reluctance for these same experts to now say "we were totally wrong" they are slowly but surely moving away from that claim and now are conceding there is no evidence of the virus being passed on to anyone via a contaminated surface. But does that mean there never was any risk, or does it mean that we all did a great job of washing our hands and being careful what we touched?

For all reasons, you shouldn't now totally neglect personal hygiene, and similarly should also keep "touch surfaces" that many people might touch at a high level of cleanliness, too.

---

[750] Would I be obsessive to say that I'd even take my own concentrator with me to the hospital? That way, if they do run out of oxygen tanks, and don't have other available equipment, I've got my own with me.

- *Disinfectant*

Three different terms are sometimes used interchangeably, but which are quite different. The three terms are cleanser, antiseptic, and disinfectant.

For our purposes, killing virus contamination, and making objects safe, you always want to use disinfectant.

The very good news is the EPA has published a list of all the approved disinfectants it considers to be suitable to disinfect areas and remove potential Covid virus contamination.[751] It is simply a case of checking to see if the product you are considering using is on the list or not.

Well, no, it isn't quite that simple, alas. The EPA requires you to key in the product's official registration number to confirm the product's approval. But what if you don't have that? Sure, it should be on the label, but maybe you're wanting to buy online and the registration number isn't mentioned in the product write-up. You should go to the "advanced search" option where you have several ways to find the product you're looking for. If all else fails, get the entire list to display at the bottom of the advance search page.

My main disinfectant is Virex II/256, which uses a quaternary ammonium active ingredient, as do many others.

It was perhaps not the best choice (it was the only highly effective product readily available when I was seeking a good disinfectant in March) because it requires ten minutes of contact time before being wiped off again. Many products seem to require much less contact time and might be a better choice, and many people don't read the fine print and realize that their disinfectant does need to sit on a surface for ten minutes.

Some interesting new products are being developed that claim to be coatings that will kill any viruses that land on coated surfaces.[752] To date, no such products have been approved by the EPA, and one, in particular, has been waiting for approval – but waiting seems to be the order of the day, with the EPA typically taking 6 – 9 months to approve submitted products. That is a dismaying

---

[751] See https://www.epa.gov/pesticide-registration/list-n-disinfectants-coronavirus-covid-19 or https://cov.cx/a1f03

[752] See https://www.dallasnews.com/business/technology/2020/06/02/a-dallas-company-touts-its-spray-on-coating-as-a-covid-19-killer-for-surfaces/ or https://cov.cx/a1f04

length of time. For now, the EPA maintains there are no approved products of this type.[753]

One more point about disinfectants, and indeed, about cleaning products in general. As mentioned above, maybe it is because of the excellent job of cleaning everything all the time that is being done everywhere at present (yes, that does sound unlikely, doesn't it!) but there have been no known cases of Covid being caught as a result of touching an infected surface.

Yes, definitely clean and disinfect, but realize that possibly this should not be your highest priority. We recommend you focus equally on getting your air as clean and safe as possible.

•   *Other Cleaning Products/Equipment*

What do you do if you have a larger possibly infected area to clean – a hotel room, a conference room, a large open-plan office, etc?

That usually calls for industrial type equipment – foggers and misters to spray an entire large area with disinfectant, and requires the person applying the spray to be in protective gear, because the disinfecting chemicals, in larger doses, are poisonous.

There is also a new type of sprayer – an electrostatic sprayer, that adds a positive charge to the droplets that are being sprayed. This charge helps the droplets to move to and then adhere to surfaces, making for better coverage.

Unfortunately, the EPA has not yet considered such methods of disinfecting areas.[754] You might well wonder why it hasn't done so, but that's a question I can't answer. In July, the EPA was promising expedited review of electrostatic sprayers,[755] but three months later, none seem to be acknowledged on its website.

There are two or three other products sometimes considered.

---

[753] See https://www.epa.gov/coronavirus/there-anything-i-can-do-make-surfaces-resistant-sars-cov-2-covid-19 or https://cov.cx/a1f05

[754] See https://www.epa.gov/coronavirus/can-i-use-fogging-fumigation-or-electrostatic-spraying-or-drones-help-control-covid-19 or https://cov.cx/a1f06

[755] See https://www.epa.gov/newsreleases/epa-takes-action-help-americans-disinfect-indoor-spaces-efficiently-and-effectively or https://cov.cx/a1f07

- *Ionizers and Ozonators*

Ionizers are sometimes claimed to do assorted magical things to the air. In theory, they add negatively charged particles to airborne contaminants, and that makes them more readily attracted to filters. Maybe there is an element of truth in that, but equally maybe, perhaps there isn't. The few scientific studies and reviews we've found tend to be neutral/negative in the sense they can't discern any benefit or change to air purity as a result of air ionization.[756]

The effectiveness of ionizers became a topic of public discussion in 2003 when a company, Sharper Image, sued Consumer Reports for the very low rating CR had given to Sharper Image's product, the Ionic Breeze. Consumer Reports decisively won the lawsuit, and subsequent class actions against Sharper Image by people who had bought Ionic Breeze units were a major factor leading to Sharper Image declaring Chapter 11 bankruptcy in 2008.[757]

Some ionizers have shown to be effective, but our sense is they tend to be the "industrial-grade" ionizers rather than residential type ionizers. Industrial-grade ionizers also tend to generate more ozone at the same time, which brings us to the second part of this section.

Ozonators generate ozone. Ozone is a special type of unstable oxygen molecule (O_3 rather than O_2) in gaseous form that "wants" to become the stable O_2 form, leaving a single oxygen atom that will attack things in its desire to settle into some type of molecule. Because it is gaseous, it can spread and reach lots of different places, very quickly.

This "attacking" can harm the things it comes into contact with, and that is a good thing if the thing it comes in contact with is a virus or bacteria. It is a very bad thing however if the thing it comes in contact with is you, your lungs, and your eyes/nose/mouth.

Hence the concept of using ozonators to disinfect areas. They have also been used to get rid of odors (attack the volatile smell compounds).

They may be good at this or not; but for your at-home and in-office purposes, they are a very bad choice indeed. Oxone is harmful to people, even in extraordinarily low concentrations. You actively do not want to have any type of device in your home or office that emits ozone.

---

[756] For example, https://www.ncbi.nlm.nih.gov/pmc/articles/PMC3848581/ or https://cov.cx/a1f08

[757] See https://www.consumeraffairs.com/news04/2008/02/sharper_image.html or https://cov.cx/a1f09

Many ionizers emit ozone as a byproduct of their ionizing process, and that can be a problem. Similarly, many UV-C purifiers also emit ozone as part of their light-generating process. This, again, is a problem.

There appear to be beneficial results of using ozone to disinfect large areas – as little as one part per million of ozone can reduce the virus count by over 99% in a matter of seconds.[758] But unless it is done with no people present, and then all the ozone thoroughly and completely flushed out, it is not suitable. The UL 867 acceptable limit for ozone is 0.05 parts per million. Other standards are set at similar levels.[759]

This article argues against buying either ozonators or ionizers.[760] While there may be specific exceptions to their generic advice, we find ourselves in general agreement.

- ### *UV-C Light Disinfecting*

You're probably familiar with ultraviolet (UV) light in general. It is what gives us sunburn, and is the type of "invisible light" emitted by blacklights in nightclubs that make our clothes fluoresce and look strange.

UV light is of higher frequencies than visible light, and because it is a higher frequency, it has higher energy in its "beam". Just like we split visible light, somewhat arbitrarily, into different colors (there is no exact point where red becomes orange and orange becomes yellow, is there) so too do we split UV light into three bands – UV-A, UV-B, and UV-C.

UV-A light is what you find in blacklights. [761] UV-B light is what causes sunburn and skin cancer.

---

[758] See https://www.randrmagonline.com/articles/88901-ozones-efficacy-in-deactivating-coronavirus-like-pathogens or https://cov.cx/a1f10

[759] See https://www.epa.gov/indoor-air-quality-iaq/ozone-generators-are-sold-air-cleaners#harmful-ozone or https://cov.cx/a1f11

[760] See https://www.inputmag.com/guides/do-not-buy-ozone-generator-for-coronavirus-covid-19 or https://cov.cx/a1f12

[761] As an unrelated but hopefully helpful comment, we urge you to avoid blacklights. This is not because of any concerns about their UV radiation causing skin cancer, but rather because of potential damage to your eyes. Because our eyes don't see UV light, and because blacklights are often in darkened rooms, our pupils are dilated to let the most amount of light in, and the blacklight floods in and can damage our eyes without

(continued on next page)

UV-C light is the highest frequency and has the shortest wavelength, and so has the most energy. It is also rarely found – although the sun emits plenty, it is absorbed by the atmosphere and almost none makes it down to ground level.

Perhaps because it is not found in nature, and so no viruses have evolved to have protection against UV-C, it has excellent abilities to kill virus particles, with the most effective killing wavelength being around 265 nm (nanometers). On the other hand, it is not so beneficial around the 185 nm wavelength, because at that wavelength, it causes normal oxygen to form ozone.

Unfortunately, the mercury vapor lights that are often used to create UV-C lights not only put out a lot of energy around 265 nm, but they also put out some around 185 nm, and so inherently tend to create ozone too, which as you'll recall from the preceding section is not a good thing. If the bulb uses regular soft or quartz glass, the 185 nm UV-C light can pass through and then interact with the oxygen in the air to form ozone. But if it has titanium in the glass, that absorbs the 185 nm light and makes the bulb much safer and not so prone to creating ozone.

UV-C light, of sufficiently high intensity, is the closest thing to a science-fiction type death-ray that there is when fighting the virus. But it has a major limitation. It won't shine around corners – like all light, it travels in straight lines. For area disinfection, it can only disinfect what it can "see". Any object or structure that creates shade on any other object or structure will reduce its coverage and effectiveness.

Generally, UV-C light is best used when integrated into an HVAC unit, to treat the air passing through it, rather than as an area disinfecting device.[762]

Personal Protective Equipment

Much has been made of the desperate shortages of personal protective equipment for healthcare workers.

Generally, you'll not need the same quantities or quality of products they use, because hopefully you're not in an environment where you might be exposed to higher concentrations of virus particles for hours at a time, but there are some things you should have.

---

our realizing it. Short exposures are okay, but avoid longer exposures, don't stare directly at the bulbs/tubes, especially when the other lighting is low.

[762] This article has a great discussion on UV-C light issues
https://www.energyvanguard.com/blog/do-uv-lamps-really-improve-indoor-air-quality or
https://cov.cx/a1f13

- *Hand Sanitizer*

Hand sanitizer was one of those almost-impossible-to-find products, like toilet paper, earlier this year. Now we see good availability on Amazon and in stores, but that availability could vanish in a flash, the same as it did earlier in the year if there's a new "panic" and a sudden surge in buying.

Amazon currently has plenty of choices and plenty of different hand sanitizer products. https://amzn.to/3lstJzU or https://cov.cx/a1f44 . I have a few small one-ounce pocket/travel-sized bottles of sanitizer located strategically around my home, office, car, coat pockets, and so on, and then I have larger 32 ounce/1 liter bulk supplies that I use to keep my small bottles topped up.

The active ingredient in hand sanitizer is almost always alcohol and nothing else.[763] There are other ingredients, but they are primarily to make the alcohol into a gel, to reduce the alcohol concentration, and to possibly add some moisturizer, some coloring, and some smell to it.

Note that the alcohol in hand sanitizer is (or, at least, should be) either ethyl alcohol (ethanol) or isopropyl alcohol (isopropanol). Isopropanol is also sometimes described as 2-propanol.

The alcohol should not be methyl alcohol (methanol) or 1-propanol. These are seriously harmful products and can be absorbed directly through your skin and end up in toxic concentrations.

Dismayingly, some companies have sold hand sanitizer that while labeled as containing ethyl or propyl alcohol, actually contain methyl alcohol. The FDA has a list of over 150 such products – if you are buying a brand you don't already know and trust, you should check their list first.[764] Their list also includes products that, while not poisonous, are simply not effective, either.

Surprisingly, the optimum alcohol concentration is not 100%. It seems to generally be stated to be around 70% - 85% concentration for the sanitizer to be most effective – the alcohol needs some water to help kill the virus. So there is such a thing as "too strong".

Much less surprisingly, there is also such a thing as "too weak". Generally, it seems that anything under 60% alcohol is not strong enough, and the range from 60% - 70% alcohol is on the low side of optimum. The lower the alcohol concentration, the longer it takes to kill the virus particles, and because the

---

[763] Rarely, you might find sanitizer that uses benzalkonium chloride.

[764] See https://www.fda.gov/drugs/drug-safety-and-availability/fda-updates-hand-sanitizers-consumers-should-not-use or https://cov.cx/a1f14 – we don't think this is a complete list, but at least it is a start.

alcohol tends to evaporate quite rapidly, at concentrations like 60% there's an increasing risk it will have evaporated before it has done its job.

There's no reason to make do with less effective 60% or 65% sanitizer these days. You have plenty of 70%+ products to choose from.

Interestingly, the CDC continues to point out that the best type of hand sanitizing is simply to wash your hands with soap and water. Hand sanitizer is not a superior approach, it is merely an easy approach when you are somewhere that doesn't allow soap and water handwashing.

- *Masks*

The two topics we dreaded discussing the most are hydroxychloroquine (now bravely discussed on page 13 and 375) and masks.

It is astonishing and dismaying to see how controversial mask-wearing has become, to the point where people are even shooting each other.

The dispassionate evidence is clear – wearing a mask protects the people around you, and also protects yourself. The protection isn't absolute, but it is substantial, as has been consistently demonstrated in many studies.[765]

Some people triumphantly claim it is scientifically impossible for a mask to work because the coronavirus size is very much smaller than the mesh screen gaps in a mask filter. On the face of it, that makes sense – if you have a coarse sieve, sugar granules will go through it, for example. But this is a case of "a little knowledge is a dangerous thing". There are two points to consider, and perhaps a bonus third point too.

The first is that virus particles seldom exist by themselves. They are usually bonded to something larger, like a water droplet. So the important measure isn't the size of the virus particle, but the overall size of it and whatever it has stuck to.

The second is that whereas sugar granules are primarily affected by gravity, when you get things as tiny and as light-weight as virus particles, other factors

---

[765] This is a nice measured article on the topic https://www.seattletimes.com/seattle-news/health/evidence-is-growing-but-what-will-it-take-to-prove-masks-slow-the-spread-of-covid-19/ or https://cov.cx/a1f15

This article looks primarily at N95 type respirator masks but has excellent material on fabric and surgical masks too https://fastlifehacks.com/n95-vs-ffp/ or https://cov.cx/a1f16

This article rebuts the myth about masks causing CO2 buildup and assorted other nonsense claims https://www.thedailybeast.com/5-myths-on-face-masks-amid-the-coronavirus-pandemic or https://cov.cx/a1f17

This site is full of excellent articles about masks and consistently shows the benefits associated with wearing one https://www.n95decon.org/ or https://cov.cx/a1f18

start to come into play. One in particular is electrostatic attraction that can "suck" up the particles flowing through a mask and cause them to move over to the mask fibers and "stick" on them.[766]

The bonus third point is simple. Never mind the explanations, just look at the results. Testing (see the previous link and others in this section too) clearly shows that masks do filter out virus particles.

Whether you care about your personal risk or not, politeness, courtesy and consideration should compel you to wear a mask for the benefit of the people around you.

This is particularly so because most people who become infected with the disease are at their most infectious before they know they're unwell. So you can't say to yourself "I'll wear a mask if I feel unwell" because, by then, it is too late. You may have already infected other people and contributed to the continued spread of the disease.

Perhaps one of the controversial elements of mask-wearing is where the ideal compromise point is between convenience and safety. Everyone has a different perception of that. But the lack of national consensus does make establishing these things much more difficult.

In Britain, as of 25 August, we have the ridiculous situation where in Scotland, school children 12 and older must wear masks on school buses, in school corridors, and other communal areas, but not in classrooms. Why not in classrooms, which in some respects may present as more risk than in corridors? Meanwhile, in England, no mask-wearing is required for school children at all, but the authorities might change their mind, and in Wales, they haven't yet decided what to do. As for Northern Ireland, masks are "strongly encouraged" but "not generally recommended for routine use".

When the public see such a mish-mash of contradictory and vague statements, it is understandably hard to draw any inference that there is a clear case for mask-wearing. This matter is made all the worse by the CDC and other authorities first saying there was no need for us to wear masks – all we had to do was wash our hands a lot and perhaps practice some social distancing too. Then they said, in effect, "Well, yes, you should wear a mask, and we lied to you before, because we wanted to keep all the masks for healthcare workers".

Although there are official standards for N95 and other types of "official" mask, there are no standards for other types of non-official mask – neither the "surgical" masks that you would normally see people wearing in operating

---

[766] This is a good article about how masks work with virus particles
https://www.usatoday.com/story/news/factcheck/2020/08/09/fact-check-masks-effective-covid-19-despite-drywall-dust-claims/3322819001/ or https://cov.cx/a1f19

theaters and elsewhere in hospitals, nor all the "fashion" and "do it yourself" masks that are now everywhere. This is all the more regrettable, not just because of the enormous variation in effectiveness, but because it can be quick, easy, and inexpensive to test a mask for its effectiveness.[767]

Imagine if there were no standards for car safety belts, and people were allowed to make their own and fit them to their cars, themselves. How well would that work? Well, currently, we've many more people dying every day from the virus than from car accidents, but while we've very detailed requirements for car safety belts (and airbags and ABS and all manner of other safety design elements) we're leaving one of the most important elements of virus safety completely undefined and allowing anything at all to masquerade as a mask.

There are no design requirements, nor any material requirements, apart from saying "should cover your mouth and nose". We see so many masks that barely reach up to the tip of a person's nose, with plenty of space on each side of the nostrils for air to travel directly in and out without going through the masks; we see masks made out of ridiculous materials that sometimes are little better than nothing, and we cringe when we read the recommendations to wash and reuse masks every day. Worst of all, we see people wearing masks with vents on them to "make breathing easier" – yes, it makes it easier to breathe, but it destroys the functionality of the mask.[768] Note that this linked article also points to the nonsensical nature of face shields – while they add some small amount of extra protection, they must never be used instead of a mask.

It isn't just that some masks are useless, it gets worse than that. Some masks may cause more harm than good. Here's an article that goes further than just saying that some masks work better than others. It says some masks are worse than useless and cause harm.[769]

As an interesting aside, another myth shattered is the concept of coughing into one's elbow rather than hand – it too does more harm than good.[770]

The good news is that the best (non-N95) masks are the cheapest ones – the three-layer surgical masks that you can these days buy at Costco or Walmart or

[767] See https://advances.sciencemag.org/content/6/36/eabd3083 or https://cov.cx/a1f20

[768] See https://www.studyfinds.org/face-shields-masks-with-valves-wont-stop-coronavirus-spread/ or https://cov.cx/a1f21

[769] See https://www.studyfinds.org/worst-face-masks-covid-19-bandanas-neck-gaiters-more-harmful-than-no-mask/ or https://cov.cx/a1f22

[770] See https://www.dailymail.co.uk/sciencetech/article-8661867/Coughing-uncovered-elbow-lets-droplets-hand.html or https://cov.cx/a1f23

online for less than 20c each.[771] Here's a link to Amazon's mask listings, with some brands offering boxes of 50 for less than $10. https://amzn.to/34Md3N2 or https://cov.cx/a1f45

Buy several boxes of them. They're readily available at present, but who knows what will happen as the virus infection rate intensifies at present.

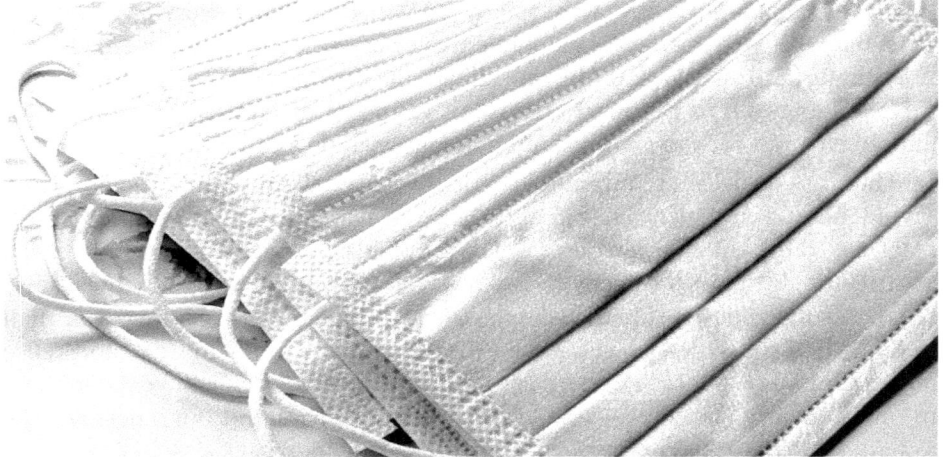

Figure 68 Low-cost surgical masks are the most effective (other than N95 specialty masks)

Something to consider with a surgical mask is there could be as many as four different ways to wear one – which side is the inside and outside, and which is the top and bottom edge?

The top and bottom are fairly simple to understand. The top has a wired strip in its middle, which is meant to shape the mask to fit closely around your nose.

As for the inside and outside, medical experts and a manufacturer say they should always be worn with the colored side outward.

To make this easy to always get right, I use a Sharpie marker and place a letter "D" (for David) on the inside top right corner. If other people are with me, I give them masks with a different letter in that place for them. That makes it easy to remember which mask belongs to which person, and how to put it on when picking it up.

Keep each person's mask separate from each other person's mask. You don't want to share/swap masks, because you might then breathe in something that

---

[771] See https://www.theguardian.com/world/2020/aug/26/non-woven-masks-better-to-stop-covid-19-says-japanese-supercomputer or https://cov.cx/a1f24

the other person breathed out and pick up either the Covid or some other infection from that person.

I mentioned washing masks. There are several problems with that, starting with the underlying need to wash a mask every day. Is that necessary? I've not seen a study to indicate that, I think it is just a reflexive thing like washing one's underwear or socks daily, too. There are also alternatives to washing – just leave the mask out in the sun for a few days and the virus particles that may be on it will all die.

But if you are going to wash anything to get rid of the virus, there are two ways you get rid of the virus. The first is by physically dislodging the virus and washing it away – in which case, be sure you don't have other clothing in the washing machine with the masks, for fear of contamination (very unlikely, but who knows).

The second way of getting rid of the virus is by killing it, and that requires water that is 140°F (60°C) or hotter. The chances are your hot water thermostat isn't set that high, and even if it is, by the time the water gets into your washing machine, the water is rapidly cooling.

As you know from washing regular clothes, the physical stress of being washed causes their fabric to thin, to stretch, and eventually to break. How many washes can a mask take before it becomes insufficiently effective? Do you know? My guess is not very many.

I use surgical masks, and I consider each one is good for about eight or so hours of use. Happily, I only need to wear them an hour or two at a time while shopping, and so a single mask can last me a week or more – even longer because there is "rest" and "recovery" time between each use.

Even after a week of use, that single 20c surgical mask might still have life in it. The virus particles die after some days, so if I was short on masks, I could put it to one side, leave it a week (ideally in the sun so some UV rays will help kill any virus particles on it), and then return to it again.

Here is a very vivid depiction of the impact masks can have on virus deaths. This projection shows three possible futures between 21 August and 1 December, depending on if there is less social distancing (red), an approach similar to what is happening at present (brown), or a cautious approach with 95% of people always wearing masks in public situations (green).[772]

---

[772] See https://covid19.healthdata.org/united-states-of-america or https://cov.cx/ihme – this chart being taken from their 21 August projections.

Daily deaths

Daily deaths is the best indicator of the progression of the pandemic, although there is generally a 17-21 day lag between infe

Scenario ○ Projection ✕ Easing ✕ Masks ✕

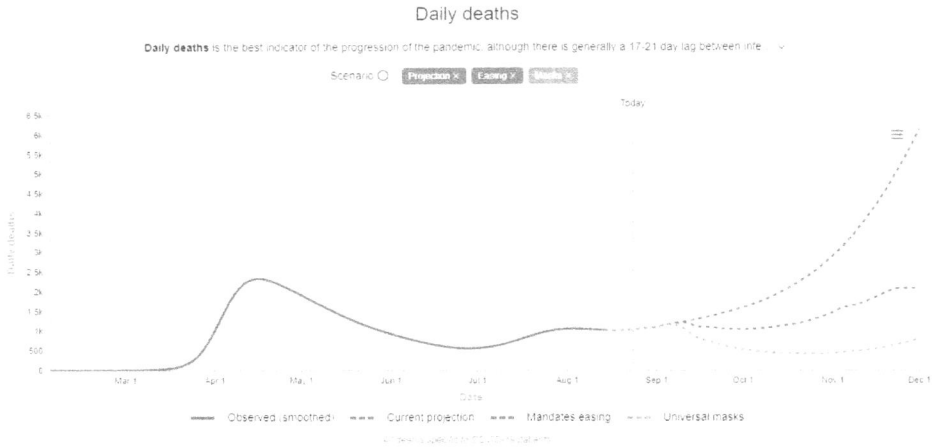

Figure 69 The effect of masks on deaths

In total, between 21 August and 1 December, the projection is guesstimating 421,000 deaths with an easing of social distancing, 310,000 with a moderate approach, or 241,000 with nearly universal mask-wearing.

In other words, 69,000 lives hang in the balance between 21 August and 1 December.[773] Masks are very impactful.

Lastly in this section, to close with some good news. It is true that current masks aren't 100% protective (but neither are seat belts, and we all wear those). However, new masks and new materials promise to be even better than current mask designs. An Israeli company, Sonovia, is developing a mask fabric that is coated with zinc oxide nano-particles that it is claimed will neutralize 99% of Covid-19 particles, even after multiple washings.[774]

---

[773] We hasten to add this is a "best guess" projection as of 21 August, and based on what the people managing the model anticipate happening both in terms of the virus activity and public health/social responses to it. It might be wildly wrong, it might be way too pessimistic, or it might be too optimistic, and of course, it might also be close to exact.

The Seattle group issuing these projections, IHME, started off with early projections that changed greatly from each release to each future release, now we notice the changes are smaller and as each month passes, have a chance to see how accurate their projections are, and their record is improving and becoming more persuasive.

[774] See https://www.reuters.com/article/us-health-coronavirus-israel-masks/israeli-mask-maker-sonovia-expects-99-coronavirus-success-after-lab-test-idUSKBN23T183 or https://cov.cx/a1f25

That's not the only possible breakthrough. In the US, scientists at Indiana University are developing a new "electroceutical" material that has embedded micro-cell silver-zinc dots that act as tiny batteries within it, and uses an electric charge to kill virus particles that pass through it.[775]

I've not seen any clear claims for its effectiveness yet and note it requires a minute of contact with the virus to "significantly lower" its viability. That seems like more time than might always be the case in real-world mask use.

- *Gloves*

We list gloves in this section not to advocate their use, but to give us a place to argue against them. We do not see any reason for normal people doing normal things to wear gloves.

Remember the disease can't penetrate your skin. You don't need any direct protection from contact, as would be the case if you were handling a dangerous acid or something like that.

Gloves instantly become unclean, the minute you touch anything with them. The protection you need is from transferring virus particles from a fomite to your face, and that is as likely to happen with gloves on as not (and these days is viewed as very unlikely in both cases). The gloves simply become the new surface for the virus to "hitch a ride on" instead of your skin.

Sure, it is easy to get safe and clean by removing the gloves (although studies show most people transfer some contamination from their gloves to their skin unless they're very skilled and careful at how to remove gloves without touching their exteriors), but it is not difficult to get safe and clean by using hand sanitizer or soap and water, either. Unless you're fastidious with how you remove your gloves and where you then discard them, there's a chance you may transfer any contamination from the gloves to your hands at that time and so should follow up with handwashing, which then makes one wonder "If I still need to wash my hands, why do I need the gloves, too?".

It could even be argued that gloves provide a false sense of safety that may encourage risky behavior. We wouldn't go that far, but we don't see any clear benefit in using gloves.

---

[775] See https://news.iu.edu/stories/2020/05/iu/releases/18-research-shows-electroceutical-fabric-eliminates-coronaviruses-on-contact.html or https://cov.cx/a1f26

- *Shields/Goggles/Glasses*

Another transmission vector may be present – becoming infected by way of virus particles landing on your eyes or possibly placed there if you get some virus particles on your hands and then touch your eyes.

This study approaches the problem positively by suggesting that maybe wearing glasses might help protect against catching the virus.[776] That's good to know, but it begs the question - how/why are eyeglass wearers protected?

There are two possible ways that glasses help. The first is by making it harder for people to touch/rub their eyes with their (possibly infected) hands. The second is to block off contaminated air from making contact with the eyes and tear ducts and allowing the virus to enter our body via that route.

The study is only weakly persuasive - it was based on a small number of observed cases, it doesn't consider other factors, and it doesn't distinguish between touching or airborne type infection. But there seems to be a possibly significant difference in infection rates between people who wear glasses all the time and people who don't.

Does that mean we should start wearing goggles? The study doesn't tell us. But if I was going into a "high-risk environment" for an extended time (ie an airplane flight) I'd definitely wear safety glasses or goggles (safety glasses or even regular glasses with plain glass lenses being a more discreet but perhaps not so effective approach).

If glasses may have a positive impact, it seems likely to infer that more comprehensive face shields would have a greater impact.

But please note that the benefit of glasses or a face shield is unrelated to that provided by a mask. Face shields provide little or any of the benefit that a face mask provides, and *should not be used as an alternate to a proper face mask.*

- *Toilet Seats with Lids*

Whenever you flush a toilet, the rushing water creates disturbances and causes a cloud of droplets and aerosol particles to erupt out of the bowl.[777] Because virus particles have been detected in feces, this can be a problem, particularly because traces can remain in the bowl for several flushes.

------

[776] See https://thehill.com/policy/healthcare/516945-eyeglasses-may-help-protect-against-coronavirus-study or https://cov.cx/a1f27

[777] See https://www.studyfinds.org/what-happens-when-you-flush-with-toilet-lid-up/ or https://cov.cx/a1f28

If your toilets have lids over their seats, you should always lower them before flushing. If they don't have lids, it is surprisingly easy to replace the seats with new seats that come with lids. No need to call a plumber, just undo two screws/nuts and bolts, remove one seat, put the new seat/lid combo in place, and do up the new screws/nuts and bolts.

Toilet seats with lids cost as little as $15 at Amazon, and there are also sure to be plenty to choose from at your local hardware store. See https://amzn.to/2I21PMq or https://cov.cx/a1f46

PART 5 : Final Comments & Appendices

In Conclusion

So, what do we really know about the virus? What should we be doing? How and when will the problems be resolved?

After reading some/most/all of this book, you're now one of the best-informed people on the planet. Sadly, many other people – including, as may now be obvious – many of the "experts" setting public health policy are not as well-informed as you have become.

But the chances are that you – like me, and, in secret truth, like the experts too – really don't have clear answers to these questions. But some things do seem clear.

Take prudent measures to keep safe. Avoid high-risk areas (especially indoor areas with few air changes and many people). Observe social distancing. Wear a mask. Consider the possible supplements and medicines to take as preventative and risk reduction measures.

If you do come down with an infection, don't just passively stay at home and wait for the virus to do the worst it can to you. Insist your doctor give you the same standard of care (but not necessarily the exact same drugs) as was given to President Trump, and talk through our list of possible medicines to take during the early stages of your infection.

When you've come out the other end of your infection, be aware that your acquired immunity may be weak rather than absolute, and may fade within a few months. Don't abandon all prudent measures.

Consider the vaccine choices carefully and understand how effective it is (or is not) for people like you (ie age and comorbidities), so you can decide if it makes sense for you and, if you take it, so you can understand how much you can rely on it and how prudent you'll need to continue to be. If you can, delay getting one until we have more choices than the two mRNA based vaccines, and a better understanding of the differences between them.

Keep up to date with the changing situation. Sign up for our free email newsletters. Follow us on Twitter.

And remember, by doing these things, you're not only improving your chance of getting through this safely, but you're also improving the chances of the people who love you and rely upon you, too. You'll not be a threat to them, and hopefully, you can encourage them to similarly adopt prudent measures and not be a threat to you.

In case public policymakers are reading, what should our national and state health services be doing? The virus will be with us for decades, maybe forever. We not only need the best vaccines, and to encourage people to be vaccinated, but we also must press on with developing treatments and cures for the people who will inevitably still become infected.

Good luck. I hope this book has been and will continue to be helpful.Appendix - Summary Chart of Treatments

The following is a summary of the material in our two chapters, "15. Non-official Treatments to Consider" and "16. Medicines, Supplements, Vitamins, etc".

We discuss the various products mentioned below in much more detail in these two chapters, including providing sources for our recommendations. You should not just plunge into this table and accept everything in it as universal received truth, and neither should you assume everything we mention is appropriate for you.

You can use it as a checklist, but be sure you understand and evaluate each item separately for yourself, and if at all possible, engage your doctor in a discussion with you about the pluses and minuses of each treatment.

Item	In General	At-Risk	If Infected
Alcohol	Go easy on the alcohol	Go easy on the alcohol	Abstain from alcohol entirely
Aspirin	Many people take a quarter aspirin every day at present (about 80 mg)	Increase to a full aspirin (about 325 mg) a day	Continue 325 mg a day
Azithromycin			500 mg on the first day, 250 mg daily for four more days
BCG TB Vaccination	As a prophylactic measure		
Budesonide		Not recommended	
Corticosteroids			Important to coordinate with your doctor
Famotidine	Optional	20 – 40 mg daily	40 mg daily
Favipiravir			1800 mg twice on day 1, 800 mg twice on days 2 - 13
Heart Monitoring		Monitor Qt interval if taking HCQ	

Item	In General	At-Risk	If Infected
Homeopathic Remedies	Maybe worth considering, but we don't recommend any in particular		
Hydrogen Peroxide		Gargle - after the risky event and nightly for a few nights	
Hydroxy-chloroquine		Optional – if you have an adequate supply, then probably wise to use some, 200 mg once or twice a day	Two doses a day for five days or longer. The first one or two doses 400 mg, then 200 mg subsequently
Ivermectin	Currently being studied as a prophylactic	Optional but maybe prudent	One single dose, possibly a second dose a day or two later if the first dose has no effect, approx 90 mcg per pound of body weight, maybe slightly less (70 mcg/lb) for a second dose
Listerine Original Mouthwash	Possibly	Yes, better than hydrogen peroxide and Povidone-Iodine	

Item	In General	At-Risk	If Infected
Melatonin	Optional up to 2 mg at night	Maybe up to 6 mg at night	If no ill effects, possibly increase to 12 mg at night
Metformin		Probably	Yes, 500 mg twice daily
Multi-vitamin	Yes, daily	Yes, daily	Yes, daily
Oxygen Level			Check regularly every day. You won't notice early declines in oxygen, so you need to check.
Povidone-Iodine		Possibly as an alternative to hydrogen peroxide.	
Propolis Spray		Before, during, and after an at-risk exposure	Perhaps continue
Quercetin		500 mg, once or twice a day	Yes, 500 mg twice a day possibly stop if hospitalized

Item	In General	At-Risk	If Infected
Rest & Sleep	Try to get enough sleep	Take things easy, don't tire yourself	Complete and total bed or couch or recliner rest, and continue to take it easy for a while after recovering to avoid a relapse
Traditional Chinese Medicine, Folk Medicines	Keep an open mind, maybe visit a TCM practitioner. No specific recommendations.		
Vitamin C	Maybe 500 mg	500 mg twice a day	At least 500 mg twice a day, maybe much more
Vitamin D	2000 IU (50 mcg)	Maybe increase to 4000 IU (100 mcg)	4000 IU (100 mcg)
Water		Be sure to drink plenty of water	Be sure to drink plenty of water or drinks with electrolyte supplements such as Gatorade
Zinc	Probably there's enough in the multi-vitamin	Increase to about 40 mg of elemental zinc or 220 mg of zinc sulfate	220 mg of zinc sulfate ie 50 mg of elemental zinc once daily

These are not our recommendations, merely reporting on what others have suggested. In most cases, there are only weak rather than definitive "proofs" of efficacy.

Please be sure to read the narrative commentaries about these medications and their possible complications before proceeding with any of them.

Appendix – About the Author

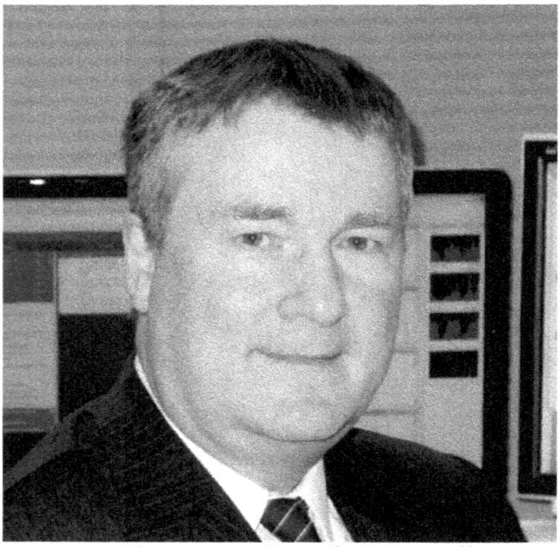

Figure 70 David M Rowell

So how did I end up spending most of 2020 obsessing over the coronavirus? During that time I've published more than 160 articles, posted I don't know how many tweets on the topic (over 1000 for sure), and of course, written this lengthy book.

Perhaps it is best to start at the beginning.

I spent my first almost 30 years in New Zealand before moving to the US in 1985; I've lived in the Seattle area most of the 35 years subsequently, with brief postings elsewhere on occasion. So I guess that gives me some perspective on both a country managing the virus about the best in the world, and, alas, a country managing the virus about the worst in the world.

I could flippantly say I spent the first half of my working life "on the dark side" and have spent my time subsequently atoning for that. By which I mean my earlier life was focused on marketing, consulting, and public relations, variously in the high tech and travel fields, with occasional forays into fields as disparate as raw meat and fish packaging, retailing (both bricks and mortar and mail-order), industrial relations, classical concert management, even furniture manufacturing.

Since 2000 my focus has been more as an iconoclastic commentator, pointing out the hypocrisies that are redolent within the travel and technology fields, and helping "normal people" make sense of the inflated uncritical nonsense, hype, and spin that surrounds these topics. I do a bit of unadvertised "dark side" work too, just to keep my hand in.

They say "it takes a thief to catch a thief". I don't know about thieving, but I see, everywhere in the media these days, the same rhetorical tricks, implications but not promises, careful word choices, obfuscations, selective data, and glosses that I formerly used myself, and feel a tingle of recognition every time I come across them.

I expect such things in political self-promotion and advertising commercial products, and these days make a career out of naming and shaming such things and translating them into truths. But imagine my surprise when, as the virus started to blow up in all our faces, I started seeing such things in medical reports, too.

I'm not a doctor, but I do understand statistics and data analysis, and as I discuss in length in the opening chapters, much of the issues to do with how to respond to and survive our Covid-19 pandemic are based on common sense, statistics, and data analysis rather than complex medical analysis of how the virus does what it does.

I've passed under-grad university classes in (among other subjects) chemistry, physics, information systems, applied maths and law, and post-graduate classes in data techniques and statistics (earning "A" passes and winning the Sheffield Prize at New Zealand's best business school). I've assorted other qualifications in fields ranging from ham radio (NZ9G) to mediation to firearms safety and self-defense. I've also a teaching English as a second language qualification (obtained with distinction) and have done volunteer teaching at middle school level on STEM subjects and also on speech and debate. I've a teenage daughter and a German Shepherd – both delightful, although one is more obedient than the other.

I never thought I'd write this book. But I'm glad I have. I hope you are pleased, too.

Appendix - Resources

I f you are unable to get the prescription medicines you need locally, there
is the slightly risky alternative of mail ordering from another country that
doesn't require prescriptions. The most common country to order from
is India. Other countries we've seen include Mexico and – perhaps surprisingly
– Fiji.

Some people claim there is a risk you'll get "bad" drugs of uncertain quality,
or expired drugs past their "use by" date, or indeed, you'll just get sugar pills
rather than the promised drugs. We're not certain there is any truth to these
stories at all, or if it is just a type of "Fear Uncertainty Doubt" tactic put out there
by people who have no actual certain evidence against using these outlets but
wish to discourage people from using them.

While we've not had a lot of experience with off-shore pharmacies, we've
never knowingly had a problem buying medicines either online or directly in the
countries that allow for US-prescription drugs to be sold without a prescription,
nor have other people we know.

In most cases, the online pharmacies are selling the exact same medications,
sourced from the exact same sources, that they and other pharmacies in those
countries are selling to the local people. These online sources are not breaking

the law in their countries. We have sometimes read some credible stories of fake medicines being sold in third world countries, but such stories are rare.[778]

I know, when I lived on and off in Russia, one could go to a local pharmacy and buy many/most types of medication without a prescription, and often would be given a choice between a Russian generic product, a generic from some other country, or a western made name brand product. There were higher prices for the generics from elsewhere and highest for the name brand product, but most of the pharmacists, while happy to sell the more expensive versions, assured me that the Russian product was just as good.

This was not a case of "breaking a law that was not enforced". It was perfectly legal and perfectly normal and common – most regular Russian people would go to a pharmacy rather than to a clinic/doctor to have their minor ailments diagnosed and treated by a pharmacist, and receiving medicines that some countries restrict and require doctors' prescriptions for, but which other countries allow to be sold by pharmacists directly.

It isn't just "very foreign" countries like Russia or India where this happens. There are significant differences between what medicines are "over-the-counter" or "prescription-only" in western countries, too.

It is hard to find off-shore online pharmacies. Google's search engine specifically refuses to link to them. Furthermore, some of the Indian sites seem to disappear and change their URLs regularly. We have a few listed below that may or may not still be up. We'll provide updated links on our website.[779]

Our suggestion is to of course pay by credit card, and if you don't get what you've ordered, dispute the charge with the credit card company.

During these difficult times, air freight services are somewhat disrupted, and shipments might be semi-randomly delayed. In other words, *order now* anything you think you might need in advance of needing it, because if you need something urgently (which is absolutely the case with antiviral medicines), there's no way that a freshly placed order and international package will get to you any time soon.

Another issue is that incoming packages of medicines may be subject to Customs seizure. It seems Customs are moderately tolerant of small quantities that are obviously for personal use, but if you decided to buy in bulk, and had hundreds of tablets all in one package, your chances of receiving it start to go

---

[778] Safely submerged in a footnote, you may be interested to guess which drug is most commonly fake. Sorry, guys, it is Viagra. See, for example, https://www.medpagetoday.org/meetingcoverage/smsna/34493 or https://cov.cx/a1f29

[779] See https://thecovidsurvivalguide.com/online-pharmacies/ or https://cov.cx/covop

down. Buy modest quantities per order, even if it means you miss out on bulk discounts and breaks on shipping costs.

We've noticed some of the online companies offer delivery insurance, which we understand to mean (but haven't confirmed) that if the package gets impounded by Customs, they'll either refund you or ship a second package at no extra cost. We've never had a package fail to arrive, but we know one person who has had that problem.

Note also that some online sources stock some medicines but not others, and availability, particularly of popular Covid-19 type medicines, is somewhat haphazard.

Prices tend to be dismayingly high compared to what you'd pay in those countries directly.   But if you need it, you need it, and if you can't get a prescription here, what are your other choices?

Some possible sources currently include

https://allinonerxmarket.com/ or https://cov.cx/a1f68 (recommended by a reader who says he has used them for many years, and never had a problem)

http://www.canadian-pharmacy-24.com/ or https://cov.cx/a1f69 (I have used)

https://mexipharmacy.mx/ or https://cov.cx/a1f70 (I know someone who has used this supplier)

https://family24rx.com/ or https://cov.cx/a1f71

https://omsi.in/ or https://cov.cx/a1f72

https://www.medicine-online.org/ or https://cov.cx/a1f73 (Seems to be European based, with many of their drugs having Russian packaging, I don't know anyone who has used them)

Appendix - References

We suggest you do your own Googling, because things are changing rapidly. Look up each medicine/supplement, perhaps adding "Covid" or a similar phrase after the name, for example

`                    Quercetin Covid`

You might want to keep an eye on our online list of helpful resources
https://thecovidsurvivalguide.com/resources/essential-sources   or
https://cov.cx/coves

One resource we respect, and which is regularly updated, is
https://www.evms.edu/media/evms_public/departments/internal_medicine/EVMS_Critical_Care_COVID-19_Protocol.pdf or https://cov.cx/a1f61 (we refer to this as **EVMS** in the document) – one of the documents linked from this parent page
https://www.evms.edu/covid-19/covid_care_for_clinicians   or
https://cov.cx/a1f62
Another regularly updated and useful list
https://www.ashp.org/-/media/assets/pharmacy-practice/resource-centers/Coronavirus/docs/ASHP-COVID-19-Evidence-Table.ashx   or
https://cov.cx/a1f63 (we refer to this as **ASHP** in the document)

This site has useful links to early treatment and prevention protocols https://c19protocols.com/ or https://cov.cx/a1f64

This is a list of physicians and facilities who are prepared to consider helping patients get early treatments, more or less as discussed in our Part Four

https://c19protocols.com/physicians-facilities-offering-early-treatment/ or https://cov.cx/a1f65

Here's another occasionally updated commentary on possible treatments

https://www.health.harvard.edu/diseases-and-conditions/treatments-for-covid-19 or https://cov.cx/a1f66

Here's a very conservative and mainstream view of many alternate treatments, and also with helpful information on possible adverse side-effects. It is helpful to at least be aware of the arguments against anything you might be considering taking, as well as the arguments for it.

https://online.epocrates.com/guidelines/10941/Herb-Supplement-Remedy-Use-in-COVID-19-epocrates-Evidence-Update or https://cov.cx/a1f67

Abbreviations Used in the Book

We've defined some of the more obscure abbreviations when using them in the book, but have omitted well-known abbreviations. Here's a complete list of everything.

ABS	Anti-lock Braking System
AHAM	Association of Home Appliance Manufacturers
AHLA	American Hotel & Lodging Association
AMA	American Medical Association
AMC	AMC Theatres aka American Entertainment Holdings, Inc
AP	Advanced Placement (education), Associated Press
ARDS	Acute Respiratory Distress Syndrome
ASHP	American Society of Health-System Pharmacists
ASHRAE Engineers	American Society of Heating, Refrigerating, and Airconditioning
BCG	The Bacillus Calmette–Guérin vaccine
BMJ	Once the British Medical Journal, now just the BMJ.
CADR	Clean Air Delivery Rate
CARB	California Air Resources Board
CDC	Centers for Disease Control and Prevention
CFM	Cubic Feet per Minute
CFR	Case Fatality Rate
CR	Consumer Reports
DCV	Demand-controlled ventilation
DV	Daily Value
ECG	Electrocardiogram
EKG	Elektrokardiogramm (the German version of ECG)
EPA	Environmental Protection Agency
EVMS	East Virginia Medical School
FDA	Food and Drug Administration
FLCCC	Frontline Covid-19 Critical Care Alliance
GDP	Gross Domestic Product
HCQ	Hydroxychloroquine
HEPA	High Efficiency Particulate Air

HMO   Health Maintenance Organization
HVAC   Heating, Ventilation, and Air Conditioning
IATA   International Air Transport Association
ICAM   A treatment plan developed by AdventHealth in Ocala, FL
ICON   Another treatment plan developed in Florida
ICU   Intensive Care Unit
IHME   Institute for Health Metrics and Evaluation, University of Washington
IR   Infrared
ISS   International Space Station
MATH   A treatment plan developed by the FLCCC (qv)
MERS   Middle East Respiratory Syndrome
MERV   Minimum Efficiency Reporting Value
MGU   Moscow State University
MI   Michigan
MSU   Moscow State University
NEJM   New England Journal of Medicine
NIAID   National Institute of Allergy and Infectious Diseases
NIH   National Institutes of Health
NV   Nevada
NYSE   New York Stock Exchange
OTC   Over-the-counter
PCR   Polymerase Chain Reaction – a type of virus test procedure
PEP   Post-exposure prophylaxis
PMA   Premarket Approval (from the FDA)
PPE   Personal Protective Equipment
PrEP   Pre-exposure prophylaxis
QT   A portion of the tracing of a heartbeat rhythm
RAID   Redundant Array of Inexpensive Disks
RDA   Recommended Dietary Amount
RNA   Ribonucleic Acid
ROI   Return on Investment
ROR   Reporting Odds Ratio
S&P   Standard & Poors (stock index)
SARS   Severe Acute Respiratory Syndrome
SD   South Dakota

TB	Tuberculosis
TCM	Traditional Chinese medicines
TSA	Transportation Security Administration
UAE	United Arab Emirates
UL	Upper Intake Level
UV	Ultraviolet
UVGI	Ultraviolet Germicidal Irradiation
WA	Washington (state)
WHO	World Health Organization
WSJ	The Wall Street Journal

Medical Abbreviations

You'll sometimes see various abbreviations when describing courses of treatment. These are often abbreviated forms of Latin phrases, so it is hard to guess what they might mean.

Here's a list of the more common terms you might encounter. They might be capitalized in part or whole, and may or may not sometimes have periods between the letters.[780]

Abbreviation	Explanation
a.c.	Ante cibum – before meals
Bds	Bis die sumendum – twice a day
Bid	Bis in die – twice a day
Gtt, gtts	Gutta(e) - drop(s)
Nocte	Nightly
Od	Omne in die – once a day

---

[780] Here's a longer list with some interesting comments.
https://en.wikipedia.org/wiki/List_of_abbreviations_used_in_medical_prescriptions or
https://cov.cx/a1f30

Abbreviation	Explanation
	(also Oculus dexter – right eye)
Pc	Post Cibum – after food
Po	Per Os – by mouth
Prn	Pro re nata – as needed
Q	Quaque – every (period of time stated next)
Q1h, Q2h, Q3h, etc	Quaque hora, etc – every 1/2/3/whatever hours
Qd	Quaque die – every day
Qh	Quaque hora - hourly
Qid	Quarter in die – four times a day
Tds	Ter die sumendum – three times a day
UT	Ut dictum – as directed

Table of Figures

www.ingramcontent.com/pod-product-compliance
Lightning Source LLC
Chambersburg PA
CBHW060303030426
42336CB00011B/921